Intravascular Ultrasound Imaging in Coronary Artery Disease

FUNDAMENTAL AND CLINICAL CARDIOLOGY

Editor-in-Chief

Samuel Z. Goldhaber, M.D.

*Harvard Medical School
and Brigham and Women's Hospital
Boston, Massachusetts*

Associate Editor, Europe

Henri Bounameaux, M.D.

*University Hospital of Geneva
Geneva, Switzerland*

1. *Drug Treatment of Hyperlipidemia*, edited by Basil M. Rifkind
2. *Cardiotonic Drugs: A Clinical Review, Second Edition, Revised and Expanded*, edited by Carl V. Leier
3. *Complications of Coronary Angioplasty*, edited by Alexander J. R. Black, H. Vernon Anderson, and Stephen G. Ellis
4. *Unstable Angina*, edited by John D. Rutherford
5. *Beta-Blockers and Cardiac Arrhythmias*, edited by Prakash C. Deedwania
6. *Exercise and the Heart in Health and Disease*, edited by Roy J. Shephard and Henry S. Miller, Jr.
7. *Cardiopulmonary Physiology in Critical Care*, edited by Steven M. Scharf
8. *Atherosclerotic Cardiovascular Disease, Hemostasis, and Endo-thelial Function*, edited by Robert Boyer Francis, Jr.
9. *Coronary Heart Disease Prevention*, edited by Frank G. Yanowitz
10. *Thrombolysis and Adjunctive Therapy for Acute Myocardial Infarction*, edited by Eric R. Bates
11. *Stunned Myocardium: Properties, Mechanisms, and Clinical Manifestations*, edited by Robert A. Kloner and Karin Przyklenk
12. *Prevention of Venous Thromboembolism*, edited by Samuel Z. Goldhaber
13. *Silent Myocardial Ischemia and Infarction: Third Edition*, Peter F. Cohn
14. *Congestive Cardiac Failure: Pathophysiology and Treatment*, edited by David B. Barnett, Hubert Pouleur, and Gary S. Francis
15. *Heart Failure: Basic Science and Clinical Aspects*, edited by Judith K. Gwathmey, G. Maurice Briggs, and Paul D. Allen

Intravascular Ultrasound Imaging in Coronary Artery Disease

edited by

Robert J. Siegel

Cedars-Sinai Medical Center and
University of California, Los Angeles, School of Medicine
Los Angeles, California

MARCEL DEKKER, INC.   NEW YORK · BASEL · HONG KONG

ISBN: 0-8247-0091-0

The publisher offers discounts on this book when ordered in bulk quantities. For more information, write to Special Sales/Professional Marketing at the address below.

This book is printed on acid-free paper.

Marcel Dekker, Inc.
270 Madison Avenue, New York, New York 10016
http://www.dekker.com

Current printing (last digit):
10 9 8 7 6 5 4 3 2 1

Printed in the United States of America

To our patients, with whom we use ultrasound to perform
intravascular imaging, a fantastic voyage
toward more accurate diagnoses and better therapies

Series Introduction

As clinical cardiologists, we have learned that coronary arteriography often tells only part of our patients' stories. The angiogram too often appears misleadingly benign. When this occurs, we can be lulled into complacency.

Robert J. Siegel and his colleagues at Cedars-Sinai have been in the forefront as pioneers in the technology of intravascular ultrasound. One benefit of Dr. Siegel's early involvement in the field is the network of internationally renowned colleagues he has enlisted as chapter authors in *Intravascular Ultrasound Imaging in Coronary Artery Disease*.

This book will be tremendously useful, not only for the interventional cardiologist but for the general cardiologist. As someone in the latter category, I plan to keep this book within arm's reach as a convenient resource for planning management strategy and reviewing conveniently a compendium of literature on this emerging and exciting topic.

Finally, Dr. Siegel's book fits well the mission of our Fundamental and Clinical Cardiology series. This 32nd volume is timely, comprehensive, practical, and scholarly. We welcome Dr. Siegel and his colleagues and thank them for furthering our education on this intriguing subject.

Samuel Z. Goldhaber

Foreword

Approximately one decade ago, a group of physician–vascular interventionalists, engineers, and hard-driving entrepreneurs created the vision of merging
the diagnostic potential of ultrasound imaging with catheter-based therapeutic
angioplasty modalities. These diverse, rather fanciful, stargazing individualists
became the pioneers of the field we now know as intravascular ultrasound
(IVUS). Pondering the early days of intravascular ultrasound forces us to relive
the agonizing era of images too crude for public display, generated via catheter
systems too bulky for safe human use. The history of vascular ultrasound, short
as it may seem, is littered with technical failures in an attempt to create
miniaturized devices with just the right combination of image clarity and
usability to accommodate the rigors of an often-treacherous intracoronary
milieu. Nevertheless, persistence has prevailed, and coronary ultrasound imaging systems have finally struck the necessary balance to provide consistent,
high-quality images of coronary pathoanatomy even under the most hostile of
circumstances. The task is then left to the clinical investigators to establish the
utility of this adjunct imaging modality as a viable tool in the rapidly changing
landscape of coronary intervention.

This volume provides the earliest glimpse at IVUS as a living, "thinking"
companion to coronary intervention in navigating the uncharted waters of new
angioplasty devices and complex lesion morphologies. Robert J. Siegel has
done a remarkable job in gathering a star-studded cast of leaders in all facets of
clinical vascular therapy, and has crafted a meaningful amalgam, starting with
a short tour through image interpretation and then emphasizing up-to-date
clinical reviews on a broad variety of topics. Different perspectives are ex-
plored, giving credence to the reality that ultrasound imaging is still "not for
everyone" but may have a meaningful role in both high- and low-volume
centers, used either in an aggressive iterative mode, or more selectively, in only

challenging or confusing clinical scenarios. IVUS is not glorified as an imaging panacea, but, rather, is examined carefully alongside standard-contrast angiographic techniques and other competitive modalities such as angioscopy and Doppler flow velocity.

Clearly, the strength of this volume is in remaining faithful to the title and in providing in-depth presentations on the use of IVUS for clinical decision-making during interventional procedures in patients with coronary artery disease. Spanning the full spectrum from "plain old" balloon angioplasty to excimer laser angioplasty, atherectomy (directional and rotational), and stent implantation, experts provide valuable clinical insights and practical tips on how IVUS can be employed to refine decision-making and enhance the results of angioplasty procedures. Less mainstream but nonetheless worthwhile topics include assessment of the cardiac transplant patient and applying IVUS to peripheral intervention. The text concludes with a critical discussion of IVUS limitations and expected future developmental enhancements.

Undoubtedly, the message of this book is "Try IVUS and you'll like it." The writing style, editing, visual presentations, and chapter organization create a logical sequence that should appeal to a broad audience from the true novice to the die-hard enthusiast. Dr. Siegel and his colleagues have provided us with the most intelligible and current text in the field of coronary IVUS. In the unpredictable arena of complex coronary intervention, where life-threatening complications can occur suddenly, unexpectedly, and with devastating consequences, perhaps IVUS has added a touch of science to the art of angioplasty decision-making. Perhaps we now have a more enlightened vision, or, as Erasmus said (referring to IVUS, no doubt), "In the land of the blind, the man with one eye is king."

Martin B. Leon

Preface

Tremendous advances in our knowledge of atherosclerotic vascular disease and catheter intervention have resulted from insight gained through the use of intravascular ultrasound (IVUS). This book, with contributions by some of the pioneers and prophets of intravascular ultrasound, is intended for practitioners of transcatheter coronary interventions. Basic concepts of atherosclerosis, intravascular ultrasound interpretation, de novo vascular remodeling, and the expected response detected by ultrasound to transcatheter therapies are described. The primary focus of this text, however, is on the practical application and value of intravascular ultrasound imaging in the coronary interventional laboratory.

The first three chapters address coronary artery disease from the viewpoints of the cardiovascular pathologist and the intravascular ultrasonographer. Similarities and correlations of histologic evaluation and ultrasound imaging of the coronary arteries and the effects of coronary atherosclerosis and vascular remodeling are delineated in Chapters 1, 2, 3, and 6. Intravascular ultrasound interpretation of arteries before and after intervention is discussed and thoroughly illustrated. The prognostic implications from IVUS with regard to restenosis, plaque burden, and stenting are detailed by the Stanford University group. In Chapters 4 and 5, investigators from Washington Hospital Center and Cedars-Sinai Medical Center describe their use of IVUS with a high volume of preinterventional ultrasound imaging and with a more selective use of IVUS imaging. The clinical benefit from each of these approaches is discussed. The informational content, diagnostic value, and utility of IVUS, compared with angiography, angioscopy, the Doppler Flowire, and three-dimensional IVUS, are extensively illustrated and specified in Chapters 7, 8, 9, and 10 by authors from the Thorax Center in Rotterdam, the Cleveland Clinic Foundation, and George Washington University. In Chapters 11 through 14, the utility of IVUS for assessing lesions before and after intervention with balloon angioplasty, excimer laser, rotational atherectomy, and stents is depicted and reviewed by investigators from high-volume interventional centers in Cleveland, Washington, D.C., and Milan. The practical and pragmatic applications of IVUS to cardiac transplant patients are characterized from the perspective of Stanford University cardiologists. Surgeons from the Arizona Heart Institute, Columbia Medical Center Phoenix, and the Royal Infirmary in Glasgow delineate the use of peripheral intervention with IVUS as an adjunctive technology. They provide extensive case examples that demonstrate IVUS applications in peripheral vascular disease. The final chapter is written by pioneers from the industry who have optimized IVUS technology. Their perspective on the limitations and future developments of IVUS addresses practical issues in the years to come.

It has been a pleasure and a great learning experience to collaborate on this text with such an experienced and distinguished group of IVUS investigators. While each author has been at the forefront of intravascular diagnostic technologies, their focus for this text has been practical and clinically oriented. It is my hope that practitioners will find this book a helpful adjunct to their use of intravascular ultrasound. As has become increasingly evident over the past decade, decision-making and intraprocedural modifications in the interventional vascular laboratory are best made when the anatomy is optimally elucidated.

Robert J. Siegel

Contents

Contributors

John E. Abele   Director, Founder, and Chairman, Boston Scientific Corporation, Natick, Massachusetts

Hans Berglund, M.D., Ph.D.   Consultant Cardiologist, Department of Cardiology, Karolinska Institutet and Huddinge Hospital, Huddinge, Sweden

Antonio Colombo, M.D.   Professor of Clinical Medicine, Department of Medicine, New York University Medical Center, New York, New York, and Columbus Hospital, Milan, Italy

Robert J. Crowley   Boston Scientific Corporation, Natick, Massachusetts

Pim J. de Feyter, M.D., Ph.D.   Director, Coronary Imaging Laboratory, Division of Cardiology, Thorax Center, University Hospital Rotterdam-Dijkzigt, Erasmus University, Rotterdam, The Netherlands

Anthony C. De Franco, M.D.   Interventional Cardiologist, The Moses H. Cone Memorial Hospital, Greensboro, and Assistant Professor of Medicine, University of North Carolina at Chapel Hill, Chapel Hill, North Carolina

Edward B. Diethrich, M.D.   Medical Director, Department of Cardiovascular and Endovascular Surgery, Arizona Heart Institute, Phoenix, Arizona

Neal L. Eigler, M.D.   Co-Director, Cardiovascular Intervention Center, Cedars-Sinai Medical Center, and Associate Professor of Medicine, University of California, Los Angeles, School of Medicine, Los Angeles, California

Michael C. Fishbein, M.D. Professor, Department of Pathology and Laboratory Medicine, University of California, Los Angeles, School of Medicine, and Cedars-Sinai Medical Center, Los Angeles, California

Peter J. Fitzgerald, M.D., Ph.D. Assistant Professor, Division of Cardiovascular Medicine, Department of Medicine, Stanford University School of Medicine, Stanford, California

Steven L. Goldberg, M.D. Associate Director, Cardiac Catheterization Laboratory, Division of Cardiology, Los Angeles County, Harbor–UCLA Medical Center, Torrance, and Assistant Professor of Medicine, University of California, Los Angeles, School of Medicine, Los Angeles, California

Rainer Hoffmann, M.D. Cardiology Fellow, Intravascular Ultrasound Imaging and Cardiac Catheterization Laboratories, Washington Cardiology Center, Washington Hospital Center, Washington, D.C.

Yue-Teh Jang, Ph.D. Boston Scientific Corporation, Natick, Massachusetts

Kenneth M. Kent, M.D., Ph.D. Director, Washington Cardiology Center, Washington Hospital Center, Washington, D.C.

Martin B. Leon, M.D. Director, Cardiovascular Research and Education, Cardiology Research Foundation, Washington, D.C.

Huai Luo, M.D. Cardiology Fellow, Division of Cardiology, Department of Internal Medicine, Cedars-Sinai Medical Center, Los Angeles, California

Maria Teresa Mallus, M.D. Research Fellow, Division of Cardiology, Thorax Center, University Hospital Rotterdam-Dijkzigt, Erasmus University, Rotterdam, The Netherlands

Peter Marx, B.S.R.T.(R)(CV) Radiology Special Procedures Technologist, Department of Cardiovascular Surgery, Columbia Medical Center Phoenix, Phoenix, Arizona

Roxana Mehran, M.D. Cardiology Fellow, Intravascular Ultrasound Imaging and Cardiac Catheterization Laboratories, Washington Cardiology Center, Washington Hospital Center, Washington, D.C.

Gary S. Mintz, M.D.   Director, Intravascular Ultrasound Program, Washington Hospital Center, Washington, D.C.

Eduardo Moreyra, M.D.   Clinical Instructor, George Washington University, Washington, D.C.

Ravi Nair, M.D.   Assistant Professor of Medicine, Case Western Reserve University, and Co-Director, Cardiac Catheterization Laboratories, University Hospitals of Cleveland, Cleveland, Ohio

Toshihiko Nishioka, M.D.   Chief, Division of Health Control Medicine, Department of Education, Ground Self-Defense Force Medical School, Tokyo, Japan

Steven E. Nissen, M.D.   Vice Chairman, and Director, Section of Clinical Cardiology, Department of Cardiology, Cleveland Clinic Foundation, Cleveland, Ohio

Augusto D. Pichard, M.D.   Washington Cardiology Center, Washington Hospital Center, Washington, D.C.

Jeffrey J. Popma, M.D.   Executive Director, Cardiology Research Foundation, Washington, D.C.

Richard L. Popp, M.D.   Professor of Medicine and Senior Associate Dean for Academic Affairs, Stanford University School of Medicine, Stanford, California

Kathleen Quealy, M.D.   Assistant Professor of Medicine, Department of Cardiology, University Hospitals of Cleveland, Cleveland, Ohio

Donald B. Reid, M.D.   Consultant Vascular Surgeon, Peripheral Vascular Surgery Unit, Royal Infirmary, Glasgow, Scotland

Lowell F. Satler, M.D.   Director, Coronary Interventions, Department of Cardiology, Washington Hospital Center, Washington, D.C.

Severin P. Schwarzacher, M.D.   Assistant Professor of Medicine, Department of Cardiology, Innsbruck University, Innsbruck, Austria

Jerome Segal, M.D.   Associate Professor of Medicine, and Director, Cardiac Catheterization Laboratory, George Washington University, Washington, D.C.

Patrick W. Serruys, M.D., Ph.D.   Professor of Interventional Cardiology, Division of Cardiology, Thorax Center, University Hospital Rotterdam-Dijkzigt, Erasmus University, Rotterdam, The Netherlands

Robert J. Siegel, M.D.   Director, Cardiac Noninvasive Laboratory, and Staff Cardiologist, Cedars-Sinai Medical Center, and Professor of Medicine in Residence, University of California, Los Angeles, School of Medicine, Los Angeles, California

Steven W. Tabak, M.D.   Assistant Clinical Professor, Department of Medicine, University of California, Los Angeles, School of Medicine, Los Angeles, California

E. Murat Tuzcu, M.D.   Director, Intravascular Core Laboratory, Department of Cardiology, Cleveland Clinic Foundation, Cleveland, Ohio

Neal G. Uren, M.D.   Interventional Fellow, Division of Cardiovascular Medicine, Department of Medicine, Stanford University School of Medicine, Stanford, California

Clemens von Birgelen, M.D.   Director, IVUS Research, Division of Cardiology, Thorax Center, University Hospital Rotterdam-Dijkzigt, Erasmus University, Rotterdam, The Netherlands

Robert Wrasper, R.T.(R)   Radiology Special Procedures Technologist, Department of Cardiovascular Surgery, Columbia Medical Center Phoenix, Phoenix, Arizona

Alan C. Yeung, M.D.   Assistant Professor of Medicine, Division of Cardiovascular Medicine, Department of Medicine, Stanford University School of Medicine, Stanford, California

Paul G. Yock, M.D.   Acting Chief of Cardiology, Division of Cardiovascular Medicine, Department of Medicine, Stanford University School of Medicine, Stanford, California

Khaled Ziada, M.D.   Cleveland Clinic Foundation, Cleveland, Ohio

Pathology of Coronary Atherosclerosis: Implications for Intravascular Ultrasound Imaging

Michael C. Fishbein   *University of California, Los Angeles, School of Medicine, and Cedars-Sinai Medical Center, Los Angeles, California*

Robert J. Siegel   *Cedars-Sinai Medical Center and University of California, Los Angeles, School of Medicine, Los Angeles, California*

I. PATHOLOGY OF ATHEROSCLEROSIS

Atherosclerosis, atheroma, and arteriosclerosis are among the terms that have been applied to lesions in coronary and other arteries which may cause luminal compromise. Arteriosclerosis is a generic term which means hardening of the arteries and includes three different lesions: Monckeberg's medial calcification, which does not cause significant luminal narrowing; arteriolosclerosis, which is small-vessel disease; and atherosclerosis, the disease responsible for over 99% of cases of ischemic heart disease (1). In 1904, Marchand introduced the term atherosclerosis to emphasize the presence of lipid in some arteriosclerotic plaques. The term atheroma had been applied by the ancient Greeks to describe arterial plaques that contained yellow pultaceous material. The arterial lesions in human epicardial coronary arteries usually contain lipid, so the terms atherosclerosis, atherosclerotic plaque, and atheroma are most appropriate.

Until recently, atherosclerosis has been classified into three basic types of lesions: the fatty streak, a flat or slightly raised yellow lesion containing lipid-laden macrophages (and smooth muscle cells); the fibrous plaque, a raised lesion in which the lipid-laden cells and extracellular lipids arc surrounded by collagen, elastic fibers, and inflammatory cells, which does not cause clinically significant disease; and the complicated plaque, an altered fibrous plaque with hemorrhage, hematoma, thrombosis, calcification, and/or cell necrosis, which is associated with medial thinning and inflammation of all vascular layers and which can cause significant luminal narrowing.

The American Heart Association Scientific Council has recently approved a new classification of atherosclerosis based on lesion composition and structure which was designed to reflect the temporal natural history of the disease (2–4). The hope is that this new classification system will be of practical value in providing a generally accepted and generally utilized standardized nomenclature (Table 1).

In this classification system, there are six types of lesions (Figs. 1–3). Types I, II, and III are early precursor lesions. Types IV, V, and VI are considered advanced lesions because of the marked disorganization of the intima caused by the abundance of extracellular lipid forming a "lipid core." In human coronary and other arteries, at sites where atherosclerosis tends to develop, the intima is often thickened by fibromuscular tissue, elastic fibers, and proteoglycans. This region is referred to as "adaptive intimal thickening." It is not apparent by angiography, but does contribute to the three-ring IVUS appearance of normal arteries. The type IV lesion is of special interest and significance because, although it may be relatively small and nonocclusive, it is thought to be vulnerable to rupture, which could result in complete thrombotic arterial occlusion. This concept of a minimally stenotic "high-risk" lesion has yet to be proven. Nonetheless, it has important clinical implications, which are especially relevant to the interpretation of intravascular imaging findings with regard to the presence of a hypoechoic lipid-containing plaque. Type V is characterized by an increase in the amount of collagen with or without calcification, while type VI is a lesion "complicated" by disruption of the surface, hematoma, hemorrhage, or thrombosis (complicated plaque of older classifications) (Fig. 4).

Regardless of whether they occur in types IV and/or V lesions, it is accepted that plaque erosions (superficial intimal injury) and fissures (tears of variable depth) with overlying microscopic mural thrombosis complicate stable, longstanding coronary atherosclerotic plaques and lead to acute ischemic events. Small plaque fissures may be found in as many as 17% of patients dying from noncardiac causes (5). If no overlying obstructive luminal thrombus develops, these small plaque defects may be of no clinical significance. However, plaque rupture (disruption of the fibrous cap) that evolves to occlusive thrombosis is clinically significant and is the lesion responsible for the majority of acute fatal coronary events: acute myocardial infarction and sudden death (6–10).

Table 1 Terms Used to Designate Different Types of Human Atherosclerotic Lesions in Pathology

Terms for atherosclerotic lesions in histological classification	Other terms for the same lesions often based on appearance with the unaided eye	
Type I lesion	Initial lesion	
Type IIa lesion	Progression-prone type II lesion	Fatty dot or streak	Early lesions
IIb	Progression-resistant type II	
Type III lesion	Intermediate lesion (preatheromal)	
Type IV lesion	Atheroma	Atheromatous plaque,
Type Va lesion	Fibroatheroma (type V lesion)	fibrolipid plaque, fibrous plaque, plaque
Vb	Calcific lesion (type VII lesion)	Calcified plaque	Advanced lesions, raised lesions
Vc	Fibrotic lesion (type VIII lesion)	Fibrous plaque
Type VI lesion	Lesion with surface defect, and/or hematoma-hemorrhage, and/or thrombotic deposit	Complicated lesion, complicated plaque

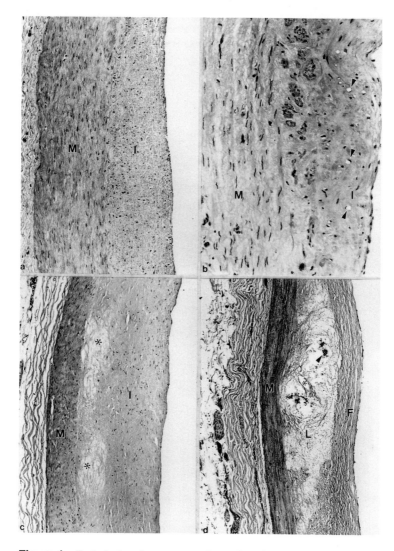

Figure 1   Early lesions in coronary atherosclerosis: (a) "adaptive intimal thickening" (I) consisting primarily of fibromuscular tissue, overlying an intact media (M); (b) early type II lesion with occasional foamy macrophages in intima (arrowheads); (c) type 3 lesion in which the intima contains small pools of extracellular lipid (asterisks); (d) a type 5 lesion in which there is thickening of the fibrous cap (F). Small calcifications are also present (arrowheads).

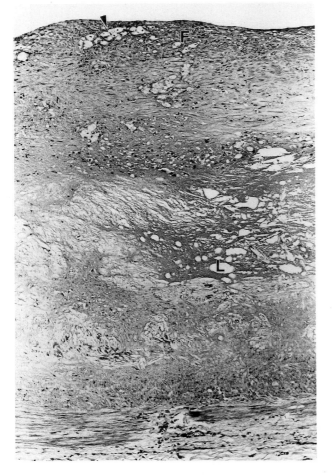

Figure 2 Lesion with some features thought to be associated with an increased risk of rupture: a large lipid pool (L), numerous macrophages, particularly infiltrating the fibrous cap (F), and numerous inflammatory cells. Shear stress, fibrous cap thinning, and the release of proteolytic enzymes may also predispose to plaque rupture.

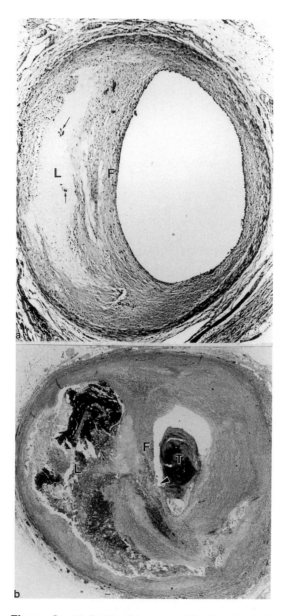

Figure 3   (a) Stable plaque, type V with a large lipid core (L), focal calcifications (arrows), and an intact fibrous cap (F); (b) ruptured plaque (arrowhead) with hemorrhage into the lipid core (L) and overlying luminal thrombosis (T).

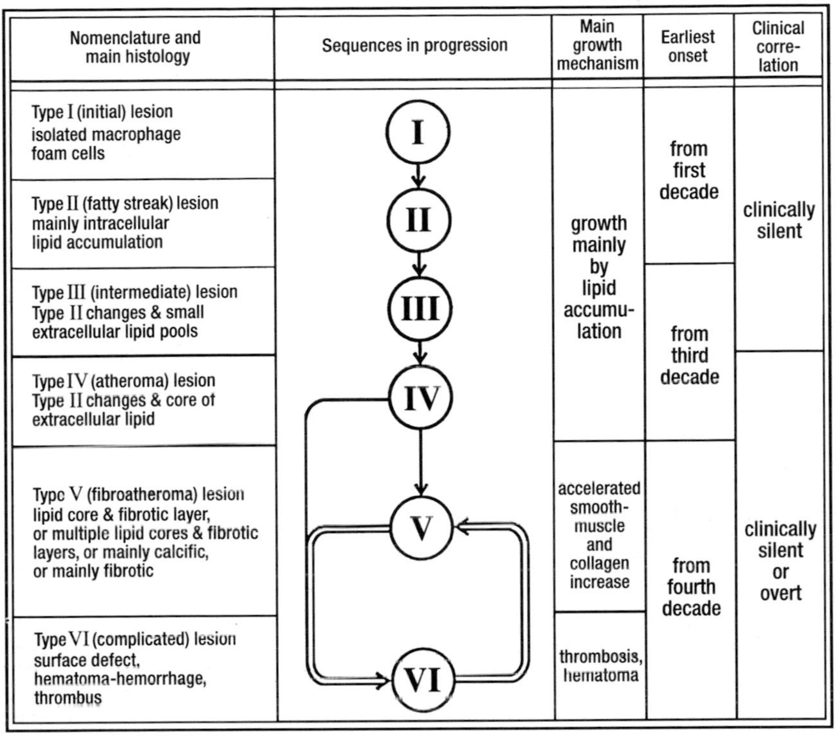

Nomenclature and main histology	Sequences in progression	Main growth mechanism	Earliest onset	Clinical correlation
Type I (initial) lesion isolated macrophage foam cells			from first decade	clinically silent
Type II (fatty streak) lesion mainly intracellular lipid accumulation		growth mainly by lipid accumulation		
Type III (intermediate) lesion Type II changes & small extracellular lipid pools			from third decade	
Type IV (atheroma) lesion Type II changes & core of extracellular lipid				
Type V (fibroatheroma) lesion lipid core & fibrotic layer, or multiple lipid cores & fibrotic layers, or mainly calcific, or mainly fibrotic		accelerated smooth-muscle and collagen increase	from fourth decade	clinically silent or overt
Type VI (complicated) lesion surface defect, hematoma-hemorrhage, thrombus		thrombosis, hematoma		

Figure 4 Flow diagram in center column indicates pathways in evolution and progression of human atherosclerotic lesions. Roman numerals indicate histologically characteristic types of lesions as defined in column at left. (From Ref. 4, with permission of authors and American Heart Association.)

II. ANGIOGRAPHY IN THE EVALUATION OF CORONARY ATHEROSCLEROSIS

Since angiography provides a "lumenogram" of the coronary arterial tree, it reveals little about the adjacent arterial wall. Acute changes such as plaque rupture and/or thrombosis may sometimes be detected. Sequential angiography before and after nonfatal myocardial infarction has shown that at the site of the complete occlusion, the preexisting, underlying plaque does not usually cause hemodynamically significant stenosis (11–18) (Table 2). Published studies have reported that nearly 50% of these lesions are at sites with less than 50% luminal diameter narrowing. Fewer than 20% of acute complete occlusions

Table 2 Severity of the Coronary Angiographic Lesions Prior to Myocardial Infarction

Study	Number of patients	Interval between 1st and 2nd angiograms (months)	% Diameter stenosis of lesion prior to MI (No. of patients)		
			<50%	50–75%	>75%
Ambrose (8)	23	18	12	6	5
Giroud (12)	92	24	72	8	12
Hacket (9)	10	21	9	1	0
Little (10)	58	24	36	15	7
Moise (14)	116	39	17	66	33
Webster (13)	30	55	16	10	4
Totals	329	30.2	162 (49%)	106 (32%)	61 (19%)

Source: *Circulation*, with permission.

occur in lesions with preexisting angiographic diameter narrowing of more than 75%. Subsequently, it has become generally accepted that most plaque ruptures that cause myocardial infarction occur in plaques that narrow the luminal diameter by less than 50%. This view has been expanded into the concept that nonstenotic, hemodynamically insignificant plaques (type IV) are those that rupture, causing occlusive thrombosis, myocardial infarction, and/or death. This is a depressing notion because it suggests that the overwhelming majority of mature males and females of the industrialized world are continuously at risk of an unpredictable, catastrophic coronary event.

Pathologic studies from patients with fatal coronary events have yielded different results. They have shown that at the sites of plaque rupture with superimposed occlusive thrombosis, the underlying abnormality is "severe" (Table 3). Morphometric studies have shown that the plaque occupied on average about 90% of the cross-sectional area (68% diameter reduction) (6–9).

III. PATHOLOGIC/ANGIOGRAPHIC DISCORDANCE

Why do these results appear so discordant? Both angiography (Table 4) and pathology (Table 5) have limitations that can result in erroneous results leading to either overestimation or underestimation of the degree of luminal narrowing by atherosclerotic plaque (19–29). However, it is likely that the most important factors responsible for the discordance between angiographic and pathologic studies are not related to poor angiographic or pathologic technique or inaccurate interpretation, but instead to two biologic variables: diffuseness of coronary atherosclerosis, and vascular remodeling.

Table 3 Severity of Underlying Stenosis by
Atherosclerotic Plaque at Sites of Occlusive Thrombosis[a]
(Cross-sectional area narrowing)

Study	<50% n	(%)	50–74% n	(%)	75–99 n	(%)	Total n	(%)
Horie (2)	4	(6)	14	(20)	51	(74)	69	(100)
Falk (3)[c]	0	(0)	1	(3)	39	(97)	40	(100)
Davies (4)[d]	3	(7)	11	(25)	30	(68)	44	(100)
Qiao (5)	7	(2)	30	(9)	298	(89)	335	(100)
Total	14	(3)	56	(11)	418	(86)	488	(100)

Source: *Circulation*, with permission.
[a]Data adapted from original articles.
[b]Equivalent to 50% or greater diameter narrowing.
[c]Arteries with occlusive thrombi.
[d]Arteries with major thrombi occluding 50–100% of lumen.

That coronary atherosclerosis is a diffuse process is well known to pathologists
(30–34), angiographers (35), and coronary ultrasonographers (36,37). In atherosclerotic coronary artery disease, it is almost impossible to find a segment of
the proximal coronary arterial wall that is completely free from atherosclerosis.
Accordingly, the concept of a focal stenosis is somewhat misleading. The
"plaque" is not a discrete lesion. It is just a segment with more severe

Table 4 Factors Contributing to Coronary Arteriographic Lesion Under- (u)
and Over- (o) Estimation

Technical	Biologic
Intra- and interobserver variability (u,o)	Vasospasm (o)
Inadequate filling of artery with contrast (u,o)	Diffuse atherosclerotic narrowing (u)
	Concentric short stenosis (u)
Inadequate angiographic projections (u)	Crescentic, slitlike, and star-shaped
Foreshortening of artery (u)	lumina (u)
Overlap or superimposition of arterial branches (u,o)	Poststenotic dilatation (o)
	Recanalized segments with multiple channels (u)
	Distal obstruction (u)
	Arterial remodeling (Glagov phenomenon) (u)

Source: *Circulation*, with permission.

Table 5 Factors Contributing to Inaccurate Pathologic Quantitation of Coronary Atherosclerosis

Postmortem collapse of arteries
Postmortem contraction of arteries
Lack of perfusion fixation at physiologic pressure
Architectural distortion and destruction in sectioning calcified arteries
Tangential sectioning of arteries
Generalized shrinkage with fixation and processing
Disproportionate dimensional changes in artery wall and lumen with fixation, processing, and sectioning
Compensatory enlargement of atherosclerotic arteries (Glagov phenomenon)

Source: *Circulation*, with permission.

involvement by a diffuse disease. This well-known fact seems to be ignored in the routine evaluation of coronary angiograms.

The second factor, vascular remodeling (38–41), has only recently begun to be appreciated. Now often called the Glagov phenomenon, this change consists of a progressive, teleologically compensatory increase in arterial cross-sectional area as the atherosclerosis progresses. The result is that while the plaque enlarges, the lumen size remains the same. Lumen size may remain normal in regions where plaques occupy 40% to 50% of the new arterial cross section. According to the work of Glagov et al. (38), only when plaques enlarge further does the lumen become compromised.

Thus, it appears that it is the diffuseness of coronary atherosclerosis and the vascular remodeling that occur that cause the major differences in the angiographic and pathologic quantification of coronary atherosclerosis. As shown in Figure 5, the angiographic stenosis is determined by comparing lumen diameter at the site of a stenosis with an adjacent site thought to be normal. Since there are no completely normal sites adjacent to severely stenotic regions in atherosclerotic coronary arteries, angiography will be comparing a severe stenosis with an adjacent milder stenosis. The volume of disease at the site of stenosis will thus be underestimated (42). Because of compensatory enlargement, a region in an artery with up to 40% involvement of the cross-sectional area by plaque may still have a lumen of normal dimensions. It is generally accepted that angiography detects a lesion only after about 50% of the arterial cross section is involved by plaque. Thus, angiography may be accurate in determining lumen size but is not an appropriate technique to determine the "volume" of atherosclerosis present.

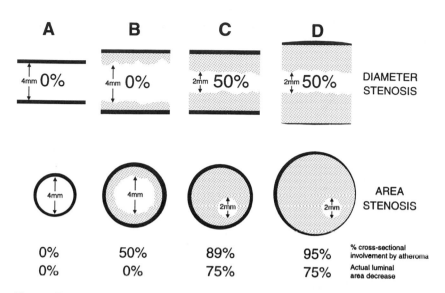

Figure 5 Top row, angiographic views; bottom row, pathologic views. Column A shows a normal artery. Column B shows an artery with "moderate" atherosclerosis. Because of remodeling, with enlargement of the vessel, the angiographer sees a normal lumen. The pathologist viewing the same artery would see the same lumen, but 50% of the cross-sectional area would be occupied by plaque. Since the pathologist has no way of knowing this lumen is still of normal size, he or she would conclude that this artery has a 50% cross-sectional area narrowing. Column C shows a more involved artery. The angiographer sees that the lumen is 50% less in diameter than the adjacent "moderate" (B) segment. This would translate into a 75% cross-sectional area narrowing, but the angiographer might conclude that this is mild or moderate disease. The pathologist sees the 2-mm lumen but a larger plaque, and measures the stenosis as an 89% narrowing. Column D shows the same situation but with even more remodeling present. The angiographer still sees a 50% diameter narrowing, even though the plaque is much larger than that in column C, and would still conclude that this is not severe disease. Because of the greater enlargement of the artery, the pathologist now measures the stenosis as a 95% cross-sectional narrowing, even though the lumen size is actually the same as that in column C. The pathologist is left with no other explanation than that the angiographer has grossly underestimated the degree of stenosis in this patient's coronary artery. (From Ref. 45, from *Circulation*, 1996, with permission.)

Pathologic evaluation can identify the percentage of cross-sectional area occupied by plaque (Fig. 5). For example, the pathologist may see a plaque that comprises 50% of the cross-sectional area of an artery. Because of the Glagov phenomenon, however, beforehand, the artery may have enlarged 50% in cross-sectional area. Thus, the lumen may actually be the same size as the original, normal lumen in spite of the growth of a substantial "plaque." The pathologist does not know the original cross-sectional area of the artery or the amount of compensatory enlargement of the artery, so, from evaluation of a single cross section of the artery at a site of stenosis, the degree of luminal narrowing of that segment cannot be determined. The pathologist quantitates the degree of stenosis by dividing the lumen area by the total area; therefore, the degree of stenosis will be "overestimated."

To summarize, the angiographer determines the degree of stenosis by comparing lumina, assuming one is normal, while the pathologist determines the degree of stenosis by comparing lumen to total plaque area. The angiographer underestimates the degree of stenosis by using a denominator that is too small. The pathologist overestimates the degree of stenosis by using a denominator that is too large.

IV. INTRAVASCULAR ULTRASOUND IN THE EVALUATION OF CORONARY ATHEROSCLEROSIS

An accurate determination of the "degree" of atherosclerosis necessitates knowledge of the state of the lumen and the plaque at the site of stenosis, and the state of the lumen and arterial wall at adjacent sites. Then, the degree of luminal narrowing and the amount of atherosclerotic plaque present at any given region can be determined.

Intravascular ultrasound (IVUS) can provide all of this information (Fig. 6). IVUS allows in vivo assessment of the arterial lumen and wall size and shape. The intima, media, and adventitia can be delineated, and the presence of calcification, lipid pools, and fibrous tissue can be determined. IVUS has been used to study remodeling in coronary arteries (43). Studies in our laboratory compared the stenosis site with a proximal reference site that had < 25% diameter narrowing by angiography, and < 50% cross-sectional area stenosis by IVUS. Compensatory enlargement was defined as a total coronary arterial cross-sectional area at the stenotic site that was greater than that at the proximal, nonstenotic site. The majority of stenotic lesions had compensatory enlargement and thus exhibited remodeling, as seen in Figure 4. In 26% of arteries, however, there was what we referred to as "inadequate" remodeling in that the total cross-sectional area at the stenotic site was less than that in the

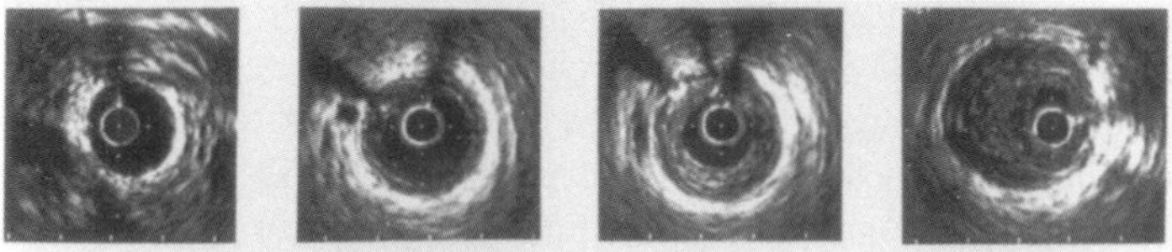

0%	0%	19%	47%	Diameter stenosis
0%	38%	69%	89%	% cross-sectional involvement by atheroma
0%	0%	34%	72%	Actual luminal area decrease

Figure 6 IVUS demonstration of coronary remodeling with atherosclerosis. The first panel shows a cross-sectional image of a normal proximal segment. The second panel shows a mild concentric lesion with 38% of the area bounded by the media involved by plaque. The lumen is actually larger than the normal segment shown in the first panel. The third panel shows a concentric plaque. Because of remodeling, when compared to the normal segment shown in the first panel, for example, there is only a 34% reduction in luminal area in spite of a lesion's occupying 69% of the cross-sectional area bounded by the media. The fourth panel shows a larger, eccentric plaque with even greater cross-sectional area involvement by atherosclerosis (89%). Because the entire vessel is larger, the actual decrease in luminal area is only 68%. Note that in spite of the considerable plaque present, diameter stenosis (as would be determined angiographically) would be considered mild: 19% in the third panel, and 47% in the fourth (all percentages determined by manual planimetry). (From Ref. 45, from *Circulation*, 1996, with permission.)

proximal and distal reference sites. Pasterkamp et al. (44) and others have referred to this phenomenon as "reverse Glagov." Unfortunately, vascular remodeling appears to be variable and inconsistent; thus, clinically significant coronary arterial narrowing by atherosclerosis may be a function of not only the amount of atherosclerosis, but also the degree or even lack of remodeling present (45).

V. WHICH LESIONS ARE PRONE TO RUPTURE?

Figure 2 shows a plaque with some features associated with rupture. According to angiographic studies, plaques such as these may rupture when there is about 50% diameter (75% area) stenosis of an artery. However, by planimetry, most pathologic studies have indicated that plaque ruptures occur at sites with an average of about 90% cross-sectional area narrowing (9). While the current consensus of opinion is that the propensity for atherosclerotic plaques to rupture is independent of plaque size, the hypothesis that small atherosclerotic plaques are the most likely to rupture, with resulting occlusive thrombosis, is unproven. In our opinion, it is not small, but rather large, plaques, which may or may not be producing significant stenosis, that undergo rupture with occlusive thrombosis, resulting in myocardial infarction and other acute ischemic events. Understanding of the angiographic, pathological, and ultrasonic images of atherosclerotic coronary arteries, and awareness of the limitations of these techniques should lead to a better understanding of the evolution and natural history of coronary atherosclerosis. It is hoped that prospective IVUS studies may provide new insights as to which coronary lesions are at the greatest risk for complications and progression to occlusion.

REFERENCES

1. Schwartz CJ, Mitchell JRA. The morphology, terminology, and pathogenesis of arterial plaques. Postgrad Med 1962; 38:25–33.
2. Stary HC, Blankenhorn DH, Chandler AB, et al. A definition of the intima of human arteries and of its atherosclerosis-prone regions. A report from the committee on vascular lesions of the Council on Arteriosclerosis, American Heart Association. Circulation 1992; 85:391–405.
3. Stary HC, Chandler AB, Glagov S, et al. A definition of initial, fatty streak, and intermediate lesions of atherosclerosis. A report from the committee on vascular lesions of the Council on Arteriosclerosis, American Heart Association. Circulation 1994; 89:2462–2478.
4. Stary HC, Chandler AB, Dinsmore RE, et al. A definition of advanced types of atherosclerotic lesions and a histologic classification of atherosclerosis. A report from the committee on vascular lesions of the Council on Arteriosclerosis, American Heart Association. Circulation 1995; 92:1355–1374.
5. Davies MJ, Bland MJ, Hangartner WR, Angelinin A, Thomas AC. Factors influencing the presence or absence of acute coronary thrombi in sudden ischemic death. Eur Heart J 1989; 10:203–208.
6. Horie T, Sekiguchi M, Hirosawa K. Coronary thrombosis in pathogenesis of acute myocardial infarction. Histopathologic study of coronary arteries in 108 necropsied cases using serial section. Br Heart J 1978; 40:153–161.
7. Falk E. Plaque rupture with severe pre-existing stenosis precipitating coronary thrombosis. Characteristics of coronary atherosclerotic plaques underlying fatal occlusive thrombi. Br Heart J 1983; 50:127–134.
8. Davies MJ, Thomas A. Thrombosis and acute coronary artery lesions in sudden cardiac ischemic death. N Engl J Med 1984; 310:1137–1140.
9. Qiao J-H, Fishbein MC. The severity of coronary atherosclerosis at sites of plaque rupture with occlusive thrombosis. J Am Coll Cardiol 1991; 17:1138–1142.
10. Richardson PD, Davies MJ, Born GVR. Influence of plaque configuration and

stress distribution on fissuring of coronary atherosclerotic plaques. Lancet 1989; 2:941–944.

11. Ambrose JA, Winters SL, Arora R, et al. Angiographic evolution of coronary artery morphology in unstable angina. J Am Coll Cardiol 1986; 7:472–478.

12. Ambrose JA, Tannenbaum MA, Alexopoulos D, et al. Angiographic progression of coronary artery disease and the development of myocardial infarction. J Am Coll Cardiol 1988; 12:56–62.

13. Hackett D, Verwilghen J, Davies G, Maseri A. Coronary stenoses before and after myocardial infarction. Am J Cardiol 1989; 63:1517–1518.

14. Little WC, Constantinescu M, Applegate RJ, et al. Can coronary angiography predict the site of a subsequent myocardial infarction in patients with mild to moderate coronary artery disease. Circulation 1988; 78:1157–1166.

15. Little WC, Downes TR, Applegate RJ. The underlying coronary lesion in myocardial infarction: implications for coronary angiography. Clin Cardiol 1991; 14: 868 874.

16. Giroud D, Li JM, Urban P, Meier B, Rutishauser W. Relation of the site of acute myocardial infarction to the most severe coronary arterial stenosis at prior angiography. Am J Cardiol 1992; 69:729–732.

17. Webster MWI, Chesebro JH, Smith HC, et al. Myocardial infarction and coronary artery occlusion: a prospective 5-year angiographic study. J Am Coll Cardiol 1990; 15:218A.

18. Moise A, Lesperance J, Therous P, Taeymans Y, Goulet C, Bourassa MG. Clinical and angiographic predictors of new total coronary occlusion in coronary artery disease: analysis of 313 nonoperated patients. Am J Cardiol 1984; 54:1176–1181.

19. Levin DC, Baltaxe HA, Lee JG, Sos TA. Potential sources of error in coronary arteriography. I. In performance of the study. Am J Roentgen Rad Ther Nucl Med 1975; 124:378–385.

20. Levin DC, Baltaxe HA, Sos TA. Potential sources of error in coronary arteriography. II. Interpretation of the study. Am J Roentgen Rad Ther Nucl Med 1975; 124: 386–393.

21. Blankenhorn DH, Curry PJ. The accuracy of arteriography and ultrasound imaging for atherosclerosis measurement. A review. Arch Pathol Lab Med 1982; 106: 483–489.

22. Trask N, Califf RM, Conley MJ, et al. Accuracy and interobserver variability of coronary cineangiography. A comparison with postmortem evaluation. J Am Coll Cardiol 1984; 3:1145–1154.

23. Grodin CM, Dyrda I, Pasternac A, Campeau L, Bourassa MG, Lesperance J. Discrepancies between cineangiographic and post mortem findings in patients with coronary disease and recent myocardial revascularization. Circulation 1974; 49:703–708.

24. Vlodaver Z, Frech R, Van Tassel RA, Edwards JE. Correlation of the antemortem coronary arteriogram and the postmortem specimen. Circulation 1973; 47:162–169.

25. Schwartz JW, Kong Y, Hackel DB, Bartel AG. Comparison of angiographic and postmortem findings in patients with coronary artery disease. Am J Cardiol 1975; 36:174–178.

26. Isner JM, Kishel J, Kent KM, Ronan JA, Ross AM, Roberts WC. Accuracy of angiographic determination of left main coronary arterial narrowing. Angiographic-histologic correlative analysis in 28 patients. Circulation 1981; 63: 1056–1064.

27. Marcus ML, Armstrong ML, Heistad DD, Mark AL. Comparison of three methods of evaluating coronary obstructive lesions: postmortem arteriography, pathologic examination and measurement of regional myocardial perfusion during maximal vasodilation. Am J Cardiol 1982; 49:1699–1706.

28. White CW, Wright CB, Doty DB, et al. Does visual interpretation of the coronary arteriogram predict the physiologic importance of a coronary stenosis? N Engl J Med 1984; 310:819–824.

29. Siegel RJ, Swan K, Edwalds G, Fishbein MC. Limitations of postmortem assessment of human coronary artery size and luminal narrowing: differential effects of tissue fixation and processing on vessels with different degrees of atherosclerosis. J Am Coll Cardiol 1985; 5:342–346.

30. Zarins CK, Zatina MA, Glagov S. Correlation of postmortem angiography with pathologic anatomy. Quantitation of atherosclerotic lesions. In: Bond MG, Insull W Jr, Glagov S, Chandler AB, Cornhill JF, eds. Clinical Diagnosis of Atherosclerosis: Quantitative Methods of Evaluation. New York: Springer-Verlag. 1983: 283–303.

31. Dietz WA, Tobis JM, Isner JM. Failure of angiography to accurately depict the extent of coronary artery narrowing in three fatal cases of percutaneous transluminal coronary angioplasty. J Am Coll Cardiol 1992; 19:1261–1270.

32. Warnes CA, Roberts WC. Sudden coronary death: Relation of amount and distribution of coronary narrowing at necropsy to previous symptoms of myocardial ischemia, left ventricular scarring and heart weight. Am J Cardiol 1984; 54:65–73.

33. Roberts WC. The coronary arteries and left ventricle in clinically isolated angina pectoris. Circulation 1976; 54:388–390.

34. Bulkley BH, Roberts WC. Atherosclerotic narrowing of the left main coronary artery. A necropsy analysis of 152 patients with fatal coronary heart disease and varying degrees of left main narrowing. Circulation 1976; 53:823–828.

35. Leung W-H, Alderman EL, Lee TC, Stadius ML. Quantitative arteriography of apparently normal coronary segments with nearby or distant disease suggests presence of occult, nonvisualized atherosclerosis. J Am Coll Cardiol 1995; 25: 311–317.

36. Coy KM, Maurer G, Siegel RJ. Intravascular ultrasound imaging. A current perspective. J Am Coll Cardiol 1991; 18:1811–1823.

37. Mintz GS, Painter JA, Pichard AD, et al. Atherosclerosis in angiographically "normal" coronary artery reference segments: an intravascular ultrasound study with clinical correlations. J Am Coll Cardiol 1995; 25:1479–1485.

38. Glagov S, Weisenberg E, Zarins CK, Stankunavicius R, Kolettis GJ. Compensa-

tory enlargement of human atherosclerotic coronary arteries. N Engl J Med 1987; 316:1371–1375.

39. Stiel GM, Stiel LSG, Schofer J, Donath K, Mathey DG. Impact of compensatory enlargement of atherosclerotic coronary arteries on angiographic assessment of coronary artery disease. Circulation 1989; 80:1603–1609.

40. Clarkson TB, Prichard RW, Morgan TM, Petrick GS, Klein KP. Remodeling of coronary arteries in human and nonhuman primates. JAMA 1994; 271:289–294.

41. Losordo DW, Rosenfield K, Kaufman J, Pieczek A, Isner JM. Focal compensatory enlargement of human arteries in response to progressive atherosclerosis. In vivo documentation using intravascular ultrasound. Circulation 1994; 89:2570–2577.

42. Mann JM, Davies MJ. Assessment of the severity of coronary disease at post-mortem examination. Are the measurements clinically valid? Br Heart J 1995; 74:528–530.

43. Nishioka T, Luo H, Berglund H, et al. Absence of focal compensatory enlargement or constriction in diseased human coronary saphenous vein bypass grafts. An intravascular ultrasound study. Circulation 1996; 93:683–690.

44. Pasterkamp G, Wensing PJ, Post MJ, Hillen B, Mali WP, Borst C. Paradoxical arterial wall shrinkage may contribute to luminal narrowing of human athero-sclerotic femoral arteries. Circulation 1995; 91:1444–1449.

45. Zarins CK, Weisenberg E, Kolettis G, Stankunavicius R, Glagov S. Differential enlargement of artery segments in response to enlarging atherosclerotic plaques. J Vasc Surg 1988; 7:386–394.

46. Fishbein MC, Siegel RJ. How big are coronary artery atherosclerotic plaques that rupture? Circulation 1996; 94:2662–2666.

2

Intravascular Ultrasound Image Interpretation: Normal Arteries, Abnormal Vessels, and Atheroma Types Pre- and Postintervention

Neal G. Uren, Paul G. Yock, and Peter J. Fitzgerald
Stanford University School of Medicine, Stanford, California

I. INTRODUCTION

Intravascular ultrasound (IVUS) has been a major development in the imaging of coronary arteries and has allowed the operator to view not only the lumen of the artery but also the wall in sequential tomographic slices. This "look inside" has emphasized the shortcomings of conventional angiography in determining whether an apparently normal coronary artery is free of coronary atherosclerosis. Clinical studies in IVUS began in 1989 with the development of catheters initially in the size 5 to 6 F size range, with the most recent catheter size miniaturized to 2.9 F (1). IVUS has permitted not only a greater understanding of plaque morphology and its response to interventional procedures but has provided accurate on-line quantitative information regarding lumen size and residual plaque load, an important predictor of restenosis. The presence of disease not only at the site of focal stenosis but also in reference segments believed by angiography to be free of disease has modified interventional practice significantly. It is likely that continued technical developments will enhance and define the role of IVUS in coronary interventional practice.

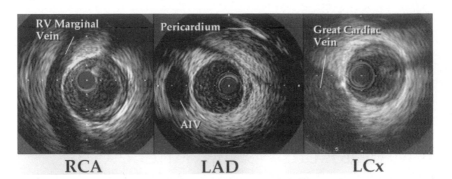

RCA   LAD   LCx

Figure 1   The left panel is an image in the mid-right coronary artery. Marginal veins cross around the artery in a horseshoe pattern, often associated with and opposite to the branch points of the right ventricular marginal arteries. Recurrent atrial branches generally emerge on the opposite side of the artery to the marginal branches.

The middle panel is an image of the proximal left anterior descending artery (LAD). The anterior interventricular vein (AIV) lies to the left of the proximal artery in the majority of people (85%), with the first two diagonal branches on the same side. In one-third of people, the anterior interventricular vein branches into two after the second diagonal to lie either side of the LAD more distally. Pericardium may be seen as a bright reflection on the anterior side of the artery. Diagonal branches emerge on the same side as the AIV. Septal branches emerge from the LAD in a perpendicular fashion to myocardium, on the opposite side to pericardium.

The right image is of the proximal left circumflex artery. Distally, the CFX is accompanied by the posterior left ventricular vein whereas in its proximal section, it is crossed and shadowed superiorly by the great cardiac vein. Recurrent atrial branches emerge from the circumflex artery toward the great cardiac vein in the opposite direction to obtuse marginal branches.

II. NORMAL CORONARY ARTERIES

An appreciation of the coronary anatomy and its relationship to the structures around it is important to the accurate interpretation of IVUS images. These spatial relations are best appreciated at the time of slow catheter pullback from distal to proximal vessel done either manually or using an automated pullback device. Advances in image quality and improved tissue penetration have allowed the use of perivascular structures in addition to side branches as reference points for tomographic and axial orientation (Fig. 1).

There are three concentric layers in the epicardial coronary arterial wall demonstrable at histology and seen by IVUS imaging (Fig. 2).

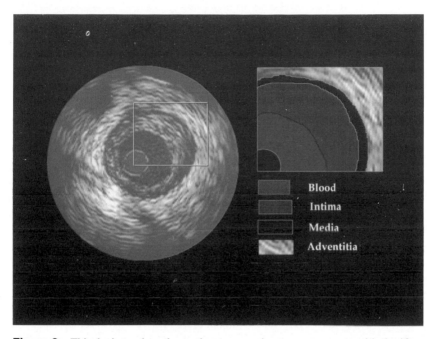

Figure 2 This depicts a three-layered appearance in a coronary artery with significant asymmetric intimal thickening. The medium is easily seen as a thin sonolucent layer between the intimal plaque and the adventitia.

1. **Intima.** The innermost layer consists of endothelial cells and the subendothelial layer of smooth-muscle cells and fibroblasts in a connective tissue matrix. The overall thickness of this layer can be just a few cells thick in childhood, expanding to 150 to 200 μm in the adult. Beneath this, there is the internal elastic lamina, which is intact in the normal state, consisting of fenestrated elastic fibers with a thickness less than 25 μm.

2. **Media.** The media consists of multiple layers of smooth muscle cells arranged helically and circumferentially around the lumen of the artery, woven through a matrix of elastic fibers and collagen. The coronary arteries are less elastic than other, similar-size arteries and thus resemble a transition toward more muscular peripheral arteries. The normal medial thickness ranges from 125 to 350 μm (mean, 200 μm), although in the presence of plaque the medial thickness may be considerably thinner, approximately 100 μm (2), or completely involuted and replaced by plaque in severe disease. The external elastic lamina encircles the medial layer. It is composed of elastin but is thinner and

more fenestrated than the internal lamina, and is not more than 20 μm in thickness.

3. **Adventitia.** This external layer is essentially fibrous tissue, i.e., collagen (type III) and elastin, with the collagen orientated longitudinally in general and to a lesser tissue density than media. It is this layer that is surrounded by the vaso vasorum, nerves, and lymphatic vessels. The adventitia can extend from 300 to 500 μm in diameter, beyond which it is considered perivascular stroma and epicardial fat.

The appearance of the three-layered appearance by IVUS occurs owing to the acoustic impedance between adjacent structures. For example, the lumen and intima are usually well delineated owing to the large acoustic impedance between fluid and tissue. The three-layered appearance of the vessel wall is dependent on the intima's being of sufficient size to be identified with the resolution of the current generation of ultrasound transducers and in the presence of a sufficient acoustic interface between media and adventitia (3). At a frequency of 30 MHz, the threshold of intimal thickening required to resolve a definite intimal layer is approximately 160 μm. Previous work has shown that there is a progressive increase in the thickness of the intimal layer with increasing age (4). In an autopsy study done to evaluate the relationship between ultrasound images and tissue histology in 16 intact hearts from subjects ranging in age from 13 to 55 years with no history of coronary artery disease, segments with a three-layered appearance had a significantly greater intimal thickness (243 ± 105 μm) than nonlayered segments (112 ± 55 μm), with a threshold between the two of 178 μm (4). As this threshold is crossed in males over the age of 30 years, it is apparent that histologically normal arteries will only have a two-layered appearance in the rare patients younger than 30 undergoing ultrasound examination.

The media appears as a thin middle layer by IVUS and is often referred to as the sonolucent zone as it is less echodense than the intima or adventitia due to a lesser collagen content. IVUS imaging was performed in vitro on six histologically normal and 104 minimally diseased arteries in patients aged 13 to 83 years to test the hypothesis that normal coronary arteries produce a three-layer image that corresponds to the histologic layers of intima, media, and adventitia (5). The results showed a very strong correlation between area of the echolucent ultrasound layer with the media and the inner echogenic layer with intimal area. In addition, a three-layer appearance was consistently seen when the internal elastic membrane was present with or without intimal hyperplasia. If the internal elastic membrane was absent, a three-layer appearance was still seen if the collagen content of the media was low. However, a two-layer appearance was observed when there was absence of the internal elastic membrane as well as a high collagen content of the media (5). In addition, the relative composition of the intimal layer also determined the ability to discriminate the three vessel wall layers. Thus, over a given coronary artery segment, the three-layered appearance may alternate with a two-layered appearance owing to the relative content of elastin and collagen. However, for the purposes of quantitation, the acoustic impedance between the combination of adventitia and external elastic lamina with the intima permits accurate measurement of plaque and vessel area. In the left main stem and at the proximal part of the right coronary artery, the three-layered appearance may be lost owing to the increase in elastin content in transition from the highly elastic aortic root.

III. ABNORMAL VESSELS

Intravascular ultrasound is the current imaging technology of choice for studying the morphology of atherosclerotic plaque in vivo. Early studies used a large 8 F catheter to correlate ultrasound appearances with histological findings in arteries collected at the time of autopsy (6). The arteries studied were a combination of an elastic, transitional (musculoelastic), and muscular types with respect to media/adventitia appearance. The results confirmed that a highly accurate measurement of luminal area was achieved comparing ultrasound to direct measurement of perfused isolated arteries. A distinct interface between media and adventitia was obtained only where there was a significant difference in the acoustic qualities of the two layers (namely, loose collagen in the adventitia of elastic arteries, or where there was a minimal smooth muscle cell component in the adventitia of transitional/muscular arteries). The interface between plaque and media was only apparent where there was a dense internal elastic lamina or a significant amount of necrotic material in the plaque.

The earliest accumulations of atherosclerotic plaque consist of crescentic intimal thickening of an intermediate echointensity. A common site for initial and increased plaque accumulation occurs at branch points and bifurcations due to the shear stress effect of blood flow. Transplant vasculopathy is a good model for the early development of coronary artery disease as these patients undergo ultrasound studies at angiographic follow-up early after transplantation. In one study, intravascular ultrasound was used to study epicardial arteries in 25 recently transplanted hearts from young donors (mean age 28 years) (7). In this unique study group, all donors under 25 years old had a homogeneous nonlayered vessel wall. Another group of donors, mean age 32 years, manifested a three-layered appearance. In five hearts, significant eccentric intimal

Table 1   Severity, Intimal Thickness, and
Circumferential Extent by Grade

	Severity	Intimal thickness	Circumferential extent
Grade I	Minimal	<300 μm	<180°
Grade II	Mild	<300 μm	>180°
Grade III	Moderate	300–500 μm	
		>500 μm	<180°
Grade IV	Severe	>1000 μm	
		>500 μm	>180°

Source: St. Goar et al., 1992 (8).

thickening, >500 μm, was shown in donors with risk factors for coronary disease, implying early coronary disease in the presence of angiographically normal arteries. Subsequent work by the same group in a larger group of transplant recipients over a long-term follow-up has shown that all 60 hearts had variable degrees of concentric intimal thickening after 1 year; 42 of the 60 had normal coronary arteries at angiography (8). From these studies, a grading system to describe the extent and severity of intimal thickening was proposed (the Stanford classification), with patients classified from their most severe site (Table 1).

With a greater accumulation of plaque, there is a greater complexity to the plaque which may be differentiated by broad ultrasound criteria. A fibrous plaque has an echodensity intermediate between less echodense media or lipid and more echodense calcification. By comparing the brightness of the tissue in question to that of the adventitia, a relative grading of the plaque may thus be obtained. Such fibrous plaques with similar brightness to adventitia may then be described as hard or soft (with respect to the gray scale), depending on the presence or absence of shadowing behind the plaque (Fig. 3). Fatty plaques are significantly more echolucent and when large may be appreciated as lipid pools. However, because shadowing in relation to a fibrous plaque may be misinterpreted as a lipid collection, there is a tendency to broadly classify plaques containing lipid as fibrofatty in nature.

Calcification is commonly seen by intravascular ultrasound as a bright echo with shadowing behind often associated with reverberation artifact in the area of the shadow due to oscillation of the ultrasound beam between calcium and transducer (Fig. 4). Calcium may be seen in relatively small plaque accumulations, indicating the age of the plaque or the site of previous plaque rupture and

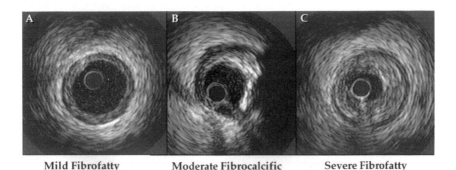

| Mild Fibrofatty | Moderate Fibrocalcific | Severe Fibrofatty |

Figure 3 These three panels demonstrate different plaque morphologies. (A) A concentric mild fibrofatty plaque which is less echodense than adventitia. (B) A more echodense eccentric plaque with an area of beam attenuation between 2 and 4 o'clock due to the presence of calcium. (C) An extensive fibrofatty plaque with echodensity similar to adventitia.

repair. In one series of patients undergoing balloon angioplasty, 82% of arterial segments exhibited small areas of calcium; these were visible by fluoroscopy in only 8% of angiograms at the lesion site or in 155 of more proximal segments (9). In the GUIDE (Guidance by Ultrasound Imaging for Decision Endpoints) trial (Phase I), 70% of target lesions had areas of calcium by ultrasound, compared to 40% of angiograms (10). Calcification may be graded from absent (0) to severe (3+) by the extent of the arc subtended by a fibrocalcific matrix (11). In general, at least 180° of calcium is required to achieve a mass of calcium identifiable by angiography (74% identification by fluoroscopy) increasing to 86% of cases identified if more than two quadrants or calcium length ≥6 mm is present (12).

By definition, plaque calcification results in shadowing of deeper structures, obscuring evaluation of underlying arterial wall components. Furthermore, shadowing may occur without any obvious calcification as the calcium may be out of plane and not visualized unless hit by the ultrasound beam in a perpendicular fashion. The calcium may be distributed in the plaque in several ways: as a deep deposit in an arc at the intima-media border, in a superficial rim at the luminal surface, or as a concretion within a fibrous plaque (Fig. 5). In one study of 110 patients, superficial calcium was present in 50%, deep calcium in 15%, and both in 35% (12). On occasion, the fibrous cap may be intensely echoreflective with shadowing extending to and around the periphery of the artery, suggesting a more uniform distribution of calcium throughout the wall. Dense

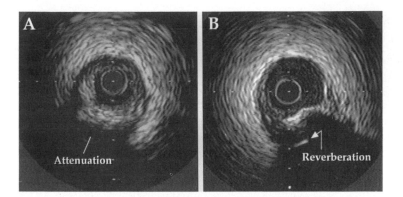

Figure 4 These two images demonstrate the ultrasound fingerprint of (A) dense fibrous plaque with gradual attenuation of the beam posterior to the plaque, and (B) a superficial fibrocalcific plaque with an acoustic shadow immediately behind the calcific rim and an acoustic reverberation in this area at 5 o'clock.

fibrotic plaques may be sufficiently underpenetrated by the ultrasound beam to cause significant shadowing; such plaques are usually referred to as fibrocalcific.

The presence of thrombus is often more difficult to establish as it is frequently mistaken for soft plaque (13). Thrombus often appears as a scintillating mass with a lobular edge; classically, it moves in an undulating manner separate from the movement of the artery. Incomplete microchannels are sometimes identified, but many intracoronary thrombi may be very difficult to differentiate as they may be relatively small and not very separate from the arterial wall. Luminal blood is characterized by a continually mobile speckled pattern. In contrast to conventional echocardiography, the gain of the intravascular ultrasound console should be set to allow its identification separate from possible thrombus. Where the flow of blood is significantly impaired, the backscatter may be sufficiently intense to mimic thrombus or soft plaque. It may be differentiated from the latter by injection of saline, converting the lumen briefly to greater echolucency. Advanced signal analysis of the radiofrequency pattern may help to provide rational and objective criteria to differentiate thrombus from fibrofatty plaque (14).

Intravascular ultrasound has confirmed the observations first made by Glagov et al. (15) that with increasing plaque accumulation, there is a remodeling process whereby the vessel expands to accommodate the plaque load. The

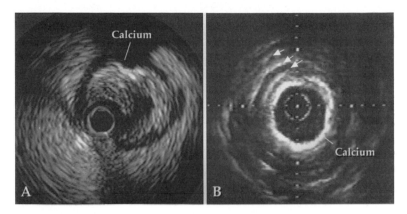

Figure 5 These images demonstrate different distributions of calcium. (A) An area of echodensity between 11 and 1 o'clock posterior to the intimal plaque, indicative of deep wall calcium. (B) A superficial ring of calcium with reverberations readily visible (arrows).

extent of remodeling in a given artery may be highly variable with segments of positive remodeling, no change, and negative remodeling (shrinkage). Even in angiographically normal segments, the average plaque burden in the normal reference segment may comprise 40% of the total vessel cross-sectional area. The inability of angiography to detect this occult disease is due to the presence of positive arterial remodeling and the diffuse nature of disease throughout the entire vessel length in many patients. It has been suggested that discrete coronary artery lesions become apparent angiographically only when the accumulation of plaque rises to above a threshold of 40% of vessel area—e.g., overcomes the ability of the vessel to expand any further (16–18).

Occasionally, image interpretation can be obscured in abnormal vessels owing to incorrect assumptions of the borders of the vessel layers traced manually. This can occur because the internal elastic lumina may not be a separate layer in the presence of plaque. Media may also appear unusually thick owing to attenuation of the ultrasound beam passing through intimal plaque. By contrast, the media layer may also be thinner than expected owing to the spread of the signal from an area of high reflectivity (plaque) to one low reflectivity (media). For these reasons, the outer border of the plaque is usually defined as being at the media/adventitia border (the external elastic lamina), which is believed to be a fair assumption given the relative contribution of media to the plaque area. It is implicit in image interpretation that frames are selected with the best image quality and selected by an experienced operator.

IV. ATHEROMA TYPES PRE- AND POSTINTERVENTION

Intravascular ultrasound has provided an invaluable insight into the characteristics of atherosclerotic plaque with an accurate on-line means for measuring the dimensions of the index artery prior to and after intervention. Furthermore, the reduction in the diameter of ultrasound catheters (to < 1 mm in diameter) and improved deliverability characteristics have allowed an assessment to be made prior to intervention and describe vessel morphology after the procedure. The technique can now be used to assess coronary lesions with respect to device sizing and selection. Additionally, it may provide additional prognostic information regarding the likelihood of acute and subacute vessel closure and longer-term restenosis.

A. Preintervention

With the development of catheters as small as 2.9 F, intravascular ultrasound may be used to assess lesions prior to intervention and direct appropriate therapy. In general, there are two major determinants of device selection— plaque load, or burden, and the extent and severity of calcification. With an extensive plaque load, a debulking strategy has become common in interventional practice. Directional coronary atherectomy has been used to debulk lesions although it is only generally successful when the lesion is free of superficial calcium. In the latter case, high-speed rotational atherectomy has become increasingly used to ablate superficial calcium in lesions with a large plaque load, either as a stand-alone procedure or in preparation for further treatment (19).

In one study, 313 target lesions underwent intravascular ultrasound, resulting in a change of therapy in 40% of cases (20). This comprised 6% of patients who underwent therapy where none had been planned owing to a significant disparity in the assessment of lesion severity between ultrasound and angiography; 7% had revascularization deferred for the same reason, and a further 13% had a change in revascularization strategy or selection including referral for bypass surgery in 1% because of demonstration of unsuspected significant unprotected left main involvement. Intravascular ultrasound detected calcium in 68% of target lesions (compared to 37% of lesions at angiography) with additional information on calcium localization and its relation to eccentric plaque distribution. Thus, intravascular ultrasound assessment of target lesion calcification, eccentricity, or unusual morphology dictated a change in strategy or device selection. A strategy for device selection was described: lesions with significant superficial calcium were treated with rotablation, excimer laser, or surgery; eccentric, noncalcified lesions underwent directional atherectomy; dissections were stented; thrombotic vein grafts were treated with thrombolysis and/or extraction atherectomy; and fibrotic vein grafts were often stented after balloon dilatation. Although the patients in this study were selected for imaging preintervention (which would exaggerate the intravascular ultrasound influence), the results still demonstrate the ability of intravascular ultrasound to characterize lesions and modify strategy accordingly when used before as well as after intervention.

B. Postintervention

One of the common indications for an intravascular ultrasound study is to assess the appearance of a coronary artery following an interventional procedure. This scan is performed for several reasons—to examine the resulting morphologic appearance from the intervention, to judge success, to complement angiographic assessment, to quantitate lumen enlargement and plaque reduction, and to consider whether or not to proceed to further intervention including stent implantation.

1. Balloon Angioplasty

Initial in vitro validation studies were done to correlate the appearance of diseased arteries at ultrasound post-balloon dilatation with histology (21). The consistent finding following balloon dilatation was tearing of the plaque with separation of the ends of the tear and an increase in lumen cross-sectional area, with some stretching of the less diseased wall. In this study, the lumen area by ultrasound and at section were similar ($r = .88$) (21). Dissection of the plaque (separation of intima from media) was a common finding which appeared as an increase in the sonolucent area corresponding to media. One feature described was the presence of arterial flaps with protrusion of plaque into the lumen, less frequently seen in vivo owing to blood flow.

The effect of balloon dilatation on plaque morphology has been described by Honye et al. (22) and classified as types A to E on the basis of extent and depth of plaque rupture. A type A morphology comprises a partial tear which does not extend to the media. Type B morphology is a tear extending through the entire plaque but not into media. Type C morphology is a complete radial tear extending behind plaque laterally to an arc less than 180°. Type D morphology extends the plaque fracture to an arc greater than 180°. The type E morphology rather than describing medial injury, describes stretching of the plaque or free wall in a concentric atherosclerotic plaque without plaque fracture (subtype E-1) or focal stretching of the free wall in an eccentric plaque (subtype E-2). Such work has confirmed that plaque compression is not a mechanism of balloon dilatation and that plaque fracture is an important component of successful balloon angioplasty.

An alternative classification system to describe the effect of angioplasty on atheromatous plaque has been described by Gerber et al. (23). A total of 48 patients were studied successfully after angioplasty. The authors identified seven distinct morphologic patterns. Types 1 to 4 were described in concentric vessels; types 6 and 7 in eccentric vessels; and type 5 in either intimal pattern. Type 1 comprised minor superficial intimal fissures only (4% of patients); type 2 described deeper tears within the intima (2%). Type 3 involved deep tearing extending to the medial border (17%), and type 4 was described as dissection through the intima extending into media (subtype a = subintimal dissection; subtype b = submedial dissection) (4%). Type 5 dissections involved subintimal dissection separating a large part of intima from media, so-called circular dissection, which were the commonest (31%). In eccentric plaques, type 6 dissections involve stretching of the plaque-free wall (13%); cf. type 1 in concentric lesions. Type 7 dissection describes plaque rupture with two subtypes (29%); cf. type 4 (subtype a = subintimal dissection; subtype b = submedial dissection) (23). In this study, 67% of lesions had calcification by ultrasound, with 83% of patients demonstrating lumen enlargement by plaque rupture or dissection. This classification was broadly similar to that proposed by Honye et al. (22); vessel stretching and superficial tears were seen less often in the series reported by Gerber et al. (23). Deep tearing and circular dissection were roughly equal in the two studies.

The presence of calcium in a coronary lesion also determines the response of the artery to balloon dilatation. In one study of patients after balloon angioplasty of peripheral and coronary vessels, intralesional calcium and the relative size of dissection for each lesion were determined (24). A total of 76% of patients had significant dissection/plaque fracture after angioplasty. In 71% of these patients, significant localized calcium deposits were identified within the plaque, and the vast majority of dissections (87%) were adjacent to the calcific portion of the wall. Comparing the relative size of dissections with respect to the neoluminal area, dissections in calcified areas were larger than those in lesions without calcium—28% vs. 11%, respectively. It was concluded that localized calcium had a direct role in promoting dissection by increasing shear stress within the plaque at the junction between tissue types with differing elastic properties (24). Given these findings, it may be that deep calcium deposits protect against deep medial injury despite a large plaque fracture by deflecting the pressure axially. Further characterization of lesion morphology with newer ultrasound catheters is required to address these issues in a clinical context.

An important use for IVUS in interventional procedures is that it can accurately measure lumen and vessel area both at the lesion site and at the reference segment, allowing the operator to size angioplasty balloons more exactly. In a key study of 223 coronary vessels treated by a Palmaz-Schatz stent, directional atherectomy, or laser balloon angioplasty, 83% of patients underwent follow-up angiography 6 months after treatment (25). The traditional dichotomous definition of restenosis ($\geq$50% diameter stenosis) was used along with a cumulative graphical method. Although the restenosis rates were 19%, 31%, and 50% for stents, directional atherectomy, and laser balloon angioplasty, respectively; the late lumen loss was equivalent across the groups. This indicated that the major procedural determinant on restenosis was the acute lumen gain (2.6, 2.2, and 2.0 mm in the three groups), leading to the "bigger is better" hypothesis (25). Accurate balloon sizing is central to achieving the largest acute lumen gain after balloon angioplasty, and with ultrasound it is possible to demonstrate arterial remodeling and vessel expansion adjacent to diseased segments. To optimize balloon angioplasty using intravascular ultrasound to size balloons safely, the CLOUT (CLinical Outcomes of Ultrasound Trial) study has been initiated with early results on 64 patients already reported (26). Ultrasound imaging is performed after successful standard "optimal" balloon angioplasty with protocol driven balloon upsizing if unsuspected reference segment atheroma is demonstrated. The balloon size is selected by measuring

(proximal reference vessel area + proximal reference lumen area)/2

and rounding up to the nearest 0.25 mm. In CLOUT, 52 $\pm$ 15% of the reference segment cross-sectional area was occupied by atheroma, leading to balloon upsizing in 82% of lesions. Major complications were seen only in 3% of patients. There was an increase in balloon : artery ratio from 1.03 $\pm$ 0.12 to 1.16 $\pm$ 0.14 after ultrasound guidance associated with an increase in minimum lumen area from 3.17 $\pm$ 1.07 to 4.52 $\pm$ 1.0 mm^2. It is hoped that follow-up will demonstrate an improvement in restenosis rate due to an improved acute lumen gain.

2. Directional Coronary Atherectomy

This plaque-debulking technique involves the use of balloon-supported directional cutting device or atherectomy catheter. The value of adjunct intravascular ultrasound imaging is that it can direct the cutting device to the area of largest plaque load and can identify the presence of superficial calcification, which is a relative contraindication to the use of the cutting device. In one study, 52 patients were enrolled where directional atherectomy was guided by intracoronary ultrasound, and in 22 patients angiographic follow-up after a mean of 6 months was available (27). The plaque reduction at the site of the smallest lumen diameter was 65 ± 21% as measured with ultrasound. This correlated well with the weight of the resected tissue but not with quantitative angiography. The plaque reduction was higher in echolucent plaques (higher fibrin and lipid content) than in echodense plaques (higher calcium and collagen content) by ultrasound assessment—76% vs. 60%, respectively. However, the echogenecity of the lesion was a predictor of the occurrence of restenosis showing a significantly higher likelihood of restenosis in lesions that were primarily echolucent (100%, compared to 33%) by ultrasound.

One recent study was performed to investigate the effect of directional atherectomy on plaque as assessed by intravascular ultrasound (28). In the in vitro arm of the study, the volume of plaque removed was calculated with intracoronary ultrasound, which correlated well with water displacement calculations. In the clinical arm to study the mechanism of lumen enlargement, the total increase in lumen gain resulted from a combination of plaque removal and vessel stretch. In this particular study 61% of the atherosclerotic lesions were removed by atherectomy, whereas 39% of the lumen gain was created by vessel stretch at the time of the procedure. It also suggested that nonconcentric cutting may occur owing to the difference in tissue quality.

Another study measured the impact of intracoronary imaging variables as predictors for the outcome following coronary atherectomy (29). A total of 170 patients with successful ultrasound-guided atherectomy were included in the study, and a multiple stepwise regression analysis was performed. The predominant factor influencing acute lumen gain was plaque removal, and to a minor extent stretching of the vessel. Stepwise linear regression showed that the arc of calcium (in degrees) and the pre-atherectomy plaque + media cross-sectional area (plaque area) by ultrasound were associated with a larger post-atherectomy percent cross-sectional narrowing. In fact, the arc of calcium was the most consistent predictor of success by any of the ultrasound criteria such as post-atherectomy lumen area, cross-sectional narrowing, or percent plaque volume removal. Thus, not only the orientation of the cutting device but the morphologic characteristics of the plaque determine the success of the procedure which is best achieved using ultrasound imaging.

Given that the amount of plaque removal leads to an increase in acute lumen and that intravascular ultrasound may be used to guide appropriate cutting, the OARS (Optimal Atherectomy Restenosis Study) was designed to

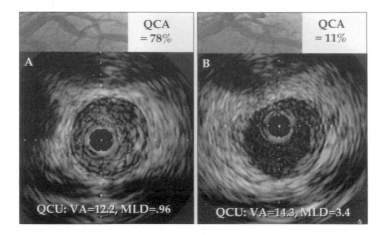

Figure 6 Two images before and after aggressive plaque debulking by directional coronary atherectomy. (A) A diameter stenosis of 78% by quantitative coronary angiography (QCA) by comparing the minimum lumen diameter (MLD) with the proximal reference segment. Quantitative coronary ultrasound (QCU) describes a vessel area (VA) of 12.2 mm^2 and an MLD of 0.96 mm (the diameter of the 2.9 F ultrasound catheter). (B) After atherectomy, the residual diameter stenosis is 11% by QCA. By QCU, the vessel area is increased to 14.3 mm^2, and the MLD is now 3.4 mm.

introduce an aggressive DCA strategy (<15% residual diameter stenosis) (Fig. 6). The study was designed to see if a lower residual plaque area by ultrasound translates into a reduced restenosis rate at follow-up. Adjunctive angioplasty was strongly encouraged, leading to a mean post-procedure diameter stenosis of 8% (19% after DCA alone) and a procedural success of 98% in the first 216 lesions, translating into a restenosis rate of 30.3% (30). A residual percent plaque area of 55.6% was achieved by this aggressive IVUS-guided approach (31).

3. High-Speed Rotational Atherectomy

Rotational atherectomy uses a rotating diamond-coated burr to abrade atherosclerotic plaque at speeds as high as 180,000 rpm. The technique works through the method of differential cutting whereby the burr selectively abrades harder tissue and is deflected away from normal vessel wall, thus removing superficial calcium and dense fibrous plaque through microembolization and pushing softer plaque away from the cutting path of the device. The appearance of vessels undergoing rotational atherectomy as a debulking strategy has been

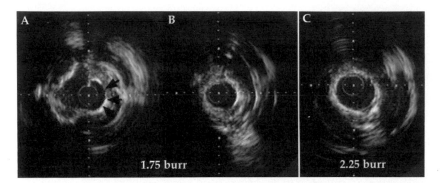

Figure 7 Three ultrasound images recorded at the time of high-speed rotational atherectomy. (A) Proximal inflow to the lesion with a characteristic signature of differential cutting of superficial calcium between 12 and 6 o'clock (arrows). (B) Midlesion at the minimum cross-sectional area with a similar appearance after a burr size of 1.75 mm. (C) Following a 2.25 mm burr, there is a marked increase in minimum lumen area in the midlesion with a round, nondissected contour to the intima-lumen interface.

described (32). In this study, 28 patients (22 calcified plaques, a third of which were circumferential) underwent ultrasound imaging after the procedure (with 71% having adjunct balloon angioplasty). Following rotablation, a distinct, circular intima-lumen interface was achieved with the lumen size 20% larger than the largest burr used (Fig. 7). Deviations from a circular geometry occurred only in areas of soft plaque or superficial tissue disruption of calcified plaque. This study confirmed that there was no significant damage to the media, and no dissections were caused by the procedure. A residual plaque load of 54% was reported indicating that atheroablation using a burr strategy of 70% to 80% of the reference vessel lumen by angiography resulted in a significant residual plaque, even with adjunctive balloon dilatation, in the majority of patients (32).

A subsequent study of sequential ultrasound imaging before and after rotational atherectomy did confirm dissection planes in 26% of cases following rotablation increasing to 76% of cases after adjunct balloon dilatation with spread of the dissection plane to areas not only with the calcified plaque but also adjacent to the plaque, in part contributing to the expansion of the lumen area (33). There was a reduction in plaque area from 15.7 ± 4.1 to 13.0 ± 4.7 mm^2 after initial rotablation but still a residual percent cross-sectional narrowing of 74%, indicating the need for adjunct balloon angioplasty to achieve an adequate final lumen area. In this study, the arc of calcium decreased significantly, with full thickness calcium removal in some patients. Even without a measurable decrease in calcium arc, significant calcium ablation occurred, as evidenced by an increase in lumen area, the uncovering of deeper calcium deposits, and the uncovering of deeper adventitial structures not seen pre-rotational atherectomy.

In everyday practice, pre-interventional ultrasound scanning can direct atheroablation appropriately. Superficial calcium not apparent by angiography is amenable to successful rotablation if the calcium arc is >180° and extends to more than half the lesion length. This preliminary debulking may then be supplemented by balloon angioplasty or intracoronary stenting.

V. CONCLUSIONS

The therapeutic approaches at the time of interventional procedures may be guided by ultrasound appearance such as the presence, severity, and extent of coronary dissection following balloon angioplasty. An aggressive burr-sizing strategy may be employed at the time of rotational atherectomy with ultrasound guidance. Adequate directional atherectomy may be guided by ultrasound, and the best debulking may be achieved through this approach. Future technical developments include transducer miniaturization, on-line tissue characterization, and three-dimensional reconstruction are likely to expand the clinical role of intravascular ultrasound as it becomes a common tool in the interventional catheter laboratory.

REFERENCES

1. Yock PG, Fitzgerald PJ, Popp RL. Intravascular ultrasound. Sci Am 1995; 2: 68–77.
2. Waller BF. The eccentric coronary atherosclerotic plaque: morphologic observations and clinical relevance. Clin Cardiol 1989; 12:14.
3. Picano E, Landini L, Lattanzi F, et al. Time domain echo pattern evaluations from normal and atherosclerotic arterial walls: a study in vitro. Circulation 1988; 3:654.
4. Fitzgerald PJ, St. Goar FG, Connolly RJ, et al. Intravascular ultrasound imaging of coronary arteries. Is three layers the norm? Circulation 1992; 86:154–158.
5. Maheswaran B, Leung CY, Gutfinger DE, et al. Intravascular ultrasound appearance of normal and mildly diseased coronary arteries—correlation with histologic specimens. Am Heart J 1995; 130:976–986.
6. Nishimura RA, Edwards WD, Warnes CA, et al. Intravascular ultrasound imaging: in vitro validation and pathologic correlation. J Am Coll Cardiol 1990; 16: 145–154.
7. St. Goar FG, Pinto FJ, Alderman EL, et al. Intracoronary ultrasound in cardiac

transplant recipients: in vivo evidence of "angiographically silent" intimal thickening. Circulation 1992; 85:979–987.

8.   St. Goar FG, Pinto FJ, Alderman EL, et al. Detection of coronary atherosclerosis in young adult hearts using intravascular ultrasound. Circulation 1992; 86:756–763.

9.   Tobis JM, Mallery J, Mahon D, et al. Intravascular ultrasound imaging of human coronary arteries in vivo: analysis of tissue characterization with comparison to in vitro histological specimens. Circulation 1991; 83:319–326.

10.   GUIDE Trial Investigators. IVUS-determined predictors of restenosis in PTCA and DCA: final report from the GUIDE trial, Phase II. J Am Coll Cardiol 1996; 27:156A. Abstract.

11.   Farb A, Virmani R, Atkinson JB, Kolodgie FD. Plaque morphology and pathologic changes in arteries from patients dying after coronary balloon angioplasty. J Am Coll Cardiol 1990; 16:1421–1429.

12.   Mintz GS, Douek P, Pichard A, et al. Target lesion calcification in coronary artery disease: an intravascular ultrasound study. J Am Coll Cardiol 1992; 20:1149–1155.

13.   Siegel RJ, Ariani M, Fishbein MC, et al. Histopathologic validation of angioscopy and intravascular ultrasound. Circulation 1991; 84:109–117.

14.   Metz JA, Preuss P, Komiyama N, et al. Discrimination of soft plaque and thrombus based on radiofrequency analysis of intravascular ultrasound. J Am Coll Cardiol 1996; 27(suppl. A):220A. Abstract.

15.   Glagov S, Weisenberg E, Zarins CK, Stankunavicius R, Kolettis GJ. Compensatory enlargement of human atherosclerotic arteries. N Engl J Med 1987; 316: 1371–1375.

16.   Kakuta T, Currier JW, Haudenschild CC, Ryan TJ, Faxon DP. Differences in compensatory vessel enlargement, not intimal formation, account for restenosis after angioplasty in the hypercholesterolemic rabbit model. Circulation 1994; 89: 2809–2815.

17.   Post MJ, Borst C, Kuntz RE. The relative importance of arterial remodeling compared with intimal hyperplasia in lumen renarrowing after balloon angioplasty. Circulation 1994; 89:2816–2821.

18.   Currier JW, Faxon DP. Restenosis after percutaneous transluminal coronary angioplasty: have we been aiming at the wrong target? J Am Coll Cardiol 1995; 25: 516–520.

19.   Ellis SG, Popma JJ, Buchbinder M, et al. Relation of clinical presentation, stenosis morphology, and operator technique to the procedural results of rotational atherectomy-facilitated angioplasty. Circulation 1994; 89:882–892.

20.   Mintz GS, Pichard AD, Kovach JA, et al. Impact of preintervention intravascular ultrasound imaging on transcatheter treatment strategies in coronary artery disease. Am J Cardiol 1994; 73:423–430.

21.   Tobis JM, Mallery JA, Gessert J, et al. Intravascular ultrasound cross-sectional arterial imaging before and after balloon angioplasty in vitro. Circulation 1989; 80:873–882.

22.   Honye J, Mahon DJ, Jain A, et al. Morphological effects of coronary balloon

angioplasty in vivo assessed by intravascular ultrasound imaging. Circulation 1992; 85:1012–1025.

23. Gerber TC, Erbel R, Görge G, Ge J, Rupprecht H-J, Meyer J. Classification of morphological effects of percutaneous transluminal coronary angioplasty assessed by intravascular ultrasound. Am J Cardiol 1992; 70:1546–1554.

24. Fitzgerald PJ, Ports TA, Yock PG. Contribution of localized calcium deposits to dissection after angioplasty: an observational study using intravascular ultrasound. Circulation 1992; 86:64–70.

25. Kuntz RE, Safian RD, Levine MJ, Reis GJ, Diver DJ, Baim DS. Novel approach to the analysis of restenosis after the use of three new coronary devices. J Am Coll Cardiol 1992; 19:1493–1499.

26. Stone GW, Linnemeier T, St. Goar FG, Mudra H, Sheehan H, Hodgson JM. Improved outcome of balloon angioplasty with intracoronary ultrasound guidance—core lab angiographic and ultrasound results from the CLOUT study. J Am Coll Cardiol 1996; 27(suppl. A):155A. Abstract.

27. De Lezo JS, Romero M, Medina A, et al. Intracoronary ultrasound assessment of directional coronary atherectomy: immediate and follow up findings. J Am Coll Cardiol 1992; 21:298–307.

28. Nakamura S, Mahon D, Leung C, et al. Intracoronary ultrasound imaging before and after directional coronary atherectomy: in vitro and clinical observations. Am Heart J 1995; 129:841–851.

29. Matar FA, Mintz GS, Pinnow E, et al. Multivariate predictors of intravascular ultrasound end points after directional coronary atherectomy. J Am Coll Cardiol 1995; 25:318–324.

30. Simonton CA, Leon MB, Kuntz RE, et al. Acute and late clinical and angiographic results of directional atherectomy in the Optimal Atherectomy Restenosis Study (OARS). Circulation 1995; 92(suppl):I-545. Abstract.

31. Popma JJ, Baim DS, Kuntz RE, et al., for the OARS Investigators. Early and late quantitative angiographic outcomes in the Optimal Atherectomy Restenosis Study (OARS). J Am Coll Cardiol 1996; 27:291A. Abstract.

32. Mintz GS, Potkin BN, Keren G, et al. Intravascular ultrasound evaluation of the effect of rotational atherectomy in obstructive atherosclerotic coronary artery disease. Circulation 1992; 86:1383–1393.

33. Kovach JA, Mintz GS, Pichard AD, et al. Sequential intravascular ultrasound characterization of the mechanisms of rotational atherectomy and adjunct balloon angioplasty. J Am Coll Cardiol 1993; 22:1024–1032.

3

Prognostic Implications of Intravascular Ultrasound Imaging After Coronary Intervention

Neal G. Uren, Paul G. Yock, and Peter J. Fitzgerald
Stanford University School of Medicine, Stanford, California

I. INTRODUCTION

Intravascular ultrasound (IVUS) permits accurate quantitation and description of coronary atherosclerotic plaque before, during, and after coronary interventional procedures. It is possible to define the change in lumen area accurately by planimetry and to document the presence of dissections and tissue flaps which may contribute to the increase in lumen area during certain device strategies. Furthermore, the effect of certain device strategies on the overall vessel size and plaque conformation can be tracked by ultrasound but not completely appreciated by conventional angiography. This accurate view from inside has modified present-day restenosis concepts by highlighting the importance of both plaque burden and overall vessel wall dynamics (vascular remodeling) and their relationship to clinical outcomes following an interventional approach. Advances in image quality, catheter miniaturization, and automatic lumen tracking will in the near future enhance the efficiency of this imaging tool in today's catheterization laboratory.

II. LIMITATIONS WITH ANGIOGRAPHY

Angiography describes a planar two-dimensional silhouette of a contrast-filled lumen. At best, an orthogonal two-dimensional image may be described, although, owing to vessel overlap, foreshortening, and disease at bifurcation points, this approach may still not give an accurate description of lesion severity, plaque distribution, or plaque composition. This is particularly common when assessing the left main stem either at its origin, which may be behind the catheter tip, or at its bifurcation, where the left anterior descending, circumflex, and intermediate vessels arise. Problems with accurate angiographic quantitation are frequently accentuated after coronary intervention due to plaque fracture and the subsequent appearance of a hazy lumen (1). Even with computer-assisted edge detection, the true lumen size may be obscured owing to extensive plaque fracture. An additional problem is the reliance on adjacent segments to characterize lesion severity as a percent stenosis. The normal reference segment is frequently diseased because of the diffuse nature of atherosclerosis (2), leading to an underestimation of disease severity. The absolute resolution of image intensifiers is also limited by radiation dose considerations and by rapid coronary artery motion, as is commonly the right coronary or atrioventricular groove arteries, leading to an image blur of up to 0.5 mm (1). In normal practice, angiography is rarely performed to achieve two projections of the index vessel orthogonal to each other and to the vessel. Thus, projections are made at different angles with the view illustrating the minimum diameter taken as the index picture of the greatest lesion severity, although this may not be in fact the case.

Despite these limitations, angiography remains the standard road map for the assessment of coronary stenoses. Following coronary intervention, the angiographic appearance is routinely used to determine the success of a procedure. Given the limitations described above, however, it has proven difficult to determine the mechanism of lumen improvement such as seen in the early randomized trials of directional coronary atherectomy, CAVEAT (Coronary Angioplasty Versus Excisional Atherectomy Trial) and CCAT (Canadian Coronary Atherectomy Trial) (3,4). Both these studies demonstrated an improvement in lumen size by angiography with debulking by directional atherectomy compared to balloon dilatation. However, despite a marginal improvement after 6 months' follow-up in these patients, death and non-Q-wave myocardial infarction were also significantly higher. These studies suggested that, to make an important prognostic assessment of the success of atherectomy, more accurate information on both lumen and residual plaque load would be required.

Other trials have suggested a disparity between angiographic result and clinical outcome. In the BENESTENT (BElgium and the NEtherlands STENT)-I trial, owing to late lumen loss, the 6-month follow-up angiogram was not significantly different in the stent group from in the angioplasty-alone group, yet there was still an improvement in clinical outcome measures in the stent group (5). Pharmacological restenosis trials have also demonstrated a disparity between angiographic and clinical outcome such as the lack of angiographic improvement with angiopeptin, a growth factor inhibitor, and yet a reduction in clinical events (6). Such findings and the major lack of change in angiographic dimensions seen in the multicenter lipid-lowering trials despite significant reductions in cardiovascular events (7) have suggested that the ability to study relatively mild (<50% diameter stenosis by angiography) but potentially unstable stenoses by intravascular ultrasound may give additional information regarding clinical outcome.

III. QUANTITATION WITH ULTRASOUND IMAGING

High-frequency catheter-based ultrasound is accurate and precise in measuring the arterial lumen and wall, which makes it unique among imaging technologies. In one extensive validation study, ultrasound images and histological sections of 54 excised human coronary arteries were analyzed using computer planimetry (8). A strong correlation ($r = .94$) was demonstrated comparing the mean vessel cross-sectional area with less good correlations shown between lumen cross-sectional area ($r = .84$) and mean percent narrowing ($r = .85$). On remeasuring 48% of the sections, mean inter- and intraobserver variabilities for vessel area were 3% and 0.5%, respectively, and for lumen area were 2% and 2%. In a similar study, a better correlation was also shown between plaque area ($r = .95$) than with lumen area ($r = .85$) (9). The poorer correlation with lumen area may reflect alterations in size between ultrasound scanning and fixing the histological sections, as the accuracy approaches unity ($r = .98$) with the measurement of lumen diameter when phantom diameters are used underlining the accuracy of the technique (10). Another study on the lumen area of excised human arteries studied on two separate occasions by the same and independent observers confirmed an intraobserver correlation coefficient of $r = .99$ and an interobserver variability of $r = .98$ (11). These early validation studies confirmed the reproducibility of the technique in defining the lumen and vessel dimensions of an artery. Concerns about catheter movement during the cardiac cycle and eccentricity have not been substantiated as significant causes of error. A small degree of interobserver variability has been confirmed in several studies, as lateral dropout and distortion of the image can cause a small difference between the interpretation of different observers ($r = .93$ to .98).

Further validation work has indicated that the most significant error in image quantitation is the actual frame for analysis chosen by each observer (12).

IV. INTRAVASCULAR ULTRASOUND AS A PROGNOSTIC TOOL

Intravascular ultrasound has been validated in phantom and in in vitro models with respect to its accuracy in determining artery dimensions. Although superior to angiography in these settings, the latter technique is still used in most interventional situations as the primary means of sizing reference arteries and lesion sites (Fig. 1). To measure its accuracy at the time of intervention, a direct comparison between intravascular ultrasound and orthogonal view quantitative coronary arteriography (QCA) was performed in 174 matched coronary seg-

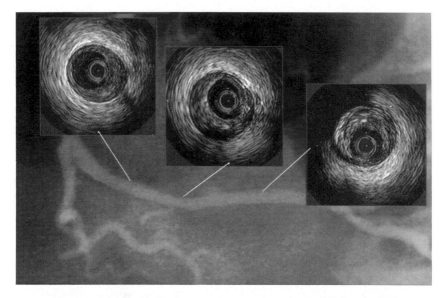

Figure 1   Three ultrasound images within the right coronary artery along the lower-right-heart border. Although there is an excellent result by angiography post-intervention, the left image indicates a significant plaque load that is even more extensive in the middle ultrasound image. The presence of disease in these images confirms the discrepancy often encountered when percent stenosis calculations are made by quantitative angiography given that proximal and distal reference segments may have a significant plaque load.

ments (13). A good correlation was achieved in angiographically normal coronary arteries ($r = .92$); however, the correlation deteriorated with mild stenoses ($r = .47$). Following angioplasty, there was a very weak correlation between the two techniques ($r = .28$). Ultrasound resulted in higher values for minimum lumen diameter than QCA in lesions <1.6 mm in diameter, and higher values in normal arteries, which is generally consistent with other studies suggesting an ultrasound lumen diameter of around 10% larger than that at angiography. This confirms the more accurate assessment of vessel architecture by intravascular ultrasound in the context of an interventional procedure where the plaque and vessel wall morphology can be quite diverse in shape (and accurate edge detection by angiography may be more difficult).

The accurate quantitation and description of coronary arteries before and after intervention permit the study of long-term changes in the vessel after intervention. There have been several studies examining the mechanisms of acute lumen gain after various coronary interventions correlating acute results and complications with lesion composition and characteristics at ultrasound imaging. In addition, other studies have examined the mechanisms of long-term changes after intervention.

A. Lesion Characteristics and the Prediction of Restenosis

Given the increased accuracy with which intravascular ultrasound can measure not only lumen dimensions but plaque load at the site of coronary intervention, the GUIDE (Guidance by Ultrasound Imaging for Decision Endpoints) trial was designed to explore the difference between intracoronary ultrasound and angiography in the assessment of lesion morphology and to attempt to identify morphologic predictors of outcome. This multicenter study randomized patients undergoing balloon angioplasty or directional coronary atherectomy to clinical or angiographic follow-up at 6 months (14). Ultrasound examination was performed using a controlled pullback through the target segment after angiography with the operator blinded to the result. In the first phase of the study, a comparison between ultrasound and angiography was performed. The ultrasound images and angiograms were analyzed at separate core facilities. Significant discrepancies were found between the two imaging modalities: lesions were classified more frequently as eccentric by ultrasound than by angiography, 77% vs. 33%. Target lesion calcification was documented in 62% of cases by ultrasound but only 35% of angiograms. After angioplasty, fracture or dissection of plaque was described in 49% of lesions by ultrasound compared to 22% of angiograms (15).

The advantage of ultrasound over angiography in quantitating lesion dimensions was also seen in the GUIDE trial. In describing acute lumen gain, it was found that the ratio of postprocedural lumen area to nominal balloon size was highest in the presence of plaque dissection. The morphologic features predicting the likelihood and location of plaque dissection were described in this study. As reported previously, areas prone to dissection are at the thinnest portion of plaque within an eccentric lesion. Other susceptible sites occur where there is differing elasticity, such as at the thin fibrous cap over a lipid pool, or at borders between soft and hard plaque, where shear forces are high. Nonetheless, the creation of a dissection leads to greater acute lumen gain than in those without dissection, which are more prone to elastic recoil.

In another study to examine the immediate and late changes after balloon angioplasty (PTCA) and directional coronary atherectomy (DCA), serial ultrasound imaging was performed in 34 patients (of 39 patients enrolled) immediately after and again 6 months after angiographically successful coronary intervention (16). A total of 19% of the 16 patients undergoing DCA had additional balloon angioplasty. Target stenoses were classified as homogeneous or mixed according to the presence of one plaque component (soft plaque, hard plaque, or calcium) or a more mixed distribution, and these were distributed similarly between the two groups. Patients undergoing DCA had a significantly larger reference diameter by angiography (3.46 ± 0.31 vs. 2.81 ± 0.66 mm). A reduction in plaque area was the main operative mechanism of DCA, accounting for 66% of acute lumen enlargement, compared to balloon angioplasty, where reduction in plaque area accounted for 52% of the increase in lumen area. There was also a significant increase in total vessel area in both groups, accounting for 48% and 34% of the acute lumen gain in PTCA and DCA groups, respectively. Fracture/dissection was seen in 67% of PTCA and in only 19% of DCA patients immediately after intervention.

Although when comparing lesion characteristics, DCA achieved a larger increase in lumen and vessel area with greater plaque reduction in soft lesions, this was not statistically significant. In the PTCA group, calcific or mixed lesions showed only a trend toward a greater increase in acute lumen gain through vessel expansion. After 6 months, clinical restenosis occurred in 39% and 25% of the PTCA and DCA groups, respectively. In the DCA group, an increase in plaque area was the predominant mechanism of late lumen loss (92%) whereas this accounted for only 33% of loss after PTCA, the remainder coming from a reduction in total vessel area. This study confirmed that plaque ablation is the main operative mechanism of DCA with particular efficacy in soft plaque, whereas PTCA is a combination of plaque redistribution/dissection and vessel expansion (16). These two interventions modify the restenosis process such that neointimal hyperplasia is the predominant component after DCA compared to the chronic recoil or vascular remodeling after PTCA.

To achieve a successful long-term outcome after angioplasty, it is imperative that the acute lumen gain immediately after the procedure be sufficiently greater than the late lumen loss such that the net lumen gain still results in a functionally nonsignificant stenosis. Previous work has suggested that acute lumen gain is both device- and lesion-dependent (17,18), whereas the late lumen loss may relate more to the response of the vessel to the extent of barotrauma or depth of atherectomy (19). This late loss is thought to be a combination of smooth-muscle cell proliferation with subsequent neointimal hyperplasia and of vascular remodeling (see below). Because intravascular ultrasound imaging enhances the assessment of plaque characteristics compared to angiography, it delivers the ability to risk-stratify lesions for a particular interventional strategy and predict the long-term outcome.

In the second phase of the GUIDE trial, angiographic restenosis occurred in 45% of cases, with clinical restenosis in 32% and major clinical events (death, infarction, and target vessel revascularization) in 21% of an enrolled pool of 480 patients (14). Angiographic restenosis was predicted in a multivariate model by the absolute or percent plaque area and the minimum lumen diameter by ultrasound but not by angiography before or after the procedure (Figs. 2, 3). Clinical restenosis was also predicted in a multivariate model by the percent plaque area by ultrasound and by the angiographic percent diameter stenosis preprocedure. Only ultrasound minimum lumen diameter predicted other clini-

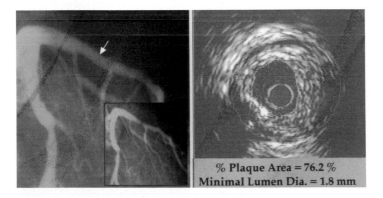

% Plaque Area = 76.2 %
Minimal Lumen Dia. = 1.8 mm

Figure 2 A patient enrolled in the GUIDE trial with a percent plaque area of 76.2% highly predictive post-intervention of restenosis despite an angiographically satisfactory result (arrow).

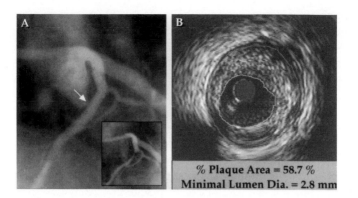

Figure 3   A patient enrolled in the GUIDE trial with a percent plaque area of 58.7% post-intervention predictive of no restenosis and with a good angiographic result (arrow).

cal events. This study, now completed, indicated the additional benefit of ultrasound in predicting future events and in the importance of reducing the plaque area in reducing the rate of restenosis. This relationship between percent plaque area and outcome has been recently corroborated by two clinical studies (20,21) and a histopathologic study (22)—in other words, the residual plaque burden following a successful intervention seems to predict restenosis.

B.   Residual Plaque Load and Directional Coronary Atherectomy

Initial experimental work suggested that intravascular ultrasound would enhance the success of the atherectomy procedure through improved characterization of intimal tissue and accurate quantitation. In one study of 52 patients, it was found that plaque reduction was greater in echolucent than in echodense plaques, which correlated with the weight of resected material (23). It was speculated that there may be increased exposure of fibrin and lipids, promoting a greater degree of platelet deposition and growth factor release. At angiographic and ultrasound follow-up in 22 patients, the restenosis rate was higher in echolucent (100%) than in echodense (33%) plaques. Another predictor of restenosis was the proportion of cellular content (compared to lipid, fibrin, and collagen) contained in the excised plaque: a higher nuclear content was found in patients with restenosis. In another study examining ultrasound predictors of successful atherectomy (a final mean diameter stenosis of 21% was achieved), the arc of calcium and pre-intervention plaque area predicted the residual lumen area and the residual cross-sectional narrowing (also predicted by lesion length). The arc of calcium also predicted the percent plaque volume removal along with the atherectomy device size (24). These findings were consistent with earlier studies indicating a reduced procedural success in calcified lesions and confirmed the greater benefit of atherectomy in larger vessels with a large plaque volume.

The Optimal Atherectomy Restenosis Study (OARS) was a prospective registry designed to test the theory that an aggressive DCA strategy achieving a <15% residual diameter stenosis would result in a better clinical outcome. Intravascular ultrasound was used to determine its value in facilitating the atherectomy technique, evaluating the mechanisms of lumen enlargement and late lumen loss, and to study procedural and anatomic predictors of restenosis. In contrast to CAVEAT and CCAT (3,4), which showed higher restenosis rates than balloon angioplasty, adjunctive angioplasty was strongly encouraged, leading to a mean post-procedure diameter stenosis of 8% (19% after DCA alone) and a procedural success of 98% in the first 216 lesions (25). The binary restenosis rate at 6 months in OARS was 30%, compared to 50% in the previous CAVEAT trial, with only 19% requiring target lesion revascularization. Using intravascular ultrasound, the area stenosis was reduced from 81% to 14% with a residual percent plaque area of 56%. This study confirmed the relationship between plaque burden and restenosis. Additionally, with aggressive debulking, adjunctive balloon angioplasty may be more effective in translating plaque both axially and circumferentially, which in OARS contributed an estimated 24% to the acute lumen gain (26). Ultrasound-guided DCA not only results in a lower postprocedure residual stenosis but is associated with infrequent angiographic complications (2%) and lower restenosis rate. However, ultrasound also indicated that despite an improved residual stenosis by angiography, leading to a reduced restenosis rate, the residual plaque burden was still surprisingly high, suggesting a future strategy of more aggressive atherectomy.

To investigate whether even more aggressive atherectomy, reducing the plaque load even further, would result in improved clinical outcome, the ABACAS (Adjunctive Balloon Angioplasty Coronary Atherectomy Study) trial was conceived. In this study, performed in Japan in patients from 12 centers, an aggressive atherectomy strategy with adjunctive balloon angioplasty was performed (Fig. 4). To date, the 3-month restenosis rate is 14% and 22% at 6-month follow-up results are under analysis. Whether these encouraging results are borne out at longer-term follow-up is eagerly awaited.

It has been suggested that one additional benefit of intravascular ultrasound

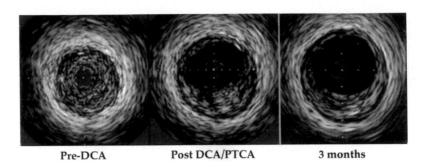

Pre-DCA   Post DCA/PTCA   3 months

Figure 4 Ultrasound images of aggressive directional coronary atherectomy from ABACAS. The left image indicates an extensive plaque load with no visible lumen around the ultrasound catheter. Following atherectomy with adjunctive balloon angioplasty (middle panel), there is a marked increase in lumen and vessel area with significant plaque debulking. The right panel demonstrates that in this patient, this benefit was sustained at three months with no late lumen loss and overall vessel wall expansion.

imaging at the time of atherectomy may be a more detailed assessment of the vessel wall. Surface irregularities including irregular cuts, small tissue flaps, and deep cuts into the media not apparent by angiography may facilitate distal embolization of debris, promote thrombus formation, and stimulate aggressive neointimal proliferation leading to adverse outcomes (increased creatine kinase levels post-procedure, non-Q-wave myocardial infarctions) (3), and a high restenosis rate despite a large lumen by angiography. It is hoped that these trials will add insight to these relationships.

Previous work has suggested that the extent of fibrous hyperplasia was related in part to the depth of tissue resection—i.e., encroachment into the medial layer (27). Because intravascular ultrasound complements successful DCA, there has been an interest in the development of a catheter that combines a cutting device with an ultrasound transducer (28). Initial in vitro studies with this combined device have suggested that orientation of the cutter toward maximal plaque load using ultrasound results in a reduction in subintimal incision from 54% to 21% with greater reduction of plaque load. It is imperative that the debulking strategy achieve an optimal tissue removal, however. In one recent study, adjunctive DCA following rotational atherectomy in 163 patients was reported (29). A total of 38 patients (23%) required target lesion revascularization over a follow-up period of 12 months. Although postintervention lumen areas were similar with or without subsequent revascularization, more aggressive tissue removal—a higher atherectomy index (Δplaque/ +Δlumen area), 84% vs. 59%—was associated with a need for revascularization. This indicates the deleterious effect of deep-wall injury with DCA.

C. Vascular Remodeling After Intervention

It has become apparent that coronary arteries may remodel following a coronary intervention not only with respect to the development of neointimal hyperplasia but also through an adaptive change in the overall vessel size. To study these changes in a prospective manner, a serial intravascular ultrasound study was conceived—the SURE (Serial Ultrasound REstenosis) trial. Ultrasound imaging was performed pre- and post-procedure, at 24 hours, and at 1 and 6 months after the balloon angioplasty or DCA. Vessel size and acute lumen gain were significantly greater in the DCA group than the angioplasty-alone group (30). There was a significant reduction in the vessel area with both techniques between 1 and 6 months from the procedure (Fig. 5). Reduction of plaque volume through either compression or removal was responsible for 57% of the acute lumen gain in the angioplasty group, compared to 71% of the DCA group. However, the time course of chronic recoil was similar in the two groups. In a complementary study, the relationship between acute lumen gain and late lumen loss was analyzed in a prospective serial ultrasound and angiographic study (31). A significant correlation was seen between acute gain and late loss. The late loss correlated closely with the reduction in vessel area and increase in plaque area. However, only the increase in vessel area was related to the acute gain, suggesting that geometric remodeling but not change in plaque volume was indicative of a generalized response to injury.

From this study and from the observations made after the GUIDE trial and the OARS and ABACAS trials, it is becoming apparent that aggressive debulking to a residual plaque load <50% of the total vessel area is likely to be of direct clinical benefit to patients (Fig. 6). Based on the observations made by Glagov et al. (32) and the recognition that the coronary artery can expand to accommodate up to a 40% plaque area (33), one hypothesis might be that such an approach may reset the mechanisms whereby adverse vessel remodeling occurs and thus contribute to a reduction in the incidence of restenosis despite neointimal hyperplasia. Many factors will modulate this resetting of remodeling including plaque type and distribution, readily documented by intravascular ultrasound. Intravascular ultrasound may help to risk-stratify the lesions in which "shrinkage" may play a dominant role in the long-term morphologic response to mechanical intervention.

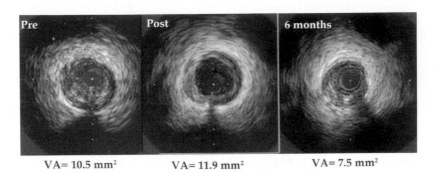

VA= 10.5 mm²　　　VA= 11.9 mm²　　　VA= 7.5 mm²

Figure 5 Images of adverse geometric remodeling following directional coronary atherectomy. The left panel is the image prior to intervention with a large plaque load and a vessel area of 10.5 mm². The middle image indicates an increase in vessel size along with a significant acute lumen gain postintervention. The right panel demonstrates that at 6 months follow-up, restenosis is primarily due to marked vessel shrinkage with a vessel area of 7.5 mm², well below that prior to intervention.

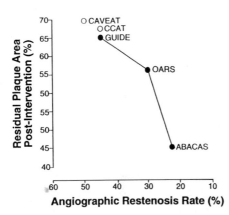

Figure 6 Plot of the projected relationship between residual plaque load and percent restenosis at 6 month angiographic follow-up in the strategy of increasingly aggressive plaque debulking with information published to date from CCAT and CAVEAT (without ultrasound), and from GUIDE, OARS, and ABACAS.

V. INTRAVASCULAR ULTRASOUND IN THE MODERN STENT ERA

In parallel with the recognized contribution of adverse vascular remodeling and shrinkage to restenosis after intervention, there has been a marked increase in the use of intracoronary stents to modify the restenosis process by achieving a larger acute lumen gain (5,34). Intravascular ultrasound has been used to guide stent deployment with the use of adjunct high-pressure balloon dilatation (mean pressure of 15 atm) and larger balloon selection to achieve superior expansion and reduce the need for formal anticoagulation (35). In one large study, subacute stent thrombosis occurred in 0.9% of lesions at 2-month follow-up, confirming the advantage of this approach and precluding the need for formal anticoagulation (35). In another study, using intravascular ultrasound to assess stent expansion when deployment at angiography was deemed perfect by visualization after high-pressure dilatation, 33% of stents were still expanded less than 90% of the distal reference area, with a further 10% demonstrating adjacent dissection or plaque protrusion (36). Given that stent underexpansion is a documented cause of subacute stent thrombosis (37), and that a lower stent volume is unlikely to result in a reduction in the restenosis rate compared to angioplasty alone (38), ultrasound imaging has been used increasingly to address this issue (Fig. 7).

Many different criteria for optimal stent expansion by ultrasound imaging have been proposed. Colombo et al. (35) first proposed that in addition to

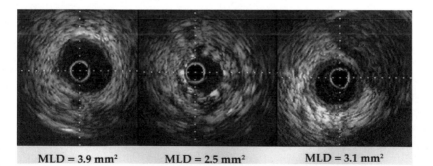

MLD = 3.9 mm²   MLD = 2.5 mm²   MLD = 3.1 mm²

Figure 7   Three ultrasound images describing significant stent underexpansion. The left and right panels demonstrate the proximal and distal reference segments with 5 mm of the stent end. The middle panel is the minimum stent area and corresponds to a stent expansion of only 71% using the average lumen area of the proximal and distal reference segments as denominator.

complete stent apposition to the vessel wall, the stent should achieve 60% of the average of proximal and distal cross-sectional lumen areas (CSA). Stricter criteria evolved such that the goal became an intrastent CSA equal to or greater than the distal reference CSA. A third criterion developed, which was that non-stented segments immediately adjacent to the stent did not reveal evidence of a significant lesion (defined as a CSA stenosis >60% relative to the reference lumen). The MUSIC (Multicenter Ultrasound guidance of Stents In Coronaries) study was designed to study the need for anticoagulation after stenting of a de novo lesion in vessels >3.0 mm in stable patients using IVUS (39). The following criteria were described to indicate optimal stent deployment: complete apposition and complete expansion (minimum stent area [MSA] >90% average of proximal + distal segments, or MSA >100% of lowest reference segment, or MSA >90% proximal segment, and subsequently revised to 80%, 90%, 80%, respectively if MSA >9 mm^2). An in-hospital subacute thrombosis rate of 0.6% was reported, with emergency bypass surgery in 1.2% and repeat angioplasty in 4.6%. However, even using the revised IVUS criteria, only 80% of patients achieved this.

In addition to adequate expansion, it is imperative that apposition to the vessel wall be achieved at the time of stent expansion. As it impossible to determine this by angiography; this and the need to achieve adequate expansion have been the driving force behind the use of intravascular ultrasound. In the Stent Treatment Region assessed by Ultrasound Tomography (STRUT) registry investigating stent deployment in the high-pressure dilatation era (40), ultrasound images from 111 patients undergoing successful stent deployment were reported. A total of 22% of patients required additional balloon inflations based on ultrasound information. Despite excellent angiographic results, 22% of cases demonstrated incomplete stent apposition. Stent area expansion <90% occurred in 68% of cases, <80% in 46%, and <70% in 28% of cases, indicating underexpansion in a significant number of cases.

Following successful stent deployment in elective or emergency situations, it has been noted that stent deployment itself may cause small tears at the margins of the stent—pocket flaps or edge tears. The mechanism of these tears occurs probably because of stent struts at the edge of the Palmaz-Schatz stent impacting in soft plaque adjacent to the stented area at the time of deployment and lifting up areas of intimal tissue. Intravascular ultrasound is the only method of documenting these tears accurately. The STRUT registry documented an incidence of edge tears in 12% of cases (40). Depending on the extent of the tear, the presence or absence of blood speckling behind the flap, and the mobility of the flap with respect to the lumen, the operator may decide either to finish the case or to proceed to further stent deployment to cover the flap (Fig. 8).

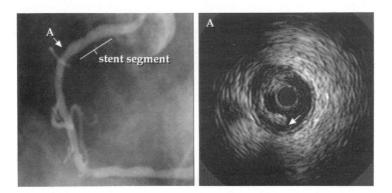

Figure 8 Angiography post-stent deployment demonstrates a small indentation in the mid-stent corresponding to the articulation site. However, the distal stent is unremarkable by angiography (arrow). The ultrasound image just distal to the stent reveals a large intimal flap or edge tear (arrow).

The BENESTENT-I and STRESS studies described a reduction in binary restenosis (>50% diameter stenosis) of 32% to 22% and from 43% to 32% in all patients randomized, respectively (5,34). These studies were performed prior to the modern era of high-pressure balloon dilatation post-deployment and the use of oversized balloons. Furthermore, intravascular ultrasound was not used to guide deployment. In-stent restenosis remains a clinical problem, and ultrasound may help guide appropriate therapy. The restenotic tissue found inside the previously deployed stent consists of a homogeneous material which, although primarily neointimal hyperplasia, is generally softer and more echolucent than atherosclerotic plaque in de novo lesions. Several strategies have evolved to deal with in-stent restenosis, such as repeat balloon angioplasty using a larger noncompliant balloon. Alternatively, an atheroablative approach using either high-speed rotational atherectomy sized within the measured minimum stent area by ultrasound or excimer laser angioplasty may be performed.

The long-term outcome after stenting is likely to improve with high-pressure dilatation and technological developments with stents themselves. The recent BENESTENT-II pilot study confirmed the safety of a regimen of aspirin and ticlopidine in a subgroup of 50 of 220 patients after stenting with heparin-coated stents resulting in no stent thrombosis, no major bleeding complications, and a restenosis rate of 6% in this subgroup (41). To evaluate objectively whether ultrasound-guided stent deployment results in an additional clinical benefit over angiography alone, the CRUISE (Can Routine

Ultrasound Impact Stent Expansion) component of the STARS (STent Anti-thrombotic Regimen Study) study is under way. This subgroup undergo ultrasound assessment after a satisfactory angiographic stent result and is divided into two groups—an ultrasound-documentary arm to assess the stent deployment without further intervention, and an ultrasound-guided arm in which further intervention may be considered on the basis of the ultrasound images. It is hoped that this study will help define the clinical benefit that may be derived from ultrasound imaging at the time of stent deployment.

VI. CONCLUSIONS

The ability to accurately assess the lesion site after coronary intervention is a major advantage of IVUS over other available imaging modalities. Initial work has suggested that the measurement of residual plaque area expressed as a percentage of the vessel area, the percent plaque area, is an accurate predictor of clinical and angiographic restenosis after balloon angioplasty and directional coronary atherectomy. Ultrasound imaging has also described an additional component to the restenotic process—adverse vascular remodeling. It is possible that more aggressive plaque debulking by atherectomy may lead to improved clinical outcome, particularly when guided by intravascular ultrasound either separately or as part of a combined device. Assessment at the end of an interventional procedure may guide the operator regarding the need for adjunct intracoronary stent deployment given the ability of the stent to achieve a greater acute lumen gain and to prevent vessel shrinkage. Improvement in overall image quality with on-line quantitative coronary ultrasound measurements and perhaps on-line tissue characterization will help refine the role of intravascular ultrasound in interventional procedures in the future.

REFERENCES

1. Topol EJ, Nissen SE. Our preoccupation with coronary luminology: the dissociation between clinical and angiographic findings in ischemic heart disease. Circulation 1995; 92:2333–2342.
2. Mintz GS, Pichard AD, Kent KM, et al. Atherosclerosis in angiographically "normal" coronary artery reference segments: an intravascular ultrasound study with clinical correlation. J Am Coll Cardiol 1995; 25:1479–1485.
3. Topol EJ, Leya F, Pinkerton CA, et al. A comparison of coronary angioplasty with directional atherectomy in patients with coronary artery disease. N Engl J Med 1993; 329:221–227.
4. Adelman AG, Cohen EA, Kimball BP, et al. A comparison of directional atherec-

tomy with balloon angioplasty for lesions of the left anterior descending coronary artery. N Engl J Med 1993; 329:228–233.

5. Serruys PW, de Jaegere P, Kiemeneij F, et al. A comparison of balloon expandable stent implantation with balloon angioplasty in patients with coronary artery disease. N Engl J Med 1994; 331:489–495.

6. Emanuelsson H, Beatt KJ, Bagger JP, et al. Long-term effects of angiopeptin treatment in coronary angioplasty. Circulation 1995; 91:1689–1696.

7. Brown BG, Zhao XQ, Sacco DE, Albers JJ. Lipid lowering and plaque regression: new insights into prevention of plaque disruption and clinical events in coronary disease. Circulation 1993; 87:1781–1790.

8. Potkin BN, Bartorelli AL, Gessert JM, et al. Coronary artery imaging with intravascular high-frequency ultrasound. Circulation 1990; 81:1575–1585.

9. Pandian N, Kreis A, Desmoyers M, et al. In vivo ultrasoundangioscopy in humans and animals: intraluminal imaging of blood vessels using a new catheter-based high resolution ultrasound probe. Circulation 1988; 78(suppl):II-22. Abstract.

10. Nishimura RA, Edwards WD, Warnes CA, et al. Intravascular ultrasound imaging: in vitro validation and pathologic correlation. J Am Coll Cardiol 1990; 16: 145–154.

11. Tobis JM, Mallery JA, Gessert J, et al. Intravascular ultrasound cross-sectional arterial imaging before and after balloon angioplasty in vitro. Circulation 1989; 80:873–882.

12. Kearney PP, Ramo P, Shaw TRD, Starkey IR, McMurray JV, Sutherland GR. The reproducibility of IVUS measurements in unselected video frames assessed in sequential catheter pullbacks and in separate analysis sessions. Circulation 1995; 92(suppl):I-78. Abstract.

13. De Scheerder I, De Man F, Herregods MC, et al. Intravascular ultrasound versus angiography for measurement of luminal diameters in normal and diseased coronary arteries. Am Heart J 1994; 127:243–251.

14. GUIDE Trial Investigators. IVUS-determined predictors of restenosis in PTCA and DCA: final report from the GUIDE trial, Phase II. J Am Coll Cardiol 1996; 27(suppl A):156A. Abstract.

15. Fitzgerald PJ, Yock PG. Mechanisms and outcomes of angioplasty and atherectomy assessed by intravascular ultrasound imaging. J Clin Ultrasound 1993; 21: 579–588.

16. Di Mario C, Gil R, Camenzind E, et al. Quantitative assessment with intracoronary ultrasound of the mechanisms of restenosis after percutaneous transluminal coronary angioplasty and directional coronary atherectomy. Am J Cardiol 1995; 75:772–777.

17. Kuntz RE, Safian RD, Levine MJ, Reis GJ, Diver DJ, Baim DS. Novel approach to the analysis of restenosis after the use of three new coronary devices. J Am Coll Cardiol 1992; 19:1493–1499.

18. Haude M, Erbel R, Issa H, Meyer J. Quantitative analysis of elastic recoil after balloon angioplasty and after intracoronary implantation of balloon-expandable Palmaz-Schatz stents. J Am Coll Cardiol 1993; 21:26–34.

19. Kuntz RE, Gibson CM, Nobuyoshi M, Baim DS. Generalized model of restenosis after conventional balloon angioplasty, stenting and directional atherectomy. J Am Coll Cardiol 1993; 21:15–25.

20. Mintz GS, Popma JJ, Pichard AD, et al. Intravascular ultrasound assessment of the mechanisms and predictors of restenosis following coronary angioplasty. J Invas Cardiol 1996; 8:1–14.

21. Gussenhoven EJ, EPISODE (Evaluation Peripheral Intravascular Sonography On Dotter Effect) Study Group. Role of intravascular ultrasound in predicting anatomic success after balloon angioplasty of the femoropopliteal artery. J Am Coll Cardiol 1996; 27(suppl A):41A. Abstract.

22. Farb A, Virmani R, Atkinson J, Kolodgie FD. Plaque morphology and pathologic changes in arteries from patients. J Am Coll Cardiol 1990; 16:1421–1429.

23. de Lezo JS, Romero M, Medina A, et al. Intracoronary ultrasound assessment of directional coronary atherectomy: immediate and follow-up findings. J Am Coll Cardiol 1993; 21:298–307.

24. Matar FA, Mintz GS, Pinnow E, et al. Multivariate predictors of intravascular ultrasound end points after directional coronary atherectomy. J Am Coll Cardiol 1995; 25:318–324.

25. Simonton CA, Leon MB, Kuntz RE, et al. Acute and late clinical and angiographic results of directional atherectomy in the Optimal Atherectomy Restenosis Study (OARS). Circulation 1995; 92(suppl):I-545. Abstract.

26. Popma JJ, Baim DS, Kuntz RE, et al. Early and late quantitative angiographic outcomes in the Optimal Atherectomy Restenosis Study (OARS). J Am Coll Cardiol 1996; 27(suppl A):291A. Abstract.

27. Garratt KN, Homes DR, Bell MR, et al. Restenosis after directional coronary atherectomy: differences between primary atheromatous and restenotic lesions and influence of subintimal tissue resection. J Am Coll Cardiol 1990; 16:1665–1671.

28. Fitzgerald PJ, Belef M, Connolly AJ, Sudhir K, Yock PG. Design and initial testing of an ultrasound-guided directional atherectomy device. Am Heart J 1995; 129:593–598.

29. Dussailant GR, Mintz GS, Pichard AD, et al. The "dark side" of overly aggressive multidevice atherectomy. J Am Coll Cardiol 1996; 27(suppl A):393A. Abstract.

30. Kimura T, Kaburagi S, Yokoi H, et al. Time course of geometric remodeling after coronary angioplasty: balloon angioplasty versus directional coronary atherectomy. J Am Coll Cardiol 1996; 27(suppl A):41A. Abstract.

31. Kimura T, Kaburagi S, Yokoi H, et al. Acute gain and late loss relationship after coronary angioplasty correlates with geometric remodeling but not with changes in plaque volume. J Am Coll Cardiol 1996; 27(suppl A):391A. Abstract.

32. Glagov S, Weisenberg E, Zarins CK, Stankunavicius R, Kolettis GJ. Compensatory enlargement of human atherosclerotic arteries. N Engl J Med 1987; 316: 1371–1375.

33. Currier JW, Faxon DP. Restenosis after percutaneous transluminal coronary angioplasty: have we been aiming at the wrong target? J Am Coll Cardiol 1995; 25: 516–520.

34. Fischman DL, Leon MB, Baim D, et al. A randomized comparison of coronary stent placement and balloon angioplasty in the treatment of coronary artery disease. N Engl J Med 1994; 331:496–501.

35. Colombo A, Hall P, Nakamura S, et al. Intracoronary stenting without anticoagulation accomplished with intravascular ultrasound guidance. Circulation 1995; 91: 1891–1897.

36. Nunez BD, Foster-Smith K, Berger PB, et al. Benefit of intravascular ultrasound guided high pressure inflations in patients with a "perfect" angiographic result: the Mayo Clinic experience. Circulation 1995; 92(suppl):I-2605. Abstract.

37. Nakamura S, Colombo A, Gaglione S, et al. Intracoronary ultrasound observations during stent implantation. Circulation 1994; 89:2026–2034.

38. Dusaillant GR, Mintz GS, Pichard AD, et al. Small stent size and intimal hyperplasia contribute to restenosis: a volumetric intravascular ultrasound analysis. J Am Coll Cardiol 1995; 26:720–724.

39. de Jaegere P, Mudra H, Almagor Y, et al. In-hospital and 1-month clinical results of an international study testing the concept of IVUS-guided optimized stent expansion alleviating the need of systemic anticoagulation. J Am Coll Cardiol 1996; 27(suppl A):137A. Abstract.

40. Metz JA, Mooney MR, Walter PD, et al. Significance of edge tears in coronary stenting: initial observations from the STRUT registry. Circulation 1995; 92 (suppl):I-546. Abstract.

41. Serruys PW, Emanuelsson H, van der Giessen W, et al. Heparin-coated Palmaz-Schatz stents in human coronary arteries. Early outcome of the Benestent-II pilot study. Circulation 1996; 93:412–422.

4

Clinical Application of Intravascular Ultrasound Imaging in a Center with High-Volume Preintervention Ultrasound Imaging

Roxana Mehran, Gary S. Mintz, Augusto D. Pichard, Kenneth M. Kent, and Lowell F. Satler *Washington Hospital Center, Washington, D.C.*

Jeffrey J. Popma and Martin B. Leon *Cardiology Research Foundation, Washington, D.C.*

I. INTRODUCTION

For the past three decades coronary angiography has been the "gold standard" for imaging the coronary arteries. However, angiography has many inherent limitations. Angiography depicts the coronary vasculature as a silhouette of a contrast-filled lumen. Therefore, any single projection may misrepresent the degree of luminal narrowing (especially in eccentric lesions). Although two orthogonal views may resolve this issue, in tortuous vessels and bifurcation lesions this may not be possible. In addition, several necropsy studies have shown that when diffuse coronary artery disease is present, accurate calculation of percent stenosis is limited (1–3). Third, at its best, angiography only analyzes the intraluminal consequences of atherosclerosis, not the disease process itself.

Conversely, intravascular ultrasound (IVUS) provides detailed, high-quality tomographic images of the coronary arteries in vivo in a manner previously not possible (4); this includes the quantitative assessment of normal and abnormal intramural anatomy (5–7). The full circumference of the vessel wall can be visualized from a single tomographic view, cross-sectional measurements of lumen and external elastic lamina area can be made, and plaque area can be calculated. These measurements have been validated in vitro (8). Furthermore, the acoustical properties of the atherosclerotic plaque allow IVUS to assess plaque morphology with some degree of accuracy (8,9). The morphology of the plaque is an important determinant of the vessel's response to transcatheter therapy.

The purpose of this chapter is to introduce the utility of routine IVUS imaging in the authors' laboratory. This tool can be used in conjunction with angiography in diagnosing coronary artery disease as well as in assessing target lesion severity and morphology before and after transcatheter therapy. However, it is also important to acknowledge the obvious current limitations of IVUS including the inability to cross all lesions, its inability to assess vessel tortuosity and lesion angulation, and its inability to measure lumen dimensions smaller than the imaging catheter.

II. INTEGRATION OF IVUS INTO THE CATHETERIZATION LAB

To develop a program of routine IVUS imaging (including routine preintervention imaging) in a busy interventional environment, certain practical issues first had to be addressed. Instrument setup, catheter preparation, etc., cannot interfere with patient care or the flow of the interventional procedures. The catheterization laboratory cannot be dependent on the availability of noninvasive laboratory personnel. Therefore, at the Washington (D.C.) Hospital Center we have created a clinical IVUS imaging service.

It is convenient for the physician who is performing the interventional procedure to have a good view of the IVUS image. We have found it useful to "wire" the labs so that the ultrasound image is displayed on one of the angiographic reference monitors. In this way the ultrasound equipment does not interfere with the interventional procedure, and the superior angiographic reference monitors are "borrowed" to display the IVUS images. (In one laboratory, we have fully integrated the equipment so that there is no free-standing IVUS unit.)

A. Personnel

There are dedicated technical personnel who are responsible for IVUS imaging. The responsible individuals are trained in performing and interpreting the studies on-line. Their responsibilities include all the practical aspects of IVUS imaging (i.e., maintaining and trouble shooting the equipment, stocking catheters and ancillary supplies, recording the studies, maintaining log books, the handling and storing of video tapes, etc.). Ideally, these individuals have technical backgrounds in both ultrasound and interventional cardiology.

B. Imaging Protocol

For both clinical and research needs, it is important to have a systematic approach to the performance of the IVUS imaging runs. This facilitates both the on-line and off-line interpretation of the IVUS studies and is essential for the systematic comparison of sequential (pre- vs. postintervention) and serial (postintervention vs. follow-up) IVUS studies. (Obviously, it is also essential for the analysis of disease progression and regression.) At the Washington Hospital Center, all imaging studies are performed in a uniform way. Under fluoroscopic guidance, the imaging catheter is advanced distal to the area of interest, imaging is started, and the videotape is set to record. Once the image is optimized, the automatic transducer pullback device (with a pullback speed of 0.5 mm/sec) is activated, and imaging is continued until the transducer reaches the aorto-ostial junction. If the run is insufficient owing to poor imaging quality or if there is a question about the pathology, then the run is repeated. Although on-line measurements can be made during imaging, we prefer to make measurements off-line (during video playback) both to minimize ischemia and procedure time and to record a complete and uninterrupted run.

Each run is annotated on screen. Annotation includes both patient and lesion demographics, the procedure performed (i.e., post-PTCA), the question being asked (i.e., is the lesion severe?), and the vessel being imaged. Voice annotation is also used to provide additional patient, procedure, and lesion information and to identify the distal reference, the target lesion(s), and the proximal reference. For example, in cases where an intervention has taken place with excellent results, it may be difficult to locate the target lesion.

C. Housekeeping Issues

Only virgin, broadcast-quality s-VHS videotapes are used. There are two simple logs. Each 2-hour videotape with its unique number contains approximately 20 cases, and each tape has a corresponding sheet in a chronologic log. Similarly, each patient and procedure is entered into a simple database to generate an alphabetical log. This allows ready identification and retrieval of any of the over 6000 studies performed to date. Finally, the tapes are copied; and the originals and copies are stored in separate, secure locations.

III. ASSESSMENT OF ATHEROSCLEROTIC PLAQUE PREINTERVENTION

Preintervention IVUS imaging is important to accurately assess the components of the plaque. Currently, IVUS is able to detect and classify lesions into calcified plaque, echogenic (but noncalcified) plaque, and echolucent plaque.

A. Calcified Plaque

Fluoroscopy is the usual method for detection of calcification in the coronary vasculature. However, only 14% to 58% of patients with documented coronary artery disease have fluoroscopic calcification, compared with 79% on pathologic examination (10–12). Moreover, fluoroscopy fails to provide information regarding the extent or location of calcium.

IVUS identification of calcium has been validated in vitro (8,13). Calcium is a powerful reflector of ultrasound; calcium prevents the penetration of ultrasound, causing shadowing of deeper arterial structures; and calcium may create concentric rings or reverberations. (Conversely, there are limitations to the ultrasound assessment of target lesion calcium. IVUS can identify only the leading edge of a calcified deposit, not its thickness. Similarly, IVUS cannot detect a deep calcific deposit behind a superficial calcific deposit. Dense fibrous tissue may attenuate the ultrasound beam to obscure or imitate deep calcium.)

IVUS can assess the arc (using a protractor centered on the lumen), length (using motorized transducer pullback), and distribution patterns (target lesion vs. reference segment and superficial vs. deep) of coronary artery calcification. In 1155 target native lesions studied by both IVUS and coronary angiography, IVUS detected lesion calcium in 73% of lesions (Fig. 1). The angiographic detection of calcium (in 38% of lesions) depended on the arc, length, and location of lesion and reference segment calcium (14).

Besides being a marker for significant coronary artery disease, target lesion calcification (especially superficial calcium) is the major determinant of the acute procedural success of many transcatheter therapies. Therefore, preintervention imaging of lesions to assess presence and degree of calcification is useful for choosing the therapeutic strategy best fit for the lesion. Recent IVUS studies have shown a relationship between coronary artery calcification and

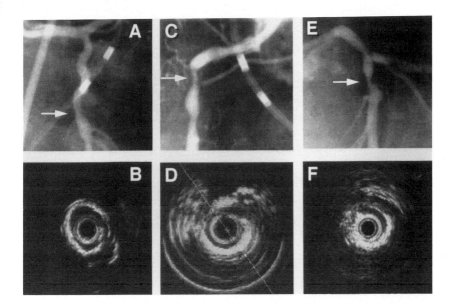

Figure 1 The coronary angiograms and IVUS studies of three target lesions are shown (panels A and B, C and D, and E and F). None of the angiograms showed calcification; the plan prior to preintervention IVUS imaging was to use directional coronary atherectomy to treat all three. Each IVUS study showed near-circumferential superficial target lesion calcium. As a result, all three lesions were treated using rotational atherectomy. The first was a stand-alone procedure (panels A and B); adjunct PTCA was used in the second (panels C and D); and adjunct directional coronary atherectomy was used in the third (panels E and F). b = Maximum plaque thickness; a = minimum plaque thickness.

coronary dissection (15,16). The final lumen dimensions, the amount of residual plaque, and the weight of tissue retrieved after directional coronary atherectomy are all related to the arc and location of IVUS target lesion calcium (17–19). Conversely, rotational atherectomy is unimpeded by even heavy lesion calcification (20,21).

B. Echogenic (Noncalcified) Plaque

Fibrous plaque has intermediate echodensity between calcium and soft, fatty plaque. The majority of the atherosclerotic plaques fall in this category. Many of these plaques have calcific elements. These fibrocalcific plaques behave less favorably to balloon angioplasty, resulting in more dissections, than softer, noncalcified plaques. Dense fibrotic plaques may attenuate the ultrasound energy.

C. Echolucent Plaque

Lipid components of the atherosclerotic plaque are poorly reflected by ultrasound (22). Therefore, soft (lipid-containing) plaques are typically echolucent. Soft lesions are more amenable to tissue removal by directional atherectomy (18,22) and may respond more favorably to balloon dilatation than fibrotic or calcified plaque. Furthermore, soft plaques may be less rigid and stents may expand more fully and more symmetrically in echolucent (vs. fibrocalcific) plaques.

Other components, like blood and thrombus, must be distinguished from echolucent plaques. Blood itself shows up in the IVUS images as a speckled, low-intensity, continuously changing pattern. However, thrombus may be very difficult to identify. Therefore, at present angioscopy is the preferred method of diagnosing thrombus (24).

IV. QUANTITATIVE ANALYSIS PREINTERVENTION

IVUS is able to delineate the boundaries of vessel wall layers in vivo (7,13,25,26). The IVUS image of young, morphologically normal coronary artery wall is homogeneous without layering (22). With advancing age, intimal thickening (early atherosclerosis) occurs, and IVUS reveals a three-layered appearance. The lumen-intima (or lumen-plaque) interface is the innermost layer. The medium contains little fibrous tissue and is hypoechoic, producing the middle layer. (The thickness of this hypoechoic zone is also dependent on the amount and type of overlying plaque; therefore, media thickness cannot be measured accurately.) Because the adventitia contains mostly fibrous tissue and is hyperechoic, the media-adventitia interface can be readily recognized; it forms the outermost layer.

Using computer planimetry, lesion site and reference segment measurements can be performed. The frequently used measurements include the following.

A. External Elastic Membrane (EEM) Cross-Sectional Areas (CSA) and Diameters

This is equivalent to the area contained within the media-adventitia border and is a reproducible measure of total arterial CSA. Limitations to the measurement of the EEM CSA include shadowing (because of calcium), attenuation, and inadequate penetration. Others have termed this the media-to-media CSA, or diameter. With plaque accumulation (either at the lesion site or within the reference), the EEM CSA tends to increase to accommodate plaque deposition (27–31).

B. Lumen CSA and Diameters

Limitations to the measurement of the lumen included stasis (in which the plaque cannot be differentiated from intense blood echoes), lumen CSA smaller than the imaging catheter, or extremely echolucent plaque. Injection of radiographic contrast, saline, or echogenic contrast may help outline the lumen, in part by overcoming stasis.

C. Plaque and Media (P+M) CSA and Plaque Burden

Because media thickness cannot be measured accurately, P+M CSA is used as a measure of atherosclerotic plaque and is calculated as EEM minus lumen CSA. Quantification of plaque burden (also called the cross-sectional narrowing or percent plaque area) may be an even more important measurement because the postintervention plaque burden has been shown to predict restenosis (32). Plaque burden is calculated as P+M divided by EEM CSA.

D. Eccentricity Index

This is the ratio of maximal to minimal P+M thickness. An index of 1.0 indicates a purely concentric plaque distribution. Because lesions are rarely purely concentric, most lesions appear to be eccentric by IVUS. However, the angiographic classification of lesion eccentricity is not related to the IVUS eccentricity index (33); rather, lesion length (influencing the amount of interpolation necessary) and the maximum plaque thickness are the major determinants of this classification (Fig. 2). The orientation of the maximum plaque thickness can be related to side branches; this is of practical use during interventional procedures.

E. Lesion Length Measurements Preintervention

Coronary artery lesion lengths as well as the longitudinal distances between lesions and major side branches or coronary ostia are important in guiding catheter-based treatment strategies such as selecting the number and length of coronary stents (34–39). Angiographic lesion length measurements are limited by the difficulty in visualizing a tortuous, three-dimensional vascular structure in two dimensions and by foreshortening. IVUS motorized transducer pullback

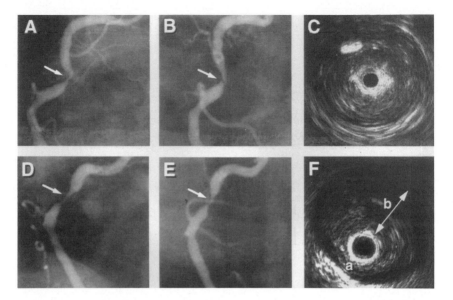

Figure 2   The left anterior oblique and right anterior oblique coronary angiograms and IVUS studies of two target lesions are shown (panels A, B, and C, and panels D, E, and F). The lesion in the top row is concentric on IVUS; there is uniform plaque thickness (panel C). The lesion in the bottom row was markedly eccentric on IVUS (panel F); b = maximum plaque thickness, a = minimum plaque thickness.

through a stationary imaging sheath enables axial length measurements; at a pullback speed of 0.5 mm/sec, each second is equal to 0.5 mm of axial length. These length measurements have been validated in vivo (40).

V. USE OF PREINTERVENTION IVUS LESION AND REFERENCE SEGMENT ASSESSMENT

A. Balloon and Device Sizing

Qualitative and quantitative measurements provide useful information regarding the target lesion and the reference vessel. For example, the quantitative measurements may be used to choose balloon and device sizes. In conventional angiography-guided PTCA, balloons are sized to the reference lumen diameter. However, IVUS studies have consistently demonstrated larger reference lumen dimensions (compared to angiography) and extensive occult reference segment disease that is hidden by the process of adaptive remodeling (27–31,41).

Even when the reference segment is selected as the least diseased anatomic cross section proximal to the lesion, the plaque burden exceeds 50%. The use of a midwall (mean of the EEM and lumen diameters) reference segment measurement may allow a significantly larger balloon to be used safely to achieve a smaller final diameter stenosis without an increased incidence of dissections (42).

In general, the proximal (but not the distal) reference is measured from the preintervention study; the distal vessel is usually underperfused and artificially small. If the distal reference is significantly smaller than the proximal reference on postintervention imaging, this may be an indication for use of a tapered balloon (43,44).

In contrast to balloons, atherectomy devices may be more appropriately sized to the lesion site EEM (or media-to-media) dimension with allowances for a margin of error to prevent perforation. This is important because in some target lesions, lumen compromise is due to vessel shrinkage rather than plaque accumulation.

B. Assessment of Lesion Severity

Preintervention IVUS may be very useful in borderline lesions (45) (Fig. 3). In conjunction with flow Doppler studies, IVUS may yield information regarding lesion severity as well as physiology.

Left main and aorto-ostial lesions in general may be difficult to evaluate by angiography alone. Therefore, careful IVUS imaging of the ostium is essential. It is important to use a slow pullback speed, to disengage the guiding catheter, and to methodically interrogate the aorto-ostial junction.

C. Assessment of Plaque Composition and Distribution

One of the advantages of the directional coronary atherectomy procedure is the ability of the catheter to be directed toward eccentric plaque. In general, eccentric lesions are best approached by appropriately matching the device to the plaque morphology. However, the most important predictor of poor tissue retrieval with directional atherectomy is the IVUS finding of calcium within the plaque. Thus, in calcified eccentric lesions, rotational atherectomy or intracoronary stent placement may be preferred.

D. Unusual Lesion Morphology

Angiographic filling defects are usually felt to be thrombus (46). Although angioscopy is the gold standard for evaluating thrombus, some angiographic filling defects represent calcified "masses" which are readily evident on preintervention IVUS (47). The pathologic process that leads to these calcified

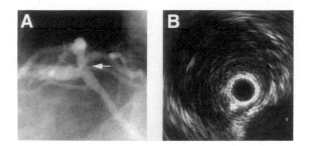

Figure 3   The coronary angiogram (panel A) and IVUS study (panel B) of an ostial
LAD lesion is shown. By quantitative coronary angiography, the reference diameter
measured 3.5 mm, the MLD measured 2.2 mm, and the diameter stenosis was calculated
to be 37%. By IVUS, the lumen was occlusive around the 1.3-mm imaging catheter.

intraluminal masses is not known. Lytic therapy and prolonged systemic anticoagulation have had little effect on these lesions.

In analyzing dissections preintervention (as well as during intervention),
important questions include the severity of the dissection (is it lumen compromising?), the location (is it superficial or does it involve the deep wall?), the
composition (is it calcified?), and is the IVUS catheter in the true or the false
lumen? A significant dissection is one that is lumen-compromising and deep-
walled. Almost all of these dissections need further treatment, usually with
endovascular stents although prolonged balloon inflation may be tried first and
the dissection reevaluated by IVUS. Dissection flaps may be excised using
directional atherectomy if the dissection flap is not calcified and if it does not
involve the deeper arterial wall. The true lumen is best recognized by the
presence of plaque elements surrounding the catheter while the false lumen is
typically adjacent to the media-adventitia border.

An aneurysm is a localized dilation of the EEM resulting in localized
dilatation of the lumen. By IVUS the internal and external elastic membranes
are intact and there is almost always significant plaque accumulation within the
aneurysm. A pseudoaneurysm is caused by localized rupture of the vessel wall
which is sealed off by thrombus which then organizes into a thin-walled fibrous
structure. By IVUS there are disruption and discontinuity of the EEM, and
there is no evidence of plaque within the aneurysm. Depending on the length
and width of the mouth of the pseudoaneurysm, treatment options include bare
or vein-covered stents. On occasion an extremely tortuous vessel with or
without an angiographic critical stenosis has proved to be an ectatic segment
with aneurysmal dilation and no evidence of lumen compromise.

IVUS imaging immediately after initial recanalization of a totally occluded vessel may be useful in guiding therapy of these difficult lesions. IVUS can identify whether the guidewire is within the true or the false lumen.

VI. IVUS USE DURING AND AFTER INTERVENTION

Routine IVUS is useful for determining the adequacy of the interventional procedure, assessing complications, and selecting the appropriate adjunct devices. The postintervention lumen dimensions can be assessed by IVUS more accurately than by angiography. During stent implantation procedures, IVUS can detect suboptimal apposition of the stent, stent underexpansion, unrecognized proximal or distal lesions, and edge dissections (48–50).

In nonstented procedures, IVUS may be able to detect the mechanism of abrupt vessel closure. Dissections and deep wall hematomas should be treated by stent implantation.

Adjunct directional coronary atherectomy can be used after rotational atherectomy to treat calcified target lesions in larger arteries (51,52). Pretreatment of calcified lesions with rotational atherectomy may render the plaque amenable to additional plaque removal by adjunct directional atherectomy. IVUS clues to the potential effectiveness of adjunct directional coronary atherectomy after rotational atherectomy are noncircumferential target lesion calcium, a decrease in the total arc of calcium after rotational atherectomy, or partial or focal penetration of the ultrasound beam after rotational atherectomy.

VII. CONCLUSION

Preintervention intravascular ultrasound imaging provides useful information regarding the target lesion and the reference vessel. Precise reference segment measurements are useful for device sizing. Characterization of the plaque, especially in determining the presence and location of calcium, is useful in device selection. The determination of lumen compromise is useful in assessing the severity of borderline lesions.

REFERENCES

1. Isner JM, Kishel J, Kent KM, et al. Accuracy of angiographic determination of left main coronary narrowing. Circulation 1981; 63:1056–1061.
2. Roberts WC, Jones AA. Quantitation of coronary arterial narrowing at necropsy in sudden coronary death: analysis of 31 patients and comparison with 25 control subjects. Am J Cardiol 1979; 44:39–44.

3. Voldaver Z, Frech R, Van Tassel RA, Edwards JE. Correlation of antemortem coronary arteriogram and the postmortem specimen. Circulation 1973; 47: 162–168.
4. Yock PG, Linker DT, Angelsen BA. Two-dimensional intervascular ultrasound: technical development and initial clinical experience. J Am Soc Echocardiogr 1989; 2:296–304.
5. Yock PG, Fitzerald PJ, Sudhir K. Intravascular ultrasound. In: Topol EJ, ed. Textbook of Interventional Cardiology. 2nd ed. Philadelphia: Saunders, 1994: 1136–1152.
6. Rosenfield K, Isner JM. Intravascular ultrasound in patients undergoing coronary and peripheral arterial revascularization. In: Topol EJ, ed. Textbook of Interventional Cardiology. 2nd ed. Philadelphia: Saunders, 1994:1153–1185.
7. Tobis JM, Mallery J, Mahon D, et al. Intravascular ultrasound imaging of human coronary arteries in vivo. Circulation 1991; 83:913–926.
8. Nishimura RA, Edwards WD, Warnes CA, et al. Intravascular ultrasound imaging: in vitro validation and pathologic correlation. J Am Coll Cardiol 1990; 16: 145–154.
9. DiMario CD, The SHK, Madretsma S, et al. Detection and characterization of vascular lesions by intravascular ultrasound: an in vitro study correlated with histology. J Am Soc Echocardiogr 1992; 5:135–146.
10. Mintz GS, Douek P, Pichard A, et al. Target lesion calcification in coronary artery disease: an intravascular ultrasound study. J Am Coll Cardiol 1992; 20:1149–1155.
11. Blackenhorn D. Coronary arterial calcification: a review. Am J Med Sci 1961; 242: 4–49.
12. Gianrossi R, Detrano R, Colombo A, Froelicher V. Cardiac fluoroscopy for the diagnosis of coronary artery disease: a meta-analytic review. Am Heart J 1990; 120:1179–1188.
13. Gussenhoven E, Essed C, Lancee C, et al. Arterial wall characteristics determined by intravascular ultrasound imaging: an in vitro study. J Am Coll Cardiol 1989; 14:947–952.
14. Mintz G, Popma J, Pichard A, et al. Patterns of calcification in coronary artery disease. A statistical analysis of intravascular ultrasound and coronary angiography in 1155 lesions. Circulation 1995; 91:1959–1965.
15. Potkin BN, Keren G, Mintz GS, et al. Arterial responses to balloon angioplasty: an intravascular ultrasound study. J Am Coll Cardiol 1992; 20:942–951.
16. Fitzgerald PJ, Ports TA, Yock PG. Contribution of localized calcium deposits to dissection after angioplasty: an observational study using intravascular ultrasound. Circulation 1992; 86:64–70.
17. Matar FA, Mintz GS, Pinnow E, et al. Multivariate predictors of intravascular ultrasound end points after directional coronary atherectomy. J Am Coll Cardiol 1995; 25:318–324.
18. Suarez de Lezo J, Romero M, Medina A, et al. Intracoronary ultrasound assess-

ment of directional coronary atherectomy: immediate and follow-up findings. J Am Coll Cardiol 1993; 21:298–307.

19. Nakamura S, Mahon DJ, Leung CY, et al. Intracoronary ultrasound imaging before and after directional coronary atherectomy: in vitro and clinical observations. Am Heart J 1995; 129:841–851.

20. Mintz GS, Potkin BN, Keren G, et al. Intravascular ultrasound evaluation of the effect of rotational atherectomy in obstructive atherosclerotic coronary artery disease. Circulation 1992; 86:1383–1393.

21. Kovach JA, Mintz GS, Pichard AD, et al. Sequential intravascular ultrasound characterization of the mechanisms of rotational atherectomy and adjunct balloon angioplasty. J Am Coll Cardiol 1993; 22:1024–1032.

22. Fitzgerald PJ, St. Goar FG, Connolly RJ, et al. Intravascular ultrasound imaging of coronary arteries. Is three layers the norm? Circulation 1992; 86:154–158.

23. Matar FA, Mintz GS, Farb A, et al. The contribution of tissue removal to lumen improvement after directional coronary atherectomy. Am J Cardiol 1994; 74:647–650.

24. Mizuno K, Satomura K, Miyamoto A, et al. Angioscopic evaluation of coronary-artery thrombi in acute coronary syndromes. N Engl J Med 1992; 326:287–291.

25. Mallery JA, Tobis JM, Griffith J, et al. Assessment of normal and atherosclerotic arterial wall thickness with an intravascular ultrasound imaging catheter. Am Heart J 1990; 119:1392–1400.

26. Nissen SE, Grines CL, Gurely JC, et al. Application of a new phased-array ultrasound imaging catheter in the assessment of vascular dimensions. In vivo comparison to cineangiography. Circulation 1990; 81:660 666.

27. Stiel GM, Ludmilla MSc, Stiel SG, et al. Impact of compensatory enlargement of atherosclerotic coronary arteries on angiographic assessment of coronary artery disease. Circulation 1989; 80:1603–1609.

28. McPherson DD, Sirna SJ, Hiratzka LF, et al. Coronary arterial remodeling studied by high-frequency epicardial echocardiography: an early compensatory mechanism in patients with obstructive coronary atherosclerosis. J Am Coll Cardiol 1991; 17:79–86.

29. Ge J, Erbel R, Zamorano J, et al. Coronary artery remodeling in atherosclerotic disease: An intravascular ultrasonic study in vivo. Cor Art Dis 1993; 4:981–986.

30. Glagov S, Weisenberg E, Zarins CK, et al. Compensatory enlargement of human atherosclerotic coronary arteries. N Engl J Med 1987; 316:1371–1375.

31. Kimura BJ, Bhargava V, DeMaria AN. Value and limitations of intravascular ultrasound imaging in characterizing coronary atherosclerotic plaque. Am Heart J 1995; 130:386–396.

32. Mintz GS, Popma JJ, Pichard AD, et al. Intravascular ultrasound predictors of restenosis following percutaneous transcatheter coronary revascularization. J Am Coll Cardiol 1996; 27:1678–1687.

33. Mintz GS, Popma JJ, Pichard AD, et al. Limitations of angiography in the assessment of plaque distribution in coronary artery disease: a systematic study of target lesion eccentricity in 1446 lesions. Circulation 1996; 93:924–931.

34. Ellis SG, Roubin GS, King SB III, et al. Angiographic and clinical predictors of acute closure after native vessel coronary angioplasty. Circulation 1988; 77: 372–379.
35. Myler RK, Shaq RE, Stertzer SH, et al. Lesion morphology and coronary angioplasty: current experience and analysis. J Am Coll Cardiol 192; 19:1641–1652.
36. Tenaglia AN, Fortin DF, Califf RM, et al. Predicting the risk of abrupt vessel closure after angioplasty in an individual patient. J Am Coll Cardiol 1994; 24: 1004–1011.
37. Ryan RJ, Faxon DP, Gunnar RP, ACC/AHA Task Force. Guidelines for percutaneous transluminal coronary angioplasty. Circulation 1988; 78:486–502.
38. Bryner JF, Khaja F, Kraft PL. Angioplasty of long or tandem coronary artery lesions using a new longer balloon dilatation catheter: a comparative study. Cathet Cardiovasc Diagn 1991; 23:84–88.
39. Cannon AD, Roubin GS, Hearn JA, et al. Acute angiographic and clinical results of long balloon percutaneous transluminal coronary angioplasty and adjuvant stenting for long narrowings. Am J Cardiol 1994; 73:635–641.
40. Fuessl RT, Mintz GS, Pichard AD, et al. In vivo validation of intravascular ultrasound length measurements using a motorized transducer pullback device. Am J Cardiol 1996; 77:1115–1118.
41. Mintz GS, Painter JA, Pichard AD, et al. Atherosclerosis in angiographically normal coronary artery reference segments: An intravascular ultrasound study with clinical correlations. J Am Coll Cardiol 1995; 25:1479–1485.
42. Stone GW, Linnemeier T, St. Goar FG, et al. Improved outcome of balloon angioplasty with intracoronary ultrasound guidance-core lab angiographic and ultrasound results from the CLOUT study. J Am Coll Cardiol 1996; 27:155A.
43. Javier S, Mintz GS, Popma JJ, et al. Intravascular ultrasound assessment of the magnitude and mechanism of coronary artery and lumen tapering. Am J Cardiol 1995; 75:177–180.
44. Banka V, Baker HI, Vermuri D, et al. Effectiveness of decremental diameter balloon catheter (tapered balloon). Am J Cardiol 1992; 69:188–193.
45. Mintz GS, Pichard AD, Kovach JA, et al. Impact of preintervention intravascular ultrasound imaging on transcatheter treatment strategies in coronary artery disease. Am J Cardiol 1994; 73:423–430.
46. Ambrose JA, Tannenbaum MA, Alexopoulos D, et al. Angiographic progression of coronary artery disease and the development of myocardial infarction. J Am Coll Cardiol 1988; 12:56–60.
47. Duissaillant GD, Mintz GS, Pichard AD, et al. Intravascular ultrasound identification of calcified intraluminal lesions misdiagnosed as thrombi by coronary angiography. Am Heart J. In press.
48. Colombo A, Hall P, Nakamura S, et al. Intracoronary stenting without anticoagulation accomplished with intravascular ultrasound guidance. Circulation 1995; 91:1676–1688.
49. Nakamura S, Colombo A, Gaglione A, et al. Intracoronary ultrasound observations during stent implantation. Circulation 1994; 89:2026–2034.

50. Goldberg SL, Colombo A, Nakamura S, et al. Benefit of intracoronary ultrasound in the deployment of Palmaz-Schatz stents. J Am Coll Cardiol 1994; 24:996–1003.

51. Mintz GS, Pichard AD, Kent KM, et al. Transcathter device synergy: preliminary experience with adjunct directional coronary atherectomy following high-speed rotational atherectomy or excimer laser angioplasty in the treatment of coronary artery disease. Cathet Cardiovasc Diagn 1993; 1:37–44.

52. Henson KD, Flood R, Javier SP, et al. Transcatheter device synergy: use of adjunct directional atherectomy after rotational atherectomy or excimer laser angioplasty. J Am Coll Cardiol 1994; 23:220A.

5

Clinical Application of IVUS Imaging in a Center with Selective Use of IVUS Imaging

Toshihiko Nishioka *Ground Self-Defense Force Medical School, Tokyo, Japan*

Huai Luo *Cedars-Sinai Medical Center, Los Angeles, California*

Neal L. Eigler and Robert J. Siegel *Cedars-Sinai Medical Center and University of California, Los Angeles, School of Medicine, Los Angeles, California*

Steven W. Tabak *University of California, Los Angeles, School of Medicine, Los Angeles, California*

I. INTRODUCTION

Two-dimensional intravascular ultrasound (IVUS) imaging provides high-quality, tomographic visualization of the coronary vessels, enabling qualitative assessment and quantitative measurement of stenosis severity and plaque composition (1–6). Before the introduction of IVUS imaging, most clinical decisions of interventional cardiologists in cardiac catheterization laboratories were based on angiographic, hemodynamic, and electrocardiographic findings along with clinical manifestations. In the early era of IVUS imaging (from the end of the 1980s to the early 1990s), it was mainly used as a research tool; the frequency with which IVUS imaging contributes to decision making during diagnostic and interventional coronary procedures is now in transition. In this chapter we describe how IVUS imaging at our institution is used as a clinical tool affecting interventional decision making in our cardiac catheterization laboratory from 1993 to 1995.

II. METHODS

A. Patients and Imaged Vessels

To maintain the uniformity of interventional decision making, only 165 patients catheterized and treated by one of the three most active interventionalists in our center were included in this study. Together they performed approximately 45% of all coronary interventions in our institution during this period. Out of 165 patients, there were three cases in which the IVUS catheter could not pass the target lesion, and four cases in which IVUS imaging was not obtained or image quality was suboptimal because of IVUS system (IVUS catheter or imaging console) failure. These seven patients have been excluded from our study. Consequently, 158 patients (men 120, women 38, mean age 67 ± 12) with known or suspected coronary artery disease were successfully studied using a single IVUS imaging system, as shown in Table 1. Informed consent was obtained from each patient before the intravascular ultrasound procedure. These patients were divided into four temporal groups, as shown in Table 2: 39 cases studied between February 1993 and December 1993 (men 29, women 10, mean age 68 ± 9); 39 cases studied between January 1994 and August 1994 (men

Table 1 Patients Studied by Treatment Modality

Patients	Number
Total	165
Failed IVUS imaging	7
IVUS catheter could not pass the lesion	3
IVUS system failure	4
Successful IVUS imaging	158
No catheter intervention	20
Medication	15
Coronary artery bypass surgery	5
Primary PTCA	45
Stent deployment	83
Plaque ablation	24
Rotablator	6
DCA	8
ELCA	10

Table 2 Population Studied February 1993 Through August 1995

	Study period				
	2/93–12/93	1/94–8/94	9/94–3/95	4/95–8/95	Total
Unsuccessful cases	4	2	1	0	7
No. of patients	39	39	40	40	158
Male/female	29/10	27/12	31/9	33/7	120/38
Age (years)	68 ± 9	67 ± 10	65 ± 11	68 ± 10	67 ± 10
Imaged vessels	39	39	40	40	158
LAD & LM	18	14	15	15	62
LCx & LM	1	3	3	6	13
RCA	13	9	6	12	40
SVG	7	13	16	7	43

27, women 12, mean age 67 ± 10); 40 cases studied between September 1994 and March 1995 (men 31, women 9, mean age 65 ± 11); and 40 cases studied between April 1995 and August 1995 (men 33, women 7, mean age 68 ± 10). The numbers of the imaged vessels are also shown in Table 2; 62 left anterior descending coronary arteries, 13 left circumflex coronary arteries, 40 right coronary arteries, and 43 saphenous vein grafts were included in this study.

B. Angiography and Transcatheter Interventions

For angiography we used a biplane system with digital acquisition at 30 frames/sec (Advantex DXC, GE Medical System, Wakeshaw, WI) using a 7-inch image intensifier field size on a $512^2 \times 8$ format. Images were displayed on 19-inch room monitors upscanned to 1024^2 pixels with extended dynamic range and spatial edge-enhancement filtration. Angiography was performed by a standard femoral approach taking multiple orthogonal views of coronary vessels. The guiding catheter was used for quantitative calibration, and the angiographically normal-appearing proximal segment adjacent to the lesion was used as a reference segment. Reference segment and lesion diameters were obtained in two orthogonal views that best displayed these vessel segments. Angiographic images were interpreted by the responsible interventional cardiologist at the time of acquisition.

Transcatheter coronary interventions being performed during this study period were balloon angioplasty (PTCA), directional atherectomy (DCA), rotational atherectomy (RCA), excimer laser angioplasty (ELCA), and stent deployment. All these interventions were performed by standard techniques.

C. Intravascular Ultrasound System and Imaging Procedure

IVUS imaging was performed following coronary angiography. The IVUS imaging system consisted of an imaging catheter (Sonicath, Boston Scientific Corporation, Watertown, MA) which has a 30-MHz single mechanically rotating piezoelectric crystal within a 3.5 F monorail catheter sheath and a SONOS Intravascular System imaging console (Hewlett-Packard, Andover, MA). Cases studied with other IVUS systems were excluded from this study to ensure uniformity in image quality.

After the completion of angiography, the imaging catheter was introduced into the native coronary arteries or saphenous vein bypass grafts through an 8 to 11 F coronary guiding catheter over a 0.014- or 0.018-inch guidewire. To prevent possible vasospasm reported in up to 3% of intravascular ultrasound studies (7,8) and to obtain maximum vasodilation, 100 to 200 μg of nitroglycerin was administered into the vessels imaged before and during the IVUS imaging. After advancing the imaging catheter across the lesion to the distal portion of the vessel under fluoroscopic guidance, continuous IVUS imaging was performed during the slow pullback (1 mm/sec) of the imaging catheter. Contrast medium was injected to enhance the ultrasound definition of the lumen in cases in which the lumen-intimal border was ambiguous. X-ray fluoroscopy was used to confirm the coaxiality of the imaging catheter at a region of interest in the coronary artery. The two-dimensional images of the vessel were displayed on a SONOS Intravascular System imaging console and recorded on a 0.5-inch Super-VHS videotape for subsequent playback, review, and quantitative analysis.

D. IVUS Image Analysis

Intravascular ultrasound images were analyzed on-line and off-line with a SONOS Intravascular System. For qualitative assessment of the vessel, degree (arc) and site (superficial or deep) of calcium deposition which was defined as bright echoes (brighter than the adventitia) with acoustic shadowing, echogenicity of noncalcified plaque (low or hyperechoic/soft or hard plaque), plaque eccentricity, identification of intimal flap, dissection (deep or superficial), and presence or absence of a thrombus were noted. When applicable, the adequacy of stent deployment (stent shape and its apposition to the vessel) and the degree of plaque removal after DCA, RCA, or ELCA was noted. For quantitative assessment of the vessel, minimum and maximum lumen diameters, lumen cross-sectional area, minimum and maximum diameters of the external lamina (EEL), EEL cross-sectional area, and plaque + media (EEL-lumen) cross-sectional area were measured at the lesion site and the reference site before and/or after interventional procedure.

1. Before Intervention

The decision making before the intervention was evaluated in three categories, as shown in Figure 1.

a. Evaluation of Stenosis Severity. Stenosis severity of the coronary vessels was evaluated by angiography before IVUS imaging. When stenosis severity of a vessel was not clearly determined by angiography, IVUS was used to identify a stenotic lesion to be treated or to exclude a significant stenosis. If there was no significant stenosis observed, the procedure was terminated and no further therapy was planned for that specific site. IVUS may also have revealed significant stenoses when it was used for other purposes. If the stenosis severity was significant, some treatment was required and planned based on IVUS findings.

b. Selection of the Optimal Therapy (i.e., medication, surgery, or catheter intervention). In cases where the significant stenosis was revealed by angiography and/or IVUS, and the lesion was not considered appropriate for catheter intervention, the patient was referred to surgery (especially in the case of left main coronary artery lesion and three-vessel disease) or medical treatment. If the interventional cardiologist decided to perform catheter intervention, the next step was considered.

c. Selection of the Type and Size of Interventional Device. When transcatheter intervention was planned, the type of interventional therapy (PTCA, stent deployment, DCA, RCA, or ELCA) and the size of the interventional

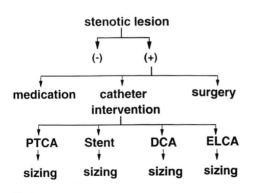

Figure 1 Decision making before intervention.

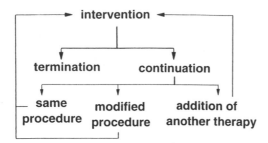

Figure 2 Decision making after intervention.

devices were selected by angiographic and/or IVUS findings. If preinterventional IVUS imaging revealed severe endoluminal calcification of the plaque, RCA or ELCA was preferred instead of PTCA and DCA.

2. After Intervention

After the interventional therapy, decision making was also classified in three categories as shown in Figure 2.

a. Termination or Continuation of the Procedure. If the interventional result was judged as acceptable by angiography and/or IVUS, the procedure was terminated. However, where the interventional result was suboptimal, the procedure was continued. There were three options: the same procedure could be repeated, or a modified procedure or surgery could be selected.

b. Modification of the Interventional Strategy. This category included increase in device size, balloon inflation pressure, and/or procedure time. The addition of different interventional procedures such as adjunctive balloon angioplasty or stent deployment after other interventional procedures was included in this category.

c. Surgery. The patient could be referred to surgery because of the failure of transcatheter intervention, acute occlusion, or rupture of the treated vessel.

Figure 3 demonstrates in detail how IVUS imaging was judged as useful or not useful in a clinical setting. Based on angiographic findings, the initial decision was usually made by the interventional cardiologist before IVUS imaging. When IVUS imaging gave some additional information that was not provided by angiography and the initial decision was altered based on the IVUS findings, IVUS imaging was considered to be useful in clinical decision making. For example, planned PTCA might be changed to RCA because IVUS revealed severe calcification which was not apparent by angiography, planned

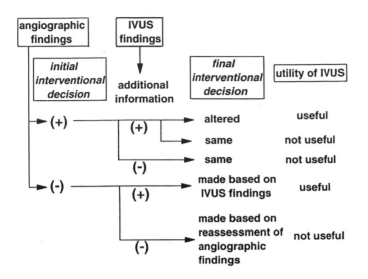

Figure 3 Definition of how IVUS imaging was judged as useful or not useful in clinical setting.

catheter intervention might be abandoned, and the patient may be referred to surgery because an angiographically silent left main coronary lesion was found by IVUS imaging or angiographically acceptable stent deployment was found to be suboptimal by IVUS and the stent was redilated by balloon. When IVUS failed to provide additional information beyond angiographic findings, it was considered not to be useful. Even though IVUS provided additional information, if that information did not change the initial decision, it was also considered not useful in clinical decision making.

In some cases the interventional cardiologist could not make an initial decision based only on angiographic findings—for example, angiographically ambiguous (moderately stenotic) ostial lesions or postinterventional lesions. In these cases, IVUS imaging was considered to have affected the decision making if it provided additional information to angiographic findings. If IVUS failed to give new information and the final decision was made based on a reassessment of angiographic findings, it was considered not to be useful.

E. Statistical Analysis

For statistical analysis, Fisher's exact test or chi-square test was performed and the difference was considered significant when the P value was $< .05$.

III. RESULTS

The intravascular ultrasound studies of human in vivo coronary arteries and saphenous vein bypass grafts were completed without major vascular complications. As shown in Table 1, of 165 patients in whom IVUS imaging was attempted, seven patients were excluded from the study because the IVUS imaging was unsuccessful. Finally, 158 cases with successful IVUS imaging were included in this study.

A. Impact of IVUS Imaging on Clinical Decision Making Throughout the Study Period

As shown in Tables 1 and 3, the 158 cases included 45 primary balloon angioplasties, 83 stent deployments, and 24 plaque ablations (6 RCAs, 8 DCAs and 10 ELCAs). Twenty patients did not receive any catheter intervention; five underwent elective coronary artery bypass surgery, and 15 patients were

Table 3 Study Results Defined as Useful

Cases or IVUS imaging	Total number	Number of cases or imaging defined as useful	Percentage of cases or imaging defined as useful
Whole cases	158	133	84.2%
No catheter intervention	20	19	95.0%
Primary PTCA cases	45	29	64.4%
Stent cases	83	81	97.6%
Plaque ablation cases	24	18	75.0%
Imaging without catheter intervention	20	19	95.0%
Preinterventional imaging	52	33	63.5%
Pre-PTCA	29	16	55.2%
Prestent	19	12	63.2%
Preplaque ablation	9	8	88.9%
Postinterventional imaging	128	99	77.3%
Post-PTCA	34	15	44.1%
Poststent	80	78	97.5%
Postplaque ablation	24	13	54.2%
Imaging for angiographically ambiguous lesion	42	42	100.0%

treated medically. Interventional decisions based on IVUS findings were made in 84.2% (133/158) of all cases. IVUS imagings were considered significantly more useful for decision making in stent cases (97.6%) than in balloon angioplasty cases (64.4%, $P < .001$) and plaque ablation cases (75.0%, $P = .0015$).

Preinterventional or diagnostic IVUS imagings were performed in 72 cases and defined as useful in 72.2% (52/72) of these cases. In this group, IVUS was used for the detection of significant stenoses (43.1%, 31/72), exclusion of significant stenoses (20.8%, 15/72), and selection or sizing of interventional devices (15.3%, 11/72).

1. **A case in which IVUS revealed significant coronary artery stenosis that was not apparent by angiography.** The patient (a 44-year-old man) presented with intermittent burning retrosternal chest discomfort. The rest thallium/stress technetium-99m sestamibi dual-isotope myocardial perfusion single-photon emission computed tomography demonstrated a moderately large and severe reversible defect involving the anterior, septal, apical, and distal inferior wall of the left ventricle consistent with ischemia caused by stenosis in the proximal left anterior descending coronary artery distribution (Fig. 4A). However, coronary angiography (Fig. 4B), despite multiple views, did not show significant stenosis of the left coronary artery. IVUS imaging was attempted and revealed an 80% calcified stenosis in the left anterior descending coronary artery close to the ostium, as shown in Figure 4C. The patient underwent coronary artery bypass surgery, and the stress myocardial perfusion study repeated 1 month later (Fig. 4D) demonstrated normal tracer uptake throughout the left ventricular myocardium both at rest and at peak stress.

2. **A case in which IVUS was used to exclude a significant stenosis.** Figure 5 shows a possible right coronary artery ostial lesion as demonstrated by coronary angiography. However, IVUS imaging showed only a mild concentric stenosis at the ostial site and PTCA was performed for distal lesions without intervention at the ostium.

Postinterventional imagings were defined as useful in 77.3% (99/128) of cases. In this group, the use of IVUS for the detection of inadequate interventional results (31.3%, 40/128) for the need of additional interventional therapy and for confirmation of adequate stent deployment (44.5%, 57/128) predominated. Balloon angioplasty results were deemed inadequate in 10 out of 34 cases in which post-PTCA IVUS imaging was performed. Among these cases, stents were placed in five cases, PTCA was repeated in four cases, and a perfusion balloon was used in one case. Stent deployment was judged as inadequate in 21 out of 80 cases in which poststent IVUS imaging was performed, and all stents were redilated by balloons with larger diameters or

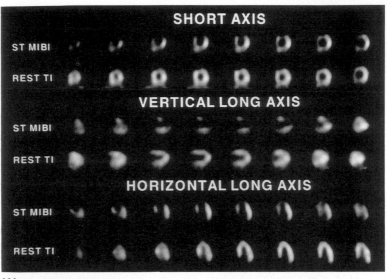

(A)

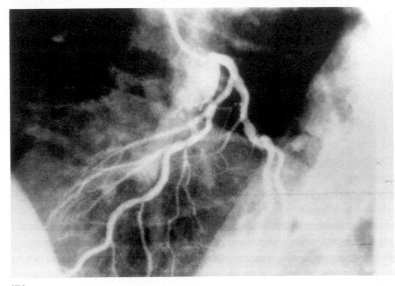

(B)

Figure 4 (A) Rest and redistribution thallium/stress technetium-99m sestamibi dual-isotope scan reveals a reversible defect involving the anterior-septal, apical, and distal inferior wall. (B) Coronary angiogram, left anterior oblique projection, does not reveal a lesion in the left anterior descending coronary artery.

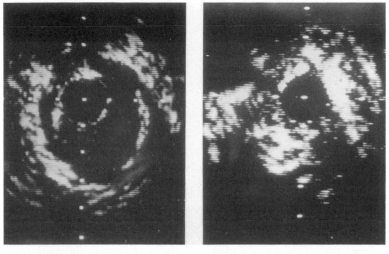

(C)

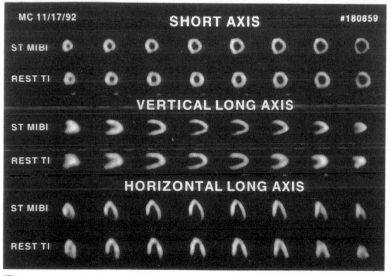

(D)

(C) The IVUS image (left panel) shows mild disease in the left anterior descending coronary artery, but IVUS images at the ostium of the left anterior descending coronary artery reveal a tight calcific lesion encircling the imaging catheter. (D) The patient underwent coronary artery bypass surgery, and the stress myocardial perfusion study repeated 1 month later demonstrates normal tracer uptake throughout the left ventricular myocardium both at rest and at peak stress. (Figures 4A, 4B, and 4C are adapted from Figures 3, 2, and 4 in Ref. 29, with permission from the authors.)

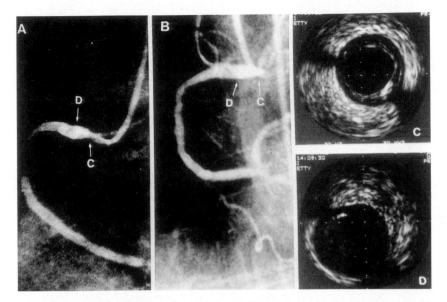

Figure 5   IVUS imaging of an apparent right coronary artery ostial lesion. The left anterior oblique (A) and right anterior oblique (B) projections showed critical stenoses at the bifurcation of the posterior descending artery and posterior lateral branch of the right coronary artery. While angiographically there appears to be a right coronary ostial lesion, IVUS demonstrates only a 30% concentric stenosis. (From Fig. 1 in Lee et al. [30], with permission from the authors.)

higher inflation pressures. Among 80 poststent imagings, 57 stents were considered to be adequately deployed.

1.   **A case in which a stent was redilated based on the IVUS finding.** Figure 6 demonstrates a case in which the interventional decision was altered by poststent IVUS imaging. Although the coronary angiogram showed satisfactory vessel dilatation of the left anterior descending coronary artery after stent (3.0 mm) deployment, IVUS imaging revealed insufficient stent expansion at its distal portion. Based on this finding, the interventional cardiologist redilated the stent with a noncompliant balloon and the maximum and minimum stent diameters increased from 2.5 × 2.0 mm to 2.5 × 2.9 mm, respectively.

2.   **A case in which DCA was terminated based on the IVUS finding.** In Figure 7 is shown a case in which IVUS demonstrated a deep incision into

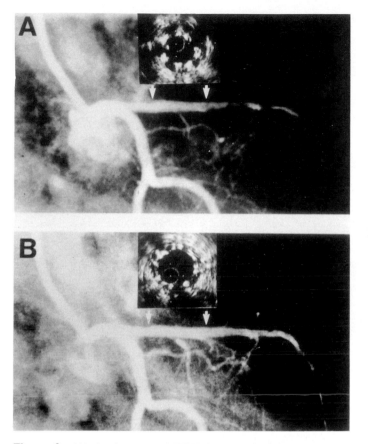

Figure 6   (A) Angiogram and IVUS images of a left anterior descending coronary artery stent thought to be optimally deployed by angiographic assessment. (B) Angiogram and IVUS image after redilatation at a higher pressure with a noncompliant balloon. (From Fig. 1 in Nishioka et al. [8], with permission from the authors.)

the adventitia with an intraluminal flap after DCA. As a consequence further DCA was discontinued and adjunctive PTCA with prolonged inflation was performed.

In some of the cases IVUS was used to evaluate more than one specific type of intervention. This accounts for the cumulative percentage of IVUS imagings exceeding 100%.

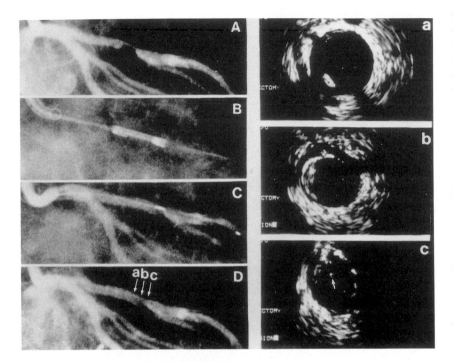

Figure 7 (A) The coronary angiogram showed an eccentric, subtotal occlusion lesion of a proximal left anterior descending coronary artery. (B) Direct coronary atherectomy was performed. (C and D) IVUS imaging revealed a patent lumen after the direct coronary atherectomy. (a) There is minimal residual plaque (8 to 10 o'clock position). (b) Deep incision (12 o'clock position) with mobile intimal flap. (c) (arrow) The direct coronary atherectomy was terminated because of depth of tissue removed at the 12 o'clock position. PTCA with a prolonged inflation was performed to "seal" intimal flap. (From Fig. 6 in Lee et al. [30], with permission from the authors.)

B. Temporal Change in Impact of IVUS Imaging on Clinical Decision Making

Table 4 and Figure 8 show temporal changes in the impact of IVUS imaging on clinical decision making and the selective use of IVUS imaging. The frequency of cases in which the interventional decision was affected by IVUS images increased significantly from 56% (22/39) in the period 2/93 to 12/93 to 100% (40/40) in the period 4/95 to 8/95 ($P < .0001$). During this time period, there were changes in the indications for IVUS imaging. Even in the early series,

Table 4 Impact of IVUS on Clinical Decision Making

	Study period				
	2/93–12/93	1/94–8/94	9/94–3/95	4/95–8/95	Total
Number of patients	39	39	40	40	158
Useful for decision	22	33	38	40	133
making	56%	85%	95%	100%	84%
Total no. of IVUS	54	49	44	53	200
imaging	26	35	40	50	151
Useful for decision					
making	48%	71%	91%	94%	76%
Diagnostic and	23	17	10	22	72
preinterventional					
imaging					
Useful for decision	12	12	8	20	52
making	52%	71%	80%	91%	72%
Postinterventional imaging	31	32	34	31	128
Useful for decision	14	23	32	30	99
making	45%	72%	94%	97%	77%
Angiographically	5	9	10	18	42
ambiguous lesion	13%	23%	25%	45%	27%
PTCA case	20	12	7	6	45
	51%	31%	18%	15%	28%
Stent case	10	17	28	28	83
	26%	67%	70%	70%	53%
Plaque ablation case	7	11	4	2	24
	18%	28%	10%	5%	15%

IVUS imaging was considered more useful for decision making in stent cases (90%) and in cases with angiographically ambiguous lesions (100%) than in balloon angioplasty cases (55%). Accordingly the three interventional cardiologists who performed all the interventions in this study began to preselect patients to be imaged by IVUS in whom the angiographic findings were limited and the IVUS images were expected to provide more definitive information. Thus imaging of stent cases increased from 26% (10/39) to 70% (28/40) ($P <$ .0001), and the imaging of angiographically ambiguous lesions including ostial segments increased from 13% (5/39) to 45% (18/40) of cases (P = .0016). IVUS imaging for balloon angioplasty cases decreased from 51% (20/39) to

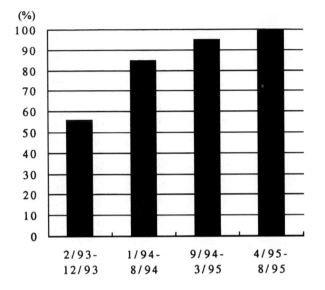

Figure 8 Bar graph showing the change in frequency of interventional decision making based on intravascular ultrasound imaging during four consecutive time periods.

15% (6/40) (P = .0006), especially for post-PTCA imaging from 44% (17/39) to 7.5% (3/40) (P = .0002).

C. Complications

There were three complications attributed to IVUS imaging. One complication involved an angiographically apparent dissection of the left anterior descending coronary artery which developed after postballoon angioplasty IVUS imaging, and which had not been observed by angiography immediately after balloon angioplasty. A coronary stent was placed in this vessel without complication. There were two cases of coronary vasospasm during IVUS imaging, which were relieved promptly by the intracoronary injection of nitroglycerin. All three cases were treated in the catheterization laboratory without further clinical sequelae.

IV. DISCUSSION

IVUS imaging affected the clinical decisions of interventionalists in 64% of PTCA cases, 75% of plaque ablation cases, and 98% of stent cases. Pre- and postinterventional imaging was considered useful for decision making in 64% and 77% of cases, respectively, and IVUS imaging for angiographically ambiguous lesions was extremely useful (100%, 42/42) for determining clinical decisions.

During this study period, IVUS imaging has become in our laboratory a useful method for supporting interventional decision making. By selecting patients undergoing stent placement and patients who have coronary angiographic lesions of uncertain severity for IVUS imaging, there has been a dramatic increase in the clinical utility of IVUS imaging in our laboratory.

A. Stenosis Severity Before Intervention

Coronary angiography has been the gold standard for the assessment of vessel lumen narrowing, and earlier IVUS studies demonstrated good correlation between angiographic and IVUS measurements (4,9,10). As angiography portrays the complex three-dimensional vessel lumen as a two-dimensional silhouette, it is inevitable that underestimation of vessel stenoses occurs, especially at a branching site, at the vessel ostium, or when its configuration is tortuous and overlapped. It is reported that angiographic and IVUS measurements sometimes show wide discrepancy (11–16). Therefore, if the angiography is ambiguous or if there is a discrepancy between clinical manifestation and angiographic findings, IVUS is very useful for decision making as shown in our data. IVUS is also useful when a significant stenosis could not be excluded because of an ostial lesion or overlapped vessels. Unnecessary catheter intervention or surgery can be avoided by excluding severe vessel narrowing using IVUS as in 15 cases out of 158 cases in our series.

B. Plaque Composition, Plaque Eccentricity, and Device Selection

Interventional device selection is influenced by the presence, severity, and location (depth) of calcification and target lesion eccentricity, both of which are better visualized by IVUS than angiography (12,17,18). It is known that calcification frequently causes vessel dissection after balloon angioplasty (19–21). Directional atherectomy does not remove a sufficient amount of plaque with the presence of endoluminal calcification (22,23), although it is suitable for eccentric noncalcified lesions (24). Conversely, rotational atherectomy can selectively ablate hard, calcified lesions (25,26), leaving soft or normal arterial tissue. Excimer laser angioplasty is also believed to be suitable for calcified plaque ablation (27). Stent deployment might be preferred to seal an intimal flap or dissection, and to treat acute and/or late recoil of the vessel (28).

C. Postinterventional IVUS Imaging

Inadequate results after balloon angioplasty include residual significant stenoses, large intimal flaps and extensive dissections. Most of these cases are treated by stent deployment or repeat balloon angioplasty.

There is a controversy in regard to whether IVUS imaging is essential after stent deployment with the use of high-pressure noncompliant balloons. In our series, IVUS imaging revealed inadequate stent deployment in 21 of 80 cases (26%), and the stents were redilated by balloon. While it is our belief that poststent IVUS imaging improves the outcome of these cases, a clinical trial to determine this is still pending.

D. Limitations to Be Overcome

In this series, the clinical utility of IVUS imaging is assessed from the viewpoint of clinical de' ision making. The patient's clinical or angiographic outcome was not compared to patients not receiving IVUS. A large randomized trial might be needed to clarify the real impact of IVUS imaging on the acute outcome as well as longer-term arterial patency.

For diagnostic or preinterventional imaging, it has not been precisely shown what constitutes a "significant" stenosis requiring treatment as defined by IVUS imaging. There are similar ambiguities after PTCA; as dissection is one of the major mechanisms of lumen enlargement, it is also difficult to define what is the optimal or acceptable result.

V. CONCLUSIONS

IVUS imaging has become a useful modality which can provide information to affect clinical decisions in the coronary interventional laboratory. During this study period, there was a significant increase in the clinical utility of IVUS imaging by the selection of patients for IVUS who have coronary angiographic lesions of uncertain severity or patients undergoing stent placement.

REFERENCES

1. Gussenhoven EJ, Essed CE, Lancee CT, et al. Arterial wall characteristics determined by intravascular ultrasound imaging: an in vitro study. J Am Coll Cardiol 1989; 14:947–952.
2. Potkin BN, Bartorelli AL, Gessert JM, et al. Coronary artery imaging with intravascular high-frequency ultrasound. Circulation 1990; 81:1575–1585.
3. Nishimura RA, Edwards WD, Warnes CA, et al. Intravascular ultrasound imaging:

in vitro validation and pathologic correlation. J Am Coll Cardiol 1990; 16: 145–154.

4. Nissen SE, Grines CL, Gurley JC, et al. Application of a new phased-array ultrasound imaging catheter in the assessment of vascular dimensions. In vivo comparison to cineangiography. Circulation 1990; 81:660–666.

5. Tobis JM, Mallery J, Mahon D, et al. Intravascular ultrasound imaging of human coronary arteries in vivo. Analysis of tissue characterizations with comparison to in vitro histological specimens. Circulation 1991; 83:913–926.

6. Siegel RJ, Ariani M, Fishbein MC, et al. Histopathologic validation of angioscopy and intravascular ultrasound. Circulation 1991; 84:109–117.

7. Hausmann D, Erbel R, Alibelli CM, et al. The safety of intracoronary ultrasound. A multicenter survey of 2207 examinations. Circulation 1995; 91:623–630.

8. Nishioka T, Luo H, Eigler N, et al. The evolving utility of intracoronary ultrasound. Am J Cardiol 1995; 75:539–541.

9. St. Goar FG, Pinto FJ, Alderman EL, et al. Intravascular ultrasound imaging of angiographically normal coronary arteries: an in vivo comparison with quantitative angiography. J Am Coll Cardiol 1991; 18:952–958.

10. Nissen SE, Gurley JC, Grines CL, et al. Intravascular ultrasound assessment of lumen size and wall morphology in normal subjects and patients with coronary artery disease. Circulation 1991; 84:1087–1099.

11. Hermiller JB, Buller CE, Tenaglia AN, et al. Unrecognized left main coronary artery disease in patients undergoing interventional procedures. Am J Cardiol 1993; 71:173–176.

12. Mintz GS, Popma JJ, Pichard AD, et al. Limitations of angiography in the assessment of plaque distribution in coronary artery disease. A systemic study of target lesion eccentricity in 1446 lesions. Circulation 1996; 93:924–931.

13. Porter TR, Sears T, Xie F, et al. Intravascular ultrasound study of angiographically mildly diseased coronary arteries. J Am Coll Cardiol 1993; 22:1858–1865.

14. Mintz GS, Painter JA, Pichard AD, et al. Atherosclerosis in angiographically "normal" coronary artery reference segments: an intravascular ultrasound study with clinical correlations. J Am Coll Cardiol 1995; 25:1479–1485.

15. Ehrlich S, Honye J, Mahon D, Bernstein R, Tobis J. Unrecognized stenosis by angiography documented by intravascular ultrasound imaging. Cathet Cardiovasc Diagn 1991; 23:198–201.

16. White CJ, Ramee SR, Collins TJ, Jain A, Mesa JE. Ambiguous coronary angiography: clinical utility of intravascular ultrasound [see comments]. Cathet Cardiovasc Diagn 1992; 26:200–203.

17. Mintz GS, Popma JJ, Pichard AD, et al. Patterns of calcification in coronary artery disease. A statistical analysis of intravascular ultrasound and coronary angiography in 1155 lesions. Circulation 1995; 91:1959–1965.

18. Mintz GS, Douek P, Pichard AD, et al. Target lesion calcification in coronary artery disease: an intravascular ultrasound study. J Am Coll Cardiol 1992; 20: 1149–1155.

19. Fitzgerald PJ, Ports TA, Yock PG. Contribution of localized calcium deposits to

dissection after angioplasty. An observational study using intravascular ultrasound [see comments]. Circulation 1992; 86:64–70.

20. Potkin BN, Keren G, Mintz GS, et al. Arterial responses to balloon coronary angioplasty: an intravascular ultrasound study. J Am Coll Cardiol 1992; 20:942–951.

21. Marsico F, Kubica J, De-Servi S, et al. Influence of plaque morphology on the mechanism of luminal enlargement after directional coronary atherectomy and balloon angioplasty. Br Heart J 1995; 74:134–139.

22. Matar FA, Mintz GS, Pinnow E, et al. Multivariate predictors of intravascular ultrasound end points after directional coronary atherectomy. J Am Coll Cardiol 1995; 25:318–324.

23. Popma JJ, Mintz GS, Satler LF, et al. Clinical and angiographic outcome after directional coronary atherectomy. A qualitative and quantitative analysis using coronary arteriography and intravascular ultrasound. Am J Cardiol 1993; 72: 55E–64E.

24. Braden GA, Herrington DM, Downes TR, Kutcher MA, Little WC. Qualitative and quantitative contrasts in the mechanisms of lumen enlargement by coronary balloon angioplasty and directional coronary atherectomy. J Am Coll Cardiol 1994; 23:40–48.

25. Mintz GS, Potkin BN, Keren G, et al. Intravascular ultrasound evaluation of the effect of rotational atherectomy in obstructive atherosclerotic coronary artery disease. Circulation 1992; 86:1383–1393.

26. Kovach JA, Mintz GS, Pichard AD, et al. Sequential intravascular ultrasound characterization of the mechanisms of rotational atherectomy and adjunct balloon angioplasty. J Am Coll Cardiol 1993; 22:1024–1032.

27. Cook SL, Eigler NL, Shefer A, Goldenberg T, Forrester JS, Litvack F. Percutaneous excimer laser coronary angioplasty of lesions not suitable for balloon angioplasty. Circulation 1991; 84:632–643.

28. Painter JA, Mintz GS, Wong SC, et al. Serial intravascular ultrasound studies fail to show evidence of chronic Palmaz-Schatz stent recoil. Am J Cardiol 1995; 75: 398–400.

29. Kiat H. Abnormal myocardial perfusion single-photon emission computed tomography and normal arteriogram: the role of intracoronary vascular ultrasound in providing diagnostic confirmation. Am Heart J 1995; 130:182–186.

30. Lee DY. Effect of intracoronary ultrasound imaging on clinical decision making. Am Heart J 1995; 129:1084–1093.

6

Intravascular Ultrasound Assessment of Regional Remodeling in Human Atherosclerotic Vessels

Hans Berglund   *Karolinska Institutet and Huddinge Hospital, Huddinge, Sweden*

Toshihiko Nishioka   *Ground Self-Defense Force Medical School, Tokyo, Japan*

Huai Luo   *Cedars-Sinai Medical Center, Los Angeles, California*

Michael C. Fishbein   *University of California, Los Angeles, School of Medicine, and Cedars-Sinai Medical Center, Los Angeles, California*

Robert J. Siegel   *Cedars-Sinai Medical Center and University of California, Los Angeles, School of Medicine, Los Angeles, California*

I.   ATHEROSCLEROTIC REMODELING IN THE ARTERY WALL

Compensatory arterial enlargement in response to plaque formation was first described in coronary arteries (1) and peripheral arteries (2) of monkeys. It was subsequently confirmed in human left main coronary arteries using postmortem histological examination (3). Histopathological studies (3,4), intraoperative high frequency epicardial coronary ultrasound imaging (5), and intracoronary ultrasound imaging (6,7) have shown that human coronary arteries enlarge in parallel with the formation of atherosclerotic plaque, suggesting that the lumen area is preserved until the progressive accumulation of plaque exceeds the compensatory mechanisms of the vessel. Similar findings have also been identified in human carotid (8) and superficial femoral arteries (9). These observations (1–9) indicate that arterial remodeling is an important factor for maintainence of the lumen in human atherosclerosis. The presence of significant atherosclerosis by IVUS criteria in angiographically normal coronary artery segments (10–13) suggests that traditional angiographic assessment of coronary artery stenosis in relation to the lumen size in a reference segment, presently used in order to guide coronary interventions, may depend on factors related to both the degree of atherosclerosis and regional compensatory mechanisms.

Conclusions derived from pathologic and IVUS studies (3,4,6,7) based on the significant correlation between plaque area and vessel area (within the external or internal elastic lamina) pooled from single measurements of different vessels of different individuals have inherent limitations (9). If the vessels from different individuals with a substantial range of sizes are analyzed together, the correlation found between the plaque area and vessel area could be due to the fact that the larger vessels tend to have more plaque area than the small vessels. IVUS provides a technique that allows identification and precise measurements of the vessel lumen, total vessel dimensions, and the vessel wall at multiple locations in the same vessel. Utilization of these unique features of IVUS therefore provides new qualitative information which may increase our understanding of atherosclerotic remodeling.

The possibility of regional or general vasoconstriction must be assessed in studies aimed at a comparison of lumen and vessel areas within or between vessels. The effect of the endothelium-independent vasodilator nitroglycerin has been shown to be relatively unaffected by atherosclerosis (14,15), and its standardized use during IVUS studies is likely to minimize the influence of vasoconstriction on the results.

II. INADEQUATE COMPENSATORY ENLARGEMENT IN STENOTIC CORONARY ARTERIES

In a landmark study by Pasterkamp and co-workers (16), combining intravascular ultrasound and pathology studies of human atherosclerotic femoral arteries, inadequate compensatory enlargement, or constriction of the arterial wall was suggested as a different mechanism associated with the development of severe arterial luminal narrowing in addition to plaque proliferation. Although arterial remodeling (recoil) in addition to intimal proliferation (17–19) has been reported to be an important determinant of restenosis after peripheral arterial balloon angioplasty (21–23) and in patients after multiple coronary transcatheter therapies (24–26), the concept of a primary failure of the artery to respond to plaque formation with enlargement warrants further exploration. We recently reported data from an IVUS study, comparing the lumen area, the vessel wall area and the vessel cross-sectional area within the same vessel in 35 de novo coronary artery lesions from 30 patients (27). The aim was to examine to what extent de novo native coronary artery stenosis is accompanied by vessel wall thickening and/or inadequate compensatory enlargement (relative vessel constriction). The vessel cross-sectional area (CSA) and lumen area (LA) were measured, and wall area (WA = CSA − LA) was calculated at the lesion site and at the proximal and distal reference sites. We defined compensatory enlargement to be present when the CSA at the lesion site was larger than the proximal reference site. We defined inadequate compensatory enlargement when CSA at the lesion site was smaller than the distal reference site, and intermediate remodeling when the CSA at the lesion site was an intermediate size between the two reference sites. Compensatory enlargement was observed in 54%, inadequate compensatory enlargement in 26%, and intermediate re-

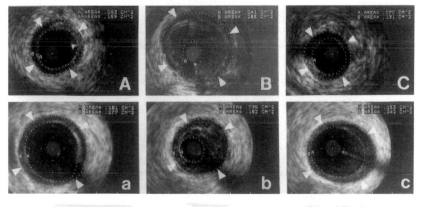

Proximal Reference   Lesion   Distal Reference

Figure 1 IVUS images from two coronary arteries. The upper panels A–C show a coronary artery in which compensatory enlargement was observed and in which lower panels a–c have inadequate compensatory enlargement. The white dotted lines show the lumen-intimal borders, and the white dotted lines accompanied by white arrowheads indicate the external elastic lamina. In upper panels A–C, the vessel cross-sectional area at the lesion site was larger than the proximal and distal reference sites (28.5 vs. 15.9 and 13.1 mm^2). In lower panels a–c, the vessel cross-sectional area at the lesion site was smaller than the proximal and distal reference sites (18.2 vs. 27.7 and 24.2 mm^2). Adapted from Ref. 27, with permission from the authors.

modeling in 20% of lesions. Representative examples of compensatory enlargement and inadequate compensatory enlargement are illustrated in Figure
1. WA and CSA at the lesion site were significantly ($P < .05$) larger in the
compensatory enlargement group than in the inadequate compensatory enlargement group. In the inadequate compensatory enlargement group, reduction of the CSA contributed to 39% of lumen reduction.

Using a 12-MHz epicardial ultrasound imaging transducer, McPherson and
co-workers (5) applied a similar approach comparing a proximal reference site
and the stenosis to study atherosclerotic human coronary arteries. They showed
that on average total arterial area increases from the proximal reference site to
the lesion site of the coronary artery. These findings are consistent with the
concept of compensatory coronary artery enlargement. Of note is that in their
study in 20% (5 of 25 coronary arteries with stenotic lesions), the total arterial
area of the vessels was actually smaller at the lesion site than at the proximal
reference site. Thus, their finding is consistent with our results.

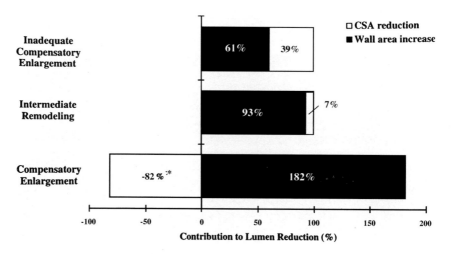

Figure 2   Bar graph shows the contribution of CSA reduction and the vessel wall area
increase to the lumen area reduction at the lesion site compared to the average lumen
areas at both reference sites. In the group with inadequate compensatory enlargement
and the group with intermediate remodeling, the CSA reduction contributed to 39% and
7% of the lumen area reduction at the lesion site, whereas the vessel wall area increase
also caused 61% and 93% of the lumen area reduction, respectively. In contrast in the
compensatory enlargement group, the vessel wall area increase (182%) markedly exceeded the lumen area reduction and was associated with a mean increase in the CSA of
82%. (Negative value of the CSA reduction represents increase in the CSA. CSA
indicates the vessel cross-sectional area.) From Ref. 27, with the permission of the
authors.

The comparison of apparently normal reference sites with the stenosis of interest is common practice in coronary angiography. Interventional decisions are based on this information. As illustrated in Figure 2, the assessment of CSA, vessel wall area, and the lumen area at the most stenotic site and reference sites provides new information which calls for a reevaluation of our concepts about coronary artery stenosis. These data indicate that inadequate compensatory enlargement (relative vessel constriction) at the lesion site should be added as a potentially important contributing factor along with plaque proliferation in approximately one-fourth of the stenotic lesions in native human coronary arteries. The awareness of the fact that the most stenotic site does not necessarily correspond to the most atherosclerotic portion of an artery may have implications for the choice of optimal treatment of each significant stenosis. These findings may also have relevance for the natural history of the coronary lesion as well as the acute and long term outcome of catheter-based coronary interventions including the restenosis process.

III. ARTERY WALL REMODELING AFTER PTCA

Clinical interventions, focused on inhibiting smooth-muscle cell proliferation to prevent restenosis, have not to date reduced the frequency of restenosis (28,29). These data suggest that the therapies designed to reduce intimal hyperplasia are ineffective or that there are additional mechanisms responsible for restenosis in humans (29,30). There are experimental data in rabbits supporting the concept of remodeling after PTCA. Lumen narrowing after balloon injury predominantly resulting from a reduction in the circumferential dimension of the entire artery has been reported, with intimal hyperplasia only a minor contributor (21). In a hypercholesterolemic rabbit model Kakuta and co-workers showed that differences in compensatory enlargement, not intimal hyperplasia, account for restenosis (22). Furthermore, Lafont and co-workers found that late residual stenosis correlated with chronic constriction ($P = .003$) but not with neointimal-medial growth or adventitial growth. Their findings suggest that factors related to arterial remodeling rather than neointimal-medial growth dominate the response to angioplasty (23).

Plaque burden and vessel size of de novo and restenosis lesions were compared by Mintz and co-workers (25) in a pooled study that included plaque debulking procedures (i.e., directional coronary atherectomy, rotational atherectomy, and excimer laser angioplasty) with and without balloon angioplasty. Since they found no large amount of myointimal tissue in the restenotic lesions they concluded that elastic recoil and change in vessel geometry may play a proportionately greater role than intimal hyperplasia in restenosis. However, the mechanisms responsible for restenosis after balloon-induced stretch and atheroma debulking may differ. This is indicated by a study comparing serial IVUS findings after directional coronary atherectomy (DCA) with those after balloon angioplasty alone (26). IVUS images were obtained during the initial intervention and at 6 months follow-up whether or not restenosis was present. In the DCA-treated lesions plaque growth predominated, whereas in the postballoon angioplasty group, remodeling accounted for most of the restenosis. However, this study was not specifically designed to evaluate clinical restenosis. Hence, the clinical restenosis rate was not reported and the average percent of diameter stenosis at follow-up was only 45% ± 11%.

Using the reference segment approach we compared CSA at the stenosis and proximal and distal reference sites in 17 restenotic PTCA treated coronary arteries (31). In addition, 14 PTCA-treated but not angiographically restenotic arterial segments served as controls. All 17 restenotic artery segments had a smaller CSA at the restenosis site as compared to the distal and proximal reference sites (Fig. 3). However, in 14 control sites without angiographic restenosis, the CSAs were similar compared to the adjacent reference sites. A representative IVUS case example is shown in Figure 4.

Our findings indicate that loss of cross-sectional area within the external elastic lamina is a major contributor to lumen loss in clinical restenosis, independent of the contribution of intimal hyperplasia. IVUS does not provide information about the cause of relative arterial narrowing. Possible mechanisms include fibrotic constriction, as demonstrated in animal data (9–11,32), and/or loss of medial mass secondary to injury-induced smooth muscle cell drop-out in the media. An equally likely cause in 20% to 25% of patients is preexisting reduction of total arterial cross-sectional area prior to angioplasty (5,27). The relative contribution of these potential factors may be clarified in the near future by an analysis of pre- and postprocedural and follow-up dimensions in the stenotic and appropriate reference segments.

IV. ATHEROSCLEROTIC REMODELING IN SAPHENOUS VEIN BYPASS GRAFTS

Saphenous vein bypass grafting is still the major approach to revascularize multivessel coronary artery disease. However, no previous data exist as to whether compensatory enlargement or vessel constriction occurs in stenotic saphenous vein bypass grafts (SVBG). A number of morphological changes in these transposed veins have the potential to influence vessel wall remodeling in response to atherosclerosis. Intimal thickening appears 1 month after implantation, increases with time, and includes intimal fibrotic proliferative lesions (33–36). The effects of vessel wall ischemia caused by the loss of vasa vasorum and denervation of the saphenous bypass vein grafts on properties of the vessel wall is unclear (37,38). In addition to fibromuscular intimal hyper-

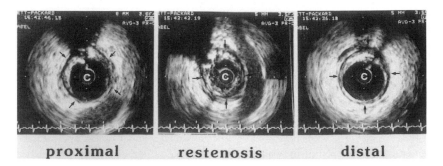

proximal   restenosis   distal

Figure 3 Total cross-sectional area at the lesion site and the proximal and distal reference sites in a coronary artery showing restenosis. Note the total CSA at the restenosis site is smaller than the proximal and distal reference site. Adapted from Ref. 31, with permission from the authors.

plasia, it has been reported that medial smooth-muscle cells are replaced, completely or in part, by fibrous tissue and collagen, and that there is a marked increase in the adventitia in fibrous tissue, with severe disruption or complete replacement of elastic fibers (37).

We addressed this issue for the first time in an IVUS study comprising 48 SVBGs from 47 consecutive patients who had not undergone previous catheter intervention, 8 to 23 (mean 12) years after coronary saphenous vein bypass

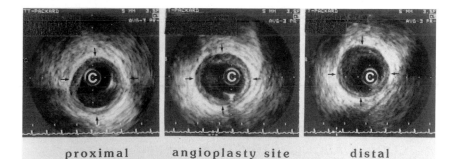

proximal   angioplasty site   distal

Figure 4 An example of a case with ultrasound assessment of coronary arteries without restenosis 6 months after PTCA, comparing the lumen area, vessel wall area, and total cross-sectional area (CSA) within the external elastic lamina at the proximal reference site, the restenotic site, and the distal site. Note that the total CSA is similar at the prior angioplasty site to the proximal and distal reference site. Adapted from Ref. 31, with permission from the authors.

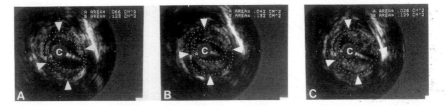

Figure 5 IVUS images on 11-year-old saphenous vein bypass graft to the right coronary artery. The white dotted lines show the lumen-intimal borders, and the white dotted lines accompanied by white arrowheads indicate the external elastic lamina. (A) At the reference site of the saphenous vein bypass graft, the lumen area was 6.6 mm² and the external EEL area was 12.3 mm². (B) At the intermediate site, the lumen area was 4.2 mm² and the EEL area was 13.2 mm². (C) At the lesion site, the lumen area was 2.8 mm² and the EEL area was 12.9 mm². In spite of the progression of disease severity from panel A to C, the EEL areas were similar and no compensatory enlargement or constriction of the saphenous vein bypass graft was observed. EEL; external elastic lamina. Adapted from Ref. 39, with permission from the authors.

grafting (39). At the time of coronary artery bypass grafting, it is the standard for our cardiac surgeons to remove the venous valves from the saphenous veins prior to their implantation as bypass grafts. Adequate intravascular ultrasound measurements were obtained from images from 43 SVBGs from 42 patients who were in this study. Lumen area, vessel wall area, and total cross-sectional area of the saphenous vein bypass graft were compared at the lesion site, the reference site, and an intermediate site. We used the total vessel cross-sectional area or the area within the external elastic lamina as an index of vessel remodeling. There was no focal compensatory enlargement or vessel constriction in the stenotic segments compared to the reference segments with the least amount of narrowing or the segments with intermediate disease (Figs. 5,6). Hence, the absence of focal compensatory enlargement in stenotic SVBGs appears to be a potentially important contributing factor associated with the progression of stenoses in coronary saphenous vein bypass grafts.

V. LOCAL VASOCONSTRICTION

Vasospasm is reported in up to 3% of IVUS studies (40,41). Such artifactual local vasoconstriction induced by the imaging procedure may influence the interpretation of the relative cross-sectional areas. Therefore, in order to obtain maximum vasodilation, 100 to 200 μg of nitroglycerin was administered directly into the coronary artery before or during the IVUS catheter imaging in

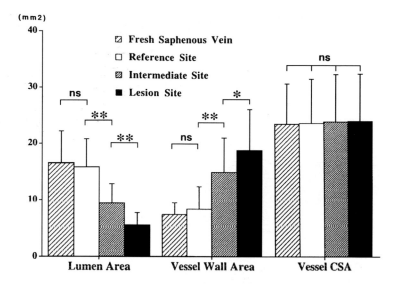

Figure 6 This bar graph demonstrates the lumen area, vessel wall area, and vessel cross-sectional area in fresh saphenous veins and saphenous vein bypass grafts at the reference site, intermediate site, and lesion site. Intravascular ultrasound measurements at the reference sites of the saphenous vein bypass grafts were similar to those of the fresh saphenous veins. In saphenous vein bypass grafts, lumen area gradually decreased and vessel wall area increased as the lumen area became smaller. The saphenous vein bypass graft cross-sectional areas were not different at the lesion site, intermediate and reference sites. CSA; cross sectional area; ns; nonsignificant; $*P < .01$, $**P < .001$. Adapted from Ref. 39, with permission from the authors.

our cited studies (27,31,39). Considering the documented vasodilatory effect of nitroglycerin, in normal and in atherosclerotic vessels (14,15), artifactual localized vasoconstriction is unlikely to have had a major impact on our conclusions. In fact, intracoronary nitroglycerin did not affect the angiographic appearance of any of the 17 restenotic segments in our study (31).

One could question whether the observed absence of total cross-sectional variation in saphenous vein grafts could be partially explained by inertness to vasoactive substances. Absence of focal compensatory enlargement seems to indicate that the atherosclerotic SVBG may be viewed as a hyperplastic passive conduit. Therefore, we addressed this issue in a separate study comparing the vasodilatory response to intracoronary nitroglycerin in moderately atherosclerotic native coronaries and equally atherosclerotic SVBGs. There was an

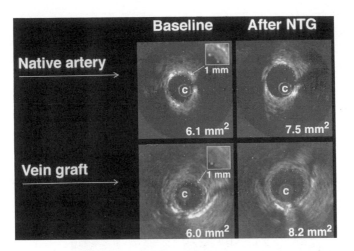

Figure 7 Vessel lumen area tracings before and after nitroglycerin. The intravascular ultrasound images show a native coronary artery in the upper panel and a saphenous vein graft in the lower panel. Baseline IVUS images and after maximum dilatation after intracoronary administration of 200 µg of nitroglycerin are shown. In the baseline images in the right upper corner an enlargement of a portion of the vessel wall (arrow) is shown. The dots define the lumen-intimal border. NTG, nitroglycerin; c, imaging catheter. From Berglund et al. (Ref. 42), with permission from the authors.

almost identical maximum increase in lumen area with nitroglycerin administration of approximately 20% in both vessel groups (42). Saphenous vein bypass grafts were 10 ± 5 years old in this study. Representative vasodilatory responses to nitroglycerin are illustrated in Figure 7. These results indicate that although compensatory enlargement in response to plaque formation does not seem to be a common phenomenon in SVBGs, we should not view these transpositioned vessels as passive conduits.

VI. LOCALIZED ATHEROSCLEROTIC ARTERY REMODELING IN THE ARTERY WALL

Atherosclerotic plaque usually appears as eccentric formations on postmortem cross sections of arteries (43,44). This irregular formation of atherosclerotic plaque can be considered a successful maintenance of a concentric lumen that requires a localized expansion of the affected portion of the artery wall. Such regional remodeling of the artery is detectable in vivo by IVUS. We therefore used IVUS to study the shape of the vessel lumen and the artery itself associated with different atherosclerotic formations in 88 atherosclerotic native coronary artery segments (45). Normal variation of lumen shape and external elastic lamina considered to represent the shape of the artery were calculated from 16 artery segments without IVUS signs of atherosclerosis. Plaque was classified as eccentric or concentric, and lumen and arterial shape as round or ovoid.

There was a strong correlation between artery wall area (an IVUS substitute for degree of atherosclerosis) and the external elastic lamina area, representing the cross sectional area of the artery itself ($r = .82$; $P < .001$; n = 104). Similar observations in previous studies have been interpreted as an indication of compensatory vessel enlargement as a response to growing plaque in arteries (3,5,6,46). The IVUS-based three-level classification system identified three patterns which accounted for 89% of all atherosclerotic artery segments (Fig. 8). These patterns were: concentric plaque with a round lumen and a round

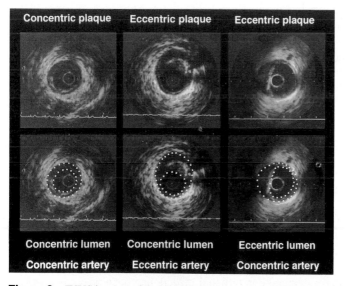

Figure 8 IVUS images of three representative artery segments in duplicate from three patients. These cases demonstrate the lumen and artery shapes most commonly found with concentric and eccentric plaque formation. The shapes of the cross-sectional areas are described as concentric or eccentric. Of the eight possible combinations of plaque, lumen, and vessel shapes, the three presented patterns accounted for 88% of the segments we have studied. Dotted lines highlight the lumen intimal border and EEL in the lower panel lines. From Ref. 45.

external elastic lamina (19%); eccentric plaque with a round lumen and an ovoid expanded external elastic lamina (40%); and eccentric plaque with an ovoid lumen and a round external elastic lamina (30%). A round lumen was preserved in 66% of all atherosclerotic artery segments. Regional remodeling was not confined to a specific coronary vessel, specific localization in the artery, or specific spatial relation to the maximum stenosis. The same individual may express compensatory remodeling and lack of this mechanism in different portions of the same coronary artery, as indicated by the 38% of patients who expressed more than one pattern of plaque-lumen-artery wall interaction in the same coronary artery. Artery segments with a round lumen in the presence of an eccentric plaque had a significantly larger lumen area than the other two main groups, indicating that regional expansion of the affected portion of the artery may help preserve lumen area. Hence, by applying geometric definitions of plaque formation in the lumen, the lumen shape, the arterial wall, and arterial circumference on our IVUS generated data, we identified a highly precise response of regional remodeling in coronary arteries which results in a virtually circular lumen in a majority of cases. Failure of this mechanism to be operant (ovoid lumens) in a certain proportion of arterial segments with eccentric plaque was associated with a smaller lumen area and a more pronounced percent lumen area stenosis as compared to coronary arteries with eccentric plaques and round lumens. Such artery segments may be prone to develop stenotic lesions.

VII. DIFFERENTIAL PATTERNS OF ATHEROSCLEROTIC REMODELING

Atherosclerotic remodeling is likely to be affected by factors such as vessel type and damage to the vessel during interventional proceedings. Localized determinants for regional adaptation in an atherosclerotic artery, such as responses to localized alterations in wall stress or degradation of underlying media and adventitia, rather than systemic factors (47) are compatible with multiple patterns of regional remodeling within the same artery (45). Although the exact mechanisms for compensatory dilatation remain unknown, a prominent role for locally mediated endothelial effects has been advocated (48).

IVUS does not provide direct information about the underlying mechanisms responsible for differential patterns of atherosclerotic remodeling. Nevertheless, the cited studies provide qualitatively new information on the interaction between plaque formation and compensatory mechanisms in the vessel wall determining the degree of lumen stenosis. Data from these studies exploring the unique features of IVUS indicate that vessel wall remodeling ranges from: compensatory enlargement at the stenosis site in native coronary arteries; to minimal remodeling in some atherosclerotic coronary arteries, stenotic saphenous vein grafts and non-restenotic post-PTCA native coronary arteries; to relative shrinkage of the external elastic lamina in PTCA treated restenotic lesions in native coronary arteries and in a proportion of primary stenoses in native coronary arteries.

The impact of differential patterns of artery remodeling with intracoronary interventions and the identification of mechanisms controlling regional vessel remodeling could lead to methods to predict restenosis rates as well as to allow prognostication for the progression of coronary artery stenoses.

REFERENCES

1. Bond MG, Adams MR, Bullock BC. Complicating factors in evaluating coronary artery atherosclerosis. Artery 1981; 9:21–29.
2. Armstrong ML, Heistad DD, Marcus ML, Megan MB, Piegors DJ. Structural and hemodynamic responses of peripheral arteries of macaque monkeys to atherogenic diet. Arteriosclerosis 1985; 5:336–346.
3. Glagov S, Weisenberg E, Zarins CK, Stankunavicius R, Kolettis GJ. Compensatory enlargement of human atherosclerotic coronary arteries. N Engl J Med 1987; 316:1371–1375.
4. Clarkson TB, Prichard RW, Morgan TM, Petrick GS, Klein KP. Remodeling of coronary arteries in human and nonhuman primates. JAMA 1994; 271:289–294.
5. McPherson DD, Sirna SJ, Hiratzka LF, et al. Coronary arterial remodeling studied by high-frequency epicardial echocardiography: an early compensatory mechanism in patients with obstructive coronary atherosclerosis. J Am Coll Cardiol 1991; 17:79–86.
6. Gerber TC, Erbel R, Görge G, Ge J, Rupprecht H-J, Meyer J. Extent of atherosclerosis and remodeling of the left main coronary artery determined by intravascular ultrasound. Am J Cardiol 1994; 73:666–671.
7. Hermiller JB, Tenaglia AN, Kisslo KB, et al. In vivo validation of compensatory enlargement of atherosclerotic coronary arteries. Am J Cardiol 1993; 71:665–668.
8. Steinke W, Els T, Hennerici M. Compensatory carotid artery dilatation in early atherosclerosis. Circulation 1994; 89:2578–2581.
9. Losordo DW, Rosenfield K, Kaufman J, Pieczek A, Isner JM. Focal compensatory enlargement of human arteries in response to progressive atherosclerosis—in vivo documentation using intravascular ultrasound. Circulation 1994; 89:2570–2577.
10. Nissen SE, Grines CL, Gurley JC, et al. Intravascular ultrasound assessment of lumen size and wall morphology in normal subjects and patients with coronary artery disease. Circulation 1991; 84:1087–1099.

11. Tobis JM, Mallery J, Mahon D, et al. Intravascular ultrasound imaging of human coronary arteries: in vivo analyses of tissue characterizations with comparison to in vitro histological specimens. Circulation 1991; 83:913–926.

12. Yock PG, Johnson EL, Linker DT. Intravascular ultrasound: development and clinical potential. Am J Card Imag 1988; 2:185–193.

13. Nissen SE, Grines CL, Gurley JC, et al. Application of new phased array ultrasound imaging catheter in the assessment of vascular dimensions: in vivo comparison with cineangiography. Circulation. 1990; 81:660–666.

14. Brown BG, Bolson E, Petersen RB, Pierce CD, Dodge HT. The mechanisms of nitroglycerin action: stenosis vasodilation as a major component of the drug response. Circulation 1981; 64:1089–1097.

15. Ku DD, Caulfield JB, Kirklin JK. Endothelium-dependent response in long-term human coronary artery bypass grafts. Circulation 1991; 83:402–411.

16. Pasterkamp G, Wensing PJW, Post MJ, Hillen B, Mali WPTM, Borst C. Paradoxical arterial wall shrinkage may contribute to luminal narrowing of human atherosclerotic femoral arteries. Circulation 1995; 91:1444–1449.

17. Clowes AW, Clowes MM. Kinetics of cellular proliferation after arterial injury. II. inhibition of smooth muscle growth by heparin. Lab Invest 1985; 52:611–616.

18. Nobuyoshi M, Kimura T, Ohishi H, et al. Restenosis after percutaneous transluminal coronary angioplasty: pathologic observations in 20 patients. J Am Coll Cardiol 1991; 17:433–439.

19. Waller BF, Pinkerton CA, Orr CM, Slack JD, VanTassel JM, Peters T. Restenosis 1 to 24 months after clinically successful coronary balloon angioplasty: a necropsy study of 20 patients. J Am Coll Cardiol 1991; 17:58B–70B.

20. Garratt KN, Holmes DR Jr, Bell MR, et al. Restenosis after directional coronary atherectomy: differences between primary atheromatous and restenosis lesions and influence of subintimal tissue resection. J Am Coll Cardiol 1990; 16:1665–1671.

21. Post MJ, Borst C, Kuntz RE. The relative importance of arterial remodeling compared with intimal hyperplasia in lumen renarrowing after balloon angioplasty: a study in the normal rabbit and the hypercholesterolemic Yucatan micropig. Circulation 1994; 89:2816–2821.

22. Kakuta T, Currier JW, Haudenschild CC, Ryan TJ, Faxon DP. Differences in compensatory vessel enlargement, not intimal formation, account for restenosis after angioplasty in the hypercholesterolemic rabbit model. Circulation 1994; 89: 2809–2815.

23. Lafont A, Guzman LA, Whitlow RL, Goormastic M, Fredrick J, Chisolm GM. Restenosis after experimental angioplasty: intimal, medial, and adventitial changes associated with constriction remodeling. Circ Res 1995; 76:996–1002.

24. Kovach JA, Mintz GS, Kent KM, et al. Serial intravascular ultrasound studies indicate that chronic recoil is an important mechanism of restenosis following transcatheter therapy. J Am Coll Cardiol 1993; 21:484A. Abstract.

25. Mintz GS, Pichard AD, Kent KM, Satler LF, Popma JJ, Leon MB. Intravascular ultrasound comparison of restenotic and de novo coronary artery narrowings. Am J Cardiol 1994; 74:1278–1280.

26. Di Mario C, Gil R, Camenzind E, et al. Quantitative assessment with intracoronary ultrasound of the mechanisms of restenosis after percutaneous transluminal coronary angioplasty and directional coronary atherectomy. Am J Cardiol 1995; 75: 772–777.

27. Nishioka T, Luo H, Eigler NL, Berglund H, Kim C-J, Siegel RJ. Contribution of inadequate compensatory enlargement to the development of human coronary artery stenosis—an in vivo intravascular ultrasound study. J Am Coll Cardiol 1996; 27:1571–1576.

28. Franklin SM, Faxon DP. Pharmacologic prevention of restenosis after coronary angioplasty: review of the randomized clinical trials. Coronary Art Dis 1993; 4: 232–242.

29. Isner JF. Vascular remodeling: honey, I think I shrunk the artery. Circulation 1994; 89:2937–2940. Editorial.

30. Currier JW, Faxon DP. Restenosis after percutaneous transluminal coronary angioplasty: have we been aiming at the wrong target? J Am Coll Cardiol 1995; 25: 516–520. Editorial.

31. Luo H, Nishioka T, Eigler NL, Berglund H, Forrester JS, Siegel RJ. Coronary artery restenosis is associated with circumferential coronary constriction. Arteriosclerosis Thromb Vasc Biol 1996; 16:1393–1398.

32. Clowes AW, Reidy MA, Clowes MM. Mechanisms of stenosis after arterial injury. Lab Invest 1983; 49:208–215.

33. Vlodaver Z, Edwards JE. Pathological changes in aortic-coronary arterial saphenous vein grafts. Circulation 1971; 47:719–728.

34. Unni KK, Kottke BA, Titus JL, Frye RL, Wallace RB, Brown AL. Pathological changes in aortocoronary saphenous vein grafts. Am J Cardiol 1974; 34:526–532.

35. Lie JT, Lawrie GM, Morris GC. Aortocoronary bypass saphenous vein graft atherosclerosis: anatomic study of 99 vein grafts from normal and hyperlipoproteinemic patients up to 75 months postoperatively. Am J Cardiol 1977; 40:906–914.

36. Campeau L, Enjalbert M, Lespérance J, Vaislic C, Grondin CM, Bourassa MG. Atherosclerosis and late closure of aortocoronary saphenous vein grafts: sequential angiographic studies at 2 weeks, 1 year, 5 to 7 years and 10 to 12 years after surgery. Circulation 1983; 68(suppl II):II-1–II-7.

37. Spray TL, Roberts WC. Changes in saphenous veins used as aortocoronary bypass grafts. Am Heart J 1977; 94:500–516.

38. Angelini GD, Newby AC. The future of saphenous vein as a coronary artery bypass conduit. Eur Heart J 1989; 10:273–280.

39. Nishioka T, Luo H, Berglund H, et al. Absence of focal compensatory enlargement or constriction in diseased human coronary saphenous vein bypass grafts. An intravascular ultrasound study. Circulation 1996; 93:683–690.

40. Nishioka T, Luo H, Eigler NL, et al. The evolving utility of intracoronary ultrasound. Am J Cardiol 1995; 75:539–541.

41. Hausmann D, Erbel R, Alibelli-Chemarin M-J, et al. The safety of intracoronary ultrasound. A multicenter survey of 2207 examinations. Circulation 1995; 91: 623–630.

42. Berglund H, Luo H, Nishioka T, et al. Preserved vasodilatory response to nitroglycerin in saphenous bypass vein grafts. Circulation 1996; 94:2871–2876.
43. Young W, Gofman JW, Tandy R, Malamud N, Waters WSG. The quantitation of atherosclerosis. I. Relationship to artery size. Am J Cardiol 1960; 6:288–293.
44. Glagov S, Zarins CK. Quantitating atherosclerosis: problems of definition. In: Bond MG, Insull W Jr, Glakov S, Chandeler AB, Cornhill JF, eds. Clinical Diagnosis of Atherosclerosis: Quantitative Methods of Evaluation. New York: Springer Verlag 1983.
45. Berglund H, Luo H, Nishioka T, Fishbein MC, Eigler NL, Tabak SW, Siegel RJ. Highly localized arterial remodeling in patients with coronary atherosclerosis: An intravascular study. Circulation 1997. In press.
46. Thomas AC, Davies MJ. Post-mortem investigation and quantification of coronary artery disease. Histopathology 1985; 9:959–976.
47. Zarin CK, Weisenberg E, Kolettis G, Stankunavicus R, Glakov S. Differential enlargement of artery segments in response to enlarging atherosclerotic plaques. J Vasc Surg 1988; 7:386–394.
48. Gibbons GH, Dzau VJ. The emerging concept of vascular remodeling. N Engl J Med 1994; 330:1431–1438.

7

Coronary Imaging: Angiography, Angioscopy, and Ultrasound

Pim J. de Feyter, Clemens von Birgelen, and Patrick W. Serruys *Thorax Center, University Hospital Rotterdam-Dijkzigt, Erasmus University, Rotterdam, The Netherlands*

I. INTRODUCTION

Coronary atherosclerosis is a worldwide disease which is the major cause of mortality in Western countries. Much has been learned about the pathogenesis of coronary atherosclerosis in the past few years, and crucial in the progression of the later stages of coronary atherosclerosis appears to be repeated plaque rupture and thrombosis leading to the development of acute coronary syndromes and the increase in the severity of a coronary lesions (1,2). In clinical practice only the advanced coronary lesions, which are either clinically stable or complicated, are subject to investigation and percutaneous treatment. Nowadays three coronary imaging techniques—angiography, intracoronary angioscopy, and ultrasound—are available during coronary intervention to characterize the coronary wall, lumen, and plaque. All three imaging techniques have their inherent strengths and limitations, but most importantly, they appear to complement each other (Tables 1, 2).

In this chapter we discuss the contribution of each imaging modality to characterize a coronary plaque, so that a better delineation of a coronary lesion may facilitate percutaneous catheter-based treatment of symptomatic ischemia-related coronary lesions.

Table 1 Coronary Plaque Imaging: Potential of Different Imaging Techniques

	Angiography	Angioscopy	Ultrasound
Lumen			
Quantification	+ +	—	+ + +
Intraluminal			
Flaps/dissection	+	+ + +	+ +
Thrombus			
Red	+	+ + +	—
White	—	+	—
Endoluminal lining			
Smooth/complex	+	+ +	—
Color	—	+ + +	—
Plaque composition			
Calcific	+	—	+ + +
Fibrous (dense)	—	—	+
Lipid	—	yellow	+ ?
Plaque quantification			
Lumen encroachment	+ +	—	+ + +
Intramural	—	—	+ + +
Total vessel area			
Quantification	—	—	+ + +
Plaque topography			
Eccentric/concentric	+	+	+ + +

II. CORONARY IMAGING TECHNIQUES

A. Angiography

The introduction of diagnostic coronary arteriography by Sones in the late 1950s was the first major step enabling the study of coronary artery disease in patients. However, it was soon recognized that coronary angiography merely is a two-dimensional shadowgram (luminogram) of the opacified coronary arteries, so that coronary lesions can only be recognized by angiography if the subintimal thickening associated with coronary atherosclerosis encroaches upon the lumen. Thus, coronary angiography provides information of the extent and severity of coronary artery disease only in the later stages of the coronary atherosclerosis. The earlier stages remain angiographically unnoticed owing to the compensatory enlargement (remodeling) of the vessel, whereby the coronary lumen is preserved.

Table 2 Coronary Imaging: Limitations of Different Imaging Techniques

	Angiography	Angioscopy	Ultrasound
Feasiblity	+++	+	++
Safety	++	+	+
Applicability			
Segments	entire coronary tree	mid-straight	prox-mid
Structure	lumen	lumen/lining	lumen/wall
Severe lesion	+++	—	—
Coronary flow	+	—	—
Collaterals	++	—	—
Ischemia during imaging	—	++	+
			(wedge imaging)
Functional field	contrast-filled	flush-filled	blood-filled
Vasomotion	+	—	+
Cost	low	high	high

Even so, coronary angiography is a formidable tool which has dramatically improved our understanding and treatment of coronary atherosclerosis. On-line and off-line computer-assisted quantification algorithms have further refined the detection and analysis of the changes of the lumen caused by coronary atherosclerosis. Coronary angiography will, for the time being, remain the mainstay of coronary imaging because it is widely available, is easily applicable, and provides information about the entire coronary tree, including the collateral circulation.

B. Intracoronary Angioscopy

Initial experience with intracoronary angioscopy dates from the early 1980s (3,4). Angioscopy provides the unique opportunity to study the endoluminal coronary surface and the presence of intraluminal structures. The greatest potential of angioscopy is its ability to detect red thrombi and yellow-colored lesions, which makes this technique particularly suitable for in vivo studying of acute coronary syndromes (4–6). Its major drawback is the difficulty to quantify the angioscopic images.

C. Intracoronary Ultrasound

Intracoronary ultrasound was developed and applied in the late 1980s during coronary intervention. The technique has the unique advantage of assessing the

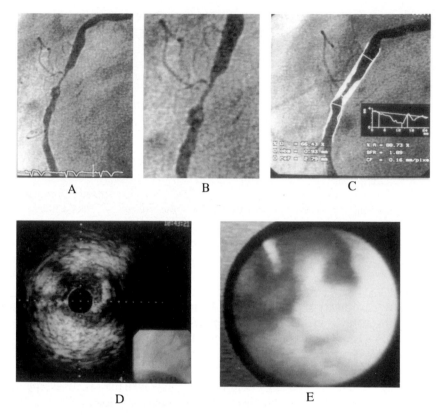

Figure 1 An example of the different image modalities "looking" at an unstable lesion. (A) Right coronary angiogram: long narrowing with post-stenotic "filling defect." (B) Blowup of A: irregular borders of stenosis and post-stenotic "filling defect." (C) Quantitative angiography: note that "poststenotic filling defect" is not detected by the contour algorithm. (D) Cross-sectional ultrasound image of lesion. Ultrasound catheter is wedged. Between 2 and 4 o'clock: calcific plaque. Between 4 and 8 o'clock: dense fibrous plaque. At 9 o'clock: guidewire artifact. At 11 o'clock: echolucent zone, possibly underlying lipid accumulation. (E) Angioscopy: irregular surface of plaque covered with red thrombus and protruding into the lumen. At 11 o'clock: guidewire in remaining lumen.

dimensions and composition of the coronary lesion and vessel wall, because it allows detection of structures beyond the endothelial lining (7). Ultrasound is also able to detect vessel wall abnormalities occurring in the earlier stages of coronary artery disease when the coronary lumen is still normal (8,9). Thus, more complete diagnostic information about the coronary plaque can be obtained by the combined use of (quantitative) coronary angiography, intracoronary angioscopy, and ultrasound (Fig. 1).

III. CHARACTERISTICS OF STABLE AND UNSTABLE PLAQUES BEFORE CORONARY INTERVENTION

We have examined 67 patients scheduled for percutaneous intracoronary intervention with both intracoronary angioscopy and ultrasound in addition to quantitative coronary angiography (10). Inadequate images were obtained in seven patients (angioscopy four patients; ultrasound three patients), and in one patient the procedure was aborted owing to insufferable ischemic pain during attempted angioscopy. These eight patients were excluded from the study. An angiographic complex lesion assumed to reflect an ulcerated thrombotic plaque was defined as a lesion that was either eccentric with irregular borders, or overhanging edges; or a lesion consisting of multiple irregularities or the presence of intraluminal defects.

Coronary angioscopy was performed with the Baxter-Edwards (Irvine, CA) monorail coronary angioscope. During angioscopic imaging the distal coronary was flushed with saline of 37°C injected with a flow of 30 to 40cc/min. Thrombi were defined as red, intraluminal masses adherent to the wall (Figs. 1E, 2). Thrombi were categorized as nonmobile-mural (closely adherent to the vessel wall), mobile-protruding into the lumen, or totally occlusive thrombi. Yellow plaques were defined as areas of homogeneous yellow color clearly identifiable from the normal white wall. Wall surface was classified as ulcerated when major disruption with lack of continuity was found. A lesion was classified as angioscopic complex if an ulcerated, thrombotic lesion was present. Ultrasound coronary imaging was performed with a 4.3 F, 30-MHz ultrasound catheter of CVIS (Cardiovascular Imaging Systems Inc., Sunnyvale, CA).

The composition of the ischemia-related lesion was classified as calcified, hard, or soft and as homogeneous or mixed (Fig. 2). A *calcific plaque* was defined as a plaque with highly echoreflective intimal thickening with acoustic shadowing. A *hard plaque* was defined as a plaque with a highly echoreflective intimal thickening without shadowing, representing dense fibrous tissue. A *soft plaque* was defined as a plaque with a poorly echoreflective intimal thickening

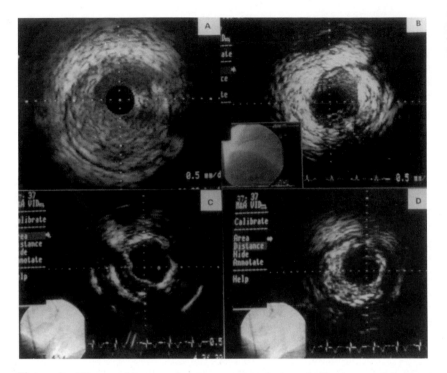

Figure 2 Ultrasound images of various coronary lesions. Left upper panel: homogenous soft plaque. Right upper panel: homogenous hard plaque. Left lower panel: calcific plaque. Right lower panel: mixed plaque—soft, fibrous, and calcific (2 to 5 o'clock).

representing soft structures such as loose fibrous tissue, lipid, and thrombus. A lesion was considered homogeneous if the plaque consisted of > 75% of one type of echoreflectivity, determined from an integrated pullback image of the entire lesion. A lesion was considered predominantly calcified if calcium occupied > 180° of the vessel circumference. A lesion was defined as mixed if it contained both highly and poorly echoreflective areas occupying > 25% of the plaque surface or if calcium deposits occupying > 30° and < 180° of the vessel circumference were present.

Quantitative measurements included measurement of lumen, total vessel area, and plaque area (Fig. 3). Total vessel area was defined as the area central to the ultrasound-defined media-adventitia boundary (EEL). Lumen area was defined as the area central to lumen-intimal boundary (IEL). Plaque area

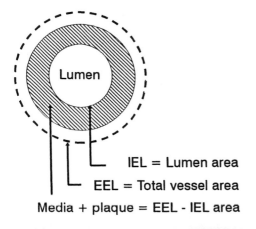

IEL = Lumen area
EEL = Total vessel area
Media + plaque = EEL - IEL area

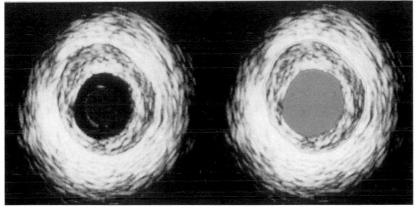

Figure 3 Schematic of ultrasound cross-sectional image of coronary plaque (top). IEL = lumen-intimal boundary; EEL = external elastic lamina. Quantitative measurements of cross-sectional ultrasound image (bottom). Total vessel area: 15.9 mm^2; lumen area: 6.2 mm^2; plaque-media area: 9.7 mm^2; area stenosis: 61%; diameter stenosis: 38%.

area was calculated as the difference between total vessel area and lumen area (EEL − IEL).

The angioscopic and ultrasound-obtained characteristics of the ischemia-related lesions are depicted in Tables 3 and 4. Angioscopy demonstrated that unstable angina patients exhibit a red thrombus in roughly two-thirds of patients, but remarkably a red thrombus is also seen in 17% of patients with

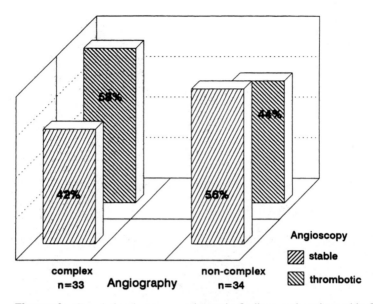

Figure 4   Correlation between angioscopic findings and angiographic findings.

Table 3   Angioscopic Characteristics of Ischemia-Related
Lesions

	Unstable angina (N = 44)	Stable angina (N = 23)	P value
Thrombus (N)	30 (68)	4 (17)	P < .001
Occlusive	2	0	
Protruding	8	1	
Mural	20	3	
Surface lesion (N)			
Ulcerated	20	3	P < .05
Rough	11	6	
Smooth	13	14	
Yellow plaque (N)	29 (66)	16 (69)	

Table 4 Intracoronary Ultrasound Characteristics of Ischemia-
Related Lesions

	Unstable angina (N = 44)	Stable angina (N = 23)
Echoreflectivity of plaque		
Homogeneous type[a] (N)	24 (55)	15 (65)
Poor	22	14
High without shadowing	1	0
High with shadowing	1	1
Mixed type (N)	20 (45)	8 (35)
Poor/high without shadowing	2	2
Poor/high with shadowing	18	6
Calcium present[b] (N)	20 (46)	7 (31)
Focal (30°–90°)	5	1
Moderate (90°–180°)	14	5
Diffuse (>180°)	1	1
Eccentric plaque (index < 0.5)	27 (61)	13 (56)
Extent plaque (mm²)	15.2 ± 5	17.0 ± 5

[a]Homogenous if the plaque induces >75% of one type of echoreflectivity.
[b]Distribution of calcium was classified according to number of degrees of vessel circumference.

stable angina. These findings are in keeping with the concept that plaque rupture and thrombosis is a continuous process occurring in different clinical situations varying from the asymptomatic state to acute myocardial infarction. We confirmed other studies (4–6) showing that angiography grossly underestimates the presence of an ulcerated thrombotic plaque if one accepts the angioscopic presence of a thrombotic ulcerated plaque as the "gold standard." The positive and negative predictive accuracy figures of angiography are 66% and 67% respectively (Figs. 4, 5). A yellow-lipid plaque was present in roughly two-thirds of both stable and unstable patients. Intracoronary ultrasound showed that the plaques were entirely soft in approximately half of the patients and were of mixed composition in the other half. Ultrasound imaging is highly sensitive to detect the presence of calcium, varying from small spots to heavily calcific lesions. In our study, we demonstrated that ultrasound images could not discriminate between a stable and unstable plaque. However, Hodgson et al. (11), using a different ultrasound catheter, were able to distinguish, although rather crudely, between a stable and an unstable plaque.

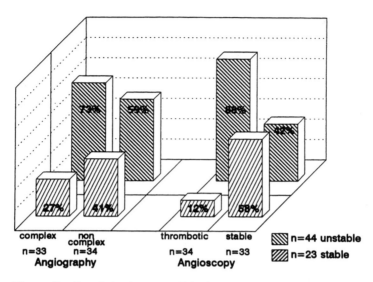

Figure 5 Correlation between clinical symptoms, angiographic findings, and angio-scopic findings.

IV. FACILITATION OF PERCUTANEOUS INTERVENTIONS

A more precise delineation of the ischemia-related lesion that can be achieved by the combined use of angiography, angioscopy, and ultrasound may provide more accurate information for device selection or use of adjunctive pharmacologic treatment (12).

A. Before Intervention

The presence and extent of coronary calcification are associated with an increased risk of dissection after balloon angioplasty, typically occurring adjacent to the calcific depositions (13). Severe calcification of the coronary plaques hampers cutting and removal of plaque during directional coronary atherectomy, particularly if the calcium is located near the luminal surface (14,15). Although angiography has a poor sensitivity to detect calcium (16) when compared to intracoronary ultrasound, it does provide useful information because it identifies patients who may or may not require intravascular ultrasound imaging before intervention. A recent study has shown that the presence of angiographically determined calcium often underlies the presence of a large calcific arch seen with ultrasound (17). Ultrasound investigation clearly identifies superficially located calcium, which is probably a contraindication for DCA, from deeply located calcium, which may not preclude the use of DCA. The use of rotational atherectomy has been recommended for treatment of severe calcific lesions, in particular in cases with superficial calcium (18,19). The absence of angiographic calcification is associated with a low likelihood of > 90° arch of superficial calcium, and routine intracoronary ultrasound examination before intervention therefore does not seem warranted (17).

An ultrasound soft plaque (associated with a high likelihood of containing lipid) may be more prone to dissection of the fibrous cap during coronary intervention. This may lead to expulsion of lipid, cholesterol clefts, or necrotic material into the distal coronary bed with the development of an acute myocardial infarction or the exposure of super-thrombogenic subintimal layers containing tissue factor to streaming blood, which may more often lead to an abrupt thrombotic occlusion. Angiography is deceptive to determine whether a lesion is truly concentric or eccentric (20). Knowledge of the true topography of a lesion may help the interventionist to select a specific device. A soft concentric lesion or an eccentric lesion with an arc of disease free wall, easily assessed with ultrasound (21) are expected to "expand" more easily and may be at greater risk of early recoil, which may require stenting (15). Focal eccentric soft lesions in large vessels may require directional coronary atherectomy. A dissection and even perforation may occur more often if one selects a concentric excimer laser catheter for treatment of an eccentric lesion that may have been prevented with the use of an eccentric laser catheter (22).

The presence of an intracoronary thrombus is associated with a high risk of acute major complications during coronary intervention due to the relatively high frequency of thrombotic abrupt occlusion (23). Intracoronary ultrasound, like angiography, in general, cannot reliably detect intracoronary thrombi. An intraluminal thrombus causes granular or finely speckled intense echoreflections that scintillate during real-time imaging while the structure appears mobile with blood flow and mural thrombus may cause a linear echogenic density along the wall of the plaque which is less dense or compact than fibrous tissue (24,25).

Angioscopy is particularly sensitive to detect intracoronary thrombi (26). Intraluminal red thrombi are often present in acute ischemic coronary syndromes, in particular in the setting of early postinfarction angina or acute myocardial infarction (4–6,10). It appears that the thrombotic burden shows a gradient from stable angina to early post-MI angina (Table 5). One can easily detect red thrombi with angioscopy, but we were unable to confirm the findings of Japanese investigators who also reported about the presence of pure white thrombi or mixed red-white thrombi (27). In our opinion it is extremely

Table 5 Angioscopic Findings in Stable, Unstable, and Early Postinfarction Patients

	Stable angina (N = 22)	Unstable angina (N = 35)	Early post-MI (N = 17)	P value
Ulcerated surface (%)	14	46	53	<.05
Red thrombus (%)	18	69	82	<.05
Thrombotic score[a]	0.6 ± 1.5	3.3 ± 3.5	4.8 ± 4.8	<.001

[a]Thrombotic score was derived from single mural, multiple mural, protruding, and occlusive thrombus; this was multiplied by the number of thrombotic sites (proximal, mid, and distal part of the lesion).

difficult to distinguish between white intimal flaps or white thrombi. However, the Japanese investigators may have used angioscopes with a higher image quality enabling them to more accurately recognize the "cotton wool" appearance of white thrombi. The distinction between white platelet thrombi, old-organized, grayish thrombi, or fresh, red fibrin thrombi may have consequences for treatment. Fresh red thrombi may require treatment with thrombolytics, whereas old-organized thrombi may be unresponsive to anticoagulant or thrombolytic treatment and pure white thrombi may be treated with new direct antithrombins or platelet glycoprotein IIb/IIIa receptor blockers (28,29). More studies are needed to confirm these speculations.

B. During and Postintervention

Directional coronary atherectomy or rotational atherectomy may be guided by ultrasound imaging to obtain optimal immediate results (30,31). Exact "directioning" of the cutter in relation to the not simultaneously obtained ultrasound images is very difficult. This problem partially has been solved by the use of the combined ultrasound-DCA device (32). An angiographically smooth, widely patent lumen is often seen after directional atherectomy. However, angioscopy often reveals dissections and bruised semicircular troughs in the vessel (Fig. 6) wall whereas incomplete removal of the plaque (unnoticed by angiography) can be observed with intracoronary ultrasound (Fig. 7) (33).

Intracoronary ultrasound imaging does play an important role in the optimal placement and deployment of a stent (34–37). Appropriate stent apposition to the vessel wall and appropriate full expansion of the stent can accurately be monitored by ultrasound whereas (quantitative) coronary angiography may be deceptive. This may prevent (sub)acute occlusion and may decrease the occurrence of restenosis. In particular three-dimensional ultrasound reconstruction,

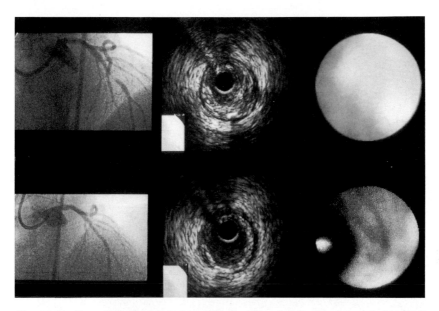

Figure 6 Example of lesion before and after directional atherectomy. Left, middle, right upper panels: angiogram, ultrasound, and angioscopy before DCA. Lower panels: after DCA.

obtained with mechanical pullback device, appears extremely useful to guide optimal intracoronary stenting (38–40) (Fig. 8). On-line techniques are currently available to help the interventionist to immediately judge the positioning and suboptimal expansion of the stent during the procedure. Ultrasound may also be helpful to investigate the proximal and distal stent artery transition zone where small dissections may occur that are often not noticed by angiography and that may require additional stenting. Coronary stenting under angioscopic guidance has been performed and in a few instances has led to a change in clinical management, in particular after visualization of thrombi in the stent (41,42). Angioscopy is able to follow the process of neointimal coverage after stent implantation, so that the duration of intense anticoagulation and antiplatelet therapy can be monitored and thus unnecessary bleeding complication may be avoided (43).

The combined use of the three techniques appears useful for comprehensive diagnosis of suboptimal post-interventional results or abrupt coronary occlusion (Table 6). Angiography clearly underestimates the presence of dissections

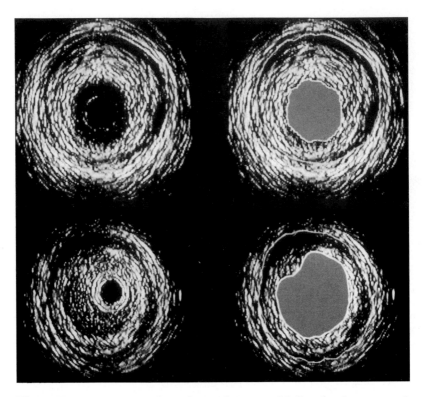

Figure 7　Pre- (upper panels) and post- (lower panels) directional coronary atherectomy. Although much plaque has been removed, a considerable rim of plaque remains. Measurements before DCA: Lumen area: 4.5 mm^2; total vessel area: 24.2 mm^2; plaque-media area: 19.7 mm^2. After DCA: Lumen area: 8.7 mm^2; total vessel area: 23.9 mm^2; plaque-media area: 15.2 mm^2.

(44,45). Ultrasound offers a better appreciation of the presence and the depth of a dissection into the media or adventitia, and angioscopy is highly suitable to detect superficial intimal tears (46,47) or new thrombus (Fig. 9). Angioscopic evaluation after various coronary interventions often shows, while the angiogram is normal, that the procedures produced intimal flaps, dissections, and intrawall bleeding. Ultrasound has confirmed previous in vitro observations that the site of a dissection often occurs at the edge between plaque and normal wall (44,48). In the future quantitative information on the composition of the plaque may be used to reconstruct computerized models of the vessel wall,

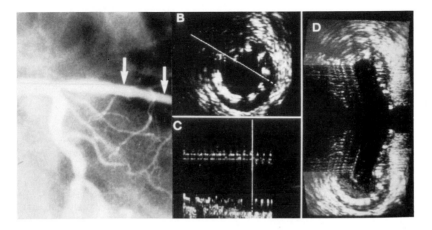

Figure 8 Post stent implantation. Left panel: angiogram shows minor irregularities of the borders at stent implantation site (arrows). Panel B: Cross-sectional ultrasound image: malapposition of stent. Panel C: Longitudinally reconstructed 3D ultrasound image demonstrating "length" of stent malapposition. Panel D: Clam shell view which provides an excellent appreciation of total area of stent malapposition.

Table 6 Postinterventional Findings: Relative Merits of the Different Imaging Techniques

	Angiography	Angioscopy	Ultrasound
Intraluminal			
Smooth/hazy	+	—	—
Thrombus	+	+++	+
Flaps/dissection	+	+++	+
Stent	+	++	+++
Endoluminal lining			
Disruption	+	++	+
Discoloration	—	+	—
bleeding	—	+	—
Lesion wall			
Dissection	+	+	+++
Lumen enlargement	+++	+	+++
"Run-off"	+++	—	—

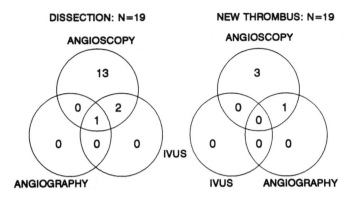

Figure 9 Complementary information obtained with angiography, angioscopy, and ultrasound in 19 patients undergoing pre- and postintervention imaging.

enabling the measurement of local wall stress in order to predict risk and site of dissection (49).

The postintervention angioscopic determined presence of a mural red thrombus may warrant prolonged heparin treatment (46,47). The mechanisms underlying abrupt coronary occlusion are often elusive using angiography. An abrupt occlusion due to a red occlusive thrombus easily recognized with angioscopy requires thrombolytic treatment whereas an occlusive intimal-medial dissection clearly assessable with angioscopy and ultrasound should be treated with bailout stent implantation (50).

V. MECHANISMS OF VARIOUS CORONARY INTERVENTIONS

Combined imaging should allow a more complete description of the mechanisms that are associated with the lumen enlargement caused by various devices (Table 7). Using all three techniques it has become clear that balloon angioplasty is often associated with both the occurrence of tears and dissections involving the media and expansion of the total vessel area (wall stretching). Directional coronary atherectomy is mainly caused by removal of plaque, but roughly one-third of the lumen enlargement is explained by total vessel expansion (33,51). Stent implantation is invariably associated with total vessel expansion. However, although initially suggested that for instance DCA, rotational atherectomy, stenting, or laser would produce of a smooth vessel wall,

Table 7 Mechanisms of Coronary Interventions

	QCA	IVUS	Angioscopy
Plaque removal	—	+ +	+
Vessel wall stretching	—	+ +	—
Dissection			
Intraluminal	+	+	+ + +
Intramural	+	+ + +	+
Normal vessel wall involvement	—	+ + +	+
Plaque distribution	—	3D	—
Plaque compression	—	+ +	—
Lumen enlargement	+ + +	+ + +	+

angioscopy has clearly revealed that there is often angiographically unnoticed vessel wall damage including intimal flaps, tears, wall bleeding, and cutting troughs (33,52,53). Whether axial plaque volume redistribution takes place can only be assessed with volumetric 3D ultrasound imaging (54,55); however, so far this has not been reported yet.

VI. SUMMARY

Intuitively it seems obvious that a more comprehensive knowledge of the pathophysiological substrate of a plaque selected for a percutaneous intervention should increase the quality of treatment. The combined information of angiography, intracoronary angioscopy, and ultrasound may allow for the selection of a specific intervention technique for a specific lesion; it may provide useful guidance during intervention; and it may suggest specific adjunctive pharmacological treatment. The data available to support this concept are preliminary, sometimes even speculative, and at this point in time one cannot draw firm conclusions about the clinical usefulness of combined imaging in stratifying patients into different therapeutic strategies. It should be appreciated that intracoronary angioscopy and ultrasound carry an albeit small, finite risk, are time-consuming and demanding for the patient, and are expensive. The clinical value of combined imaging during percutaneous interventions should be evaluated in large studies to determine if the expected benefit outweighs the additional cost before widespread use of this approach can be advocated.

REFERENCES

1. Fuster V, Badimon L, Badimon JJ, Chesebro JH. The pathogenesis of coronary artery disease and the acute coronary syndromes. N Engl J Med 1992; 326:242–250, 310–318.

2. Ross R. The pathogenesis of atherosclerosis: a perspective for the 1990's. Nature 1993; 362:801–809.

3. Spears JR, Marais J, Serur J, et al. In vivo coronary angioscopy. J Am Coll Cardiol 1983; 1:1311–1314.

4. Sherman CT, Litvack F, Grundfest W, et al. Coronary angioscopy in patients with unstable angina pectoris. N Engl J Med 1986; 315:913–919.

5. Uchida Y, Tomaru T, Nakamura F, Furuse A, Fujimori Y, Hasegawa K. Percutaneous coronary angioscopy in patients with ischemic heart disease. Am Heart J 1987; 14:1216–1222.

6. Mizuno K, Miyamoto A, Satomura K, et al. Angioscopic coronary macromorphology in patients with acute coronary disorders. Lancet 1991; 337:809–812.

7. Yock PG, Linker DT. Intravascular ultrasound. Looking below the surface of vascular disease. Circulation 1990; 81:1715–1718.

8. Yamagishi M, Miyataka K, Tamai J, Nakatani S, Koyama J, Nissen SE. Intravascular ultrasound detection of atherosclerosis at the site of focal vasospasm in angiographically normal or minimally narrowed coronary segments. J Am Coll Cardiol 1994; 23:352–357.

9. Porter TS, Sears T, Xie F, et al. Intravascular ultrasound study of angiographically mildly diseased coronary arteries. J Am Coll Cardiol 1993; 22:1858–1865.

10. de Feyter PJ, Ozaki Y, Baptista J, et al. Ischemia-related lesion characteristics in patients with stable or unstable angina. A study with intracoronary angioscopy and ultrasound. Circulation 1995; 92:1408–1413.

11. Hodgson J, Reddy K, Suneja R, Nair R, Lesnefsky E, Sheehan H. Intracoronary ultrasound imaging: correlation of plaque morphology with angiography, clinical syndrome and procedural results in patients undergoing coronary angioplasty. J Am Coll Cardiol 1993; 21:35–44.

12. Lee DY, Eigler N, Luo H, et al. Effect of intracoronary ultrasound imaging on clinical decision making. Am Heart J 1995; 129:1084–1093.

13. Fitzgerald PJ, Ports TA, Yock PG. Contribution of localized calcium deposits to dissection after angioplasty. An observational study using intravascular ultrasound. Circulation 1992; 86:64–70.

14. Mintz GS, Pichard AD, Popma JJ, Kent KM, Satler LF, Leon MB. Preliminary experience with adjunct directional coronary atherectomy after high-speed rotational atherectomy in the treatment of calcific coronary artery disease. Am J Cardiol 1993; 71:799–804.

15. Mintz GS, Pichard AD, Kovach JA, et al. Impact of preintervention intravascular ultrasound imaging on transcatheter treatment strategies in coronary artery disease. Am J Cardiol 1994; 73:423–430.

16. Mintz GS, Popma JJ, Pichard AD, et al. Patterns of calcification in coronary artery

disease. A statistical analysis of intravascular ultrasound and coronary angiography in 1155 lesions. Circulation 1995; 91:1959–1965.

17. Tuzcu ME, Berkalp B, De Franco AC, et al. The dilemma of diagnosing coronary calcification: angiography versus intravascular ultrasound. J Am Coll Cardiol 1996; 27:832–838.

18. Mintz GS, Potkin BN, Satler LF, et al. Intravascular ultrasound evaluation of the effect of rotational atherectomy in obstructive atherosclerotic coronary artery disease. Circulation 1992; 86:1383–1393.

19. Kovach JA, Mintz GS, Pichard AD, et al. Sequential intravascular ultrasound characterization of the mechanisms of rotational atherectomy and adjunct balloon angioplasty. J Am Coll Cardiol 1993; 22:1024–1032.

20. Topol EJ, Nissen SE. Our preoccupation with coronary lumenology. Circulation 1995; 92:2333–2342.

21. Hausmann D, Lundkvist A, Friedrich G, Sudhir K, Fitzgerald P, Yock P. Lumen and plaque shape in atherosclerotic coronary arteries assessed by invivo intracoronary ultrasound. Am J Cardiol 1994; 74:857–863.

22. Mintz GS, Kovach JA, Pichard AD, et al. Mechanisms of lumen enlargement after excimer laser angioplasty: an intravascular study. Circulation 1995; 92: 3408–3414.

23. de Feyter PJ, Ruygrok PN. Coronary intervention: risk stratification and management of abrupt coronary occlusion. Eur Heart J 1995; 16(suppl L):97–103.

24. Chemarin-Alibelli MJ, Pieraggi MT, Elbaz M, et al. Identification of coronary thrombus after myocardial infarction by intracoronary ultrasound compared with histology of tissues sampled by atherectomy. Am J Cardiol 1996; 77:344–349.

25. Frimerman A, Miller H, Hallman M, Laniado S, Keren G. Intravascular ultrasound characterization of thrombi of different composition. Am J Cardiol 1994; 73: 1053–1057.

26. Teirstein PS, Schatz RA, De Nardo SJ, Jensen EE, Johnson AD. Angioscopic versus angiographic detection of thrombus during coronary interventional procedures. Am J Cardiol 1995; 75:1083–1087.

27. Mizuno K, Satomura K, Miyamoto A, et al. Angioscopic evaluation of coronary artery thrombi in acute coronary syndromes. N Engl J Med 1992; 326:287–291.

28. EPIC Investigators. Use of a monoclonal antibody directed against the platelet glycoprotein IIb/IIIa receptor in high-risk coronary angioplasty. N Engl J Med 1994; 330:956–961.

29. Serruys PW, Herrman JPR, Simon R, et al. A comparison of hirudin with heparin in the prevention of restenosis after coronary angioplasty. N Engl J Med 1995; 333:757–763.

30. Mintz GS, Pichard AD, Kovach JA, et al. Impact of preinterventional intravascular ultrasound imaging on transcatheter treatment strategies in coronary artery disease. Am J Cardiol 1994; 73:423–430.

31. Tenaglia AN, Buller CE, Kisslo KB, Stack RS, Davidson ChJ. Mechanisms of balloon angioplasty and directional coronary atherectomy as assessed by intracoronary ultrasound. J Am Coll Cardiol 1992; 20:685–691.

32. Fitzgerald PJ, Belef M, Connolly AJ, Sudhir K, Yock PG. Design and initial testing of an ultrasound-guided directional atherectomy device. Am Heart J 1995; 129:593–598.
33. Umans VA, Baptista J, Di Mario C, et al. Angiographic, ultrasonic, and angioscopic assessment of the coronary artery wall and lumen area configuration after directional atherectomy: the mechanism revisited. Am Heart J 1995; 130: 217–227.
34. Colombo A, Hall P, Nakamura S, et al. Intracoronary stenting without anticoagulantion accomplished with intravascular ultrasound guidance. Circulation 1995; 91:1676–1688.
35. Gorge G, Haude M, Ge J, et al. Intravascular ultrasound after low and high inflation pressure coronary artery stent implantation. J Am Coll Cardiol 1995; 26: 725–730.
36. Nissen SE, De Franco AC, Tuczu EM, Moliterno DJ. Coronary intravascular ultrasound: diagnostic and interventional applications. Coronary Artery Dis 1995; 6:355–367.
37. Hall P, Nakamura S, Maiello et al. A randomized comparison of combined ticlopidine and aspirin therapy versus aspirin therapy alone after successful intravascular ultrasound-guided stent implantation. Circulation 1996; 93:215–222.
38. von Birgelen C, Kutryk MJB, Gil R, et al. Quantification of the minimal luminal cross-sectional area after coronary stenting by two-dimensional and three-dimensional intravascular ultrasound versus edge detection and videodensitometry. Am J Cardiol 1996; 78:520–525.
39. Roelandt JRTC, Di Mario C, Pandian NG, et al. Three-dimensional reconstruction of intracoronary ultrasound images. Rationale, approaches, problems and directions. Circulation 1994; 90:1044–1055.
40. von Birgelen C, Gil R, Ruygrok P, et al. Optimized expansion of the Wallstent compared to the Palmaz-Schatz stent: on-line observations with two- and three-dimensional intracoronary ultrasound after angiographic guidance. Am Heart J 1996; 131:1067–1075.
41. Teirstein PS, Schatz RA, Wong SC, Rocha-Singh KJ. Coronary stenting with angioscopic guidance. Am J Cardiol 1995; 15:344–347.
42. Strumpf R, Heuser R, Eagan J. Angioscopy: a valuable tool in the deployment and evaluation of intracoronary stents. Am Heart J 1993; 126:1204–1210.
43. Ueda Y, Nanto S, Komamura K, Kodama K. Neointimal coverage of stents in human coronary arteries observed by angioscopy. J Am Coll Cardiol 1994; 23: 341–346.
44. Honye J, Mahon DJ, Jain A, et al. Morphological effects of coronary balloon angioplasty in vivo assessed by intravascular ultrasound imaging. Circulation 1992; 85:1012–1025.
45. Pandian NG, Kreis A, Brockway B, Sacharoff A, Caro R. Intravascular high frequency two-dimensional ultrasound detection of arterial dissections and intimal flaps. Am J Cardiol 1990; 65:1278–1280.

46. Sassower MA, Abela GS, Kocha JM, et al. Angioscopic evaluation of periprocedural and postprocedural abrupt closure after percutaneous coronary angioplasty. Am Heart J 1993; 126:444–450.
47. den Heijer P, van Dijk RB, Hillege HL, Pentiga ML, Serruys PW, Lie KI. Serial angioscopic and angiographic observations during the first hour after successful coronary angioplasty: a preamble to a multicenter trial addressing angioscopic markers for restenosis. Am Heart J 1994 128:656–663.
48. Potkin BN, Keren C, Mintz GS, et al. Arterial responses to balloon coronary angioplasty: an intravascular ultrasound study. J Am Coll Cardiol 1992; 20:942–951.
49. Lee RT, Grodzinsky AJ, Frank EH, Kamm RD, Schoen FJ. Structure-dependent dynamic mechanical behaviour of fibrous cap from human atherosclerotic plaques. Circulation 1991; 83:1764–1770.
50. White CJ, Ramee SR, Collins TJ, Jain SP, Escobar A. Coronary angioscopy of abrupt occlusion after angioplasty. J Am Coll Cardiol 1995; 25:1681–1684.
51. Baptista J, Di Mario C, Escaned J, et al. Intracoronary two-dimensional ultrasound imaging in the assessment of plaque morphologic features and the planning of coronary interventions. Am Heart J 1995; 129:177–187.
52. Nakamura F, Kvasnicka J, Uchida Y, Geschwind HJ. Percutaneous angioscopic evaluation of luminal changes induced by excimer laser angioplasty. Am Heart J 1992; 124:1467–1472.
53. Uchida Y, Hasegawa K, Kawamura K, Shibuya I. Angioscopic observation of the coronary luminal changes induced by percutaneous transluminal coronary angioplasty. Am Heart J 1989; 117:769–776.
54. von Birgelen C, van der Lugt A, Nicosia A, et al. Computerized assessment of coronary lumen and atherosclerotic plaque dimensions in three-dimensional intravascular ultrasound correlated with histomorphometry. Am J Cardiol 1996; 78: 1202–1209.
55. von Birgelen C, de Vrey EA, Mintz GS, et al. ECG-gated three-dimensional intravascular ultrasound: feasibility and reproducibility of an automated analysis of coronary lumen and atherosclerotic plaque dimensions in humans. Circulation. In press.

8

Detection and Quantification of the Atherosclerotic Lesion: Comparison of Angiography and Intravascular Ultrasound

Steven E. Nissen and E. Murat Tuzcu   *Cleveland Clinic Foundation, Cleveland, Ohio*

I. INTRODUCTION

Accurate detection, classification, and quantification of coronary atherosclerosis in vivo represents an important, although daunting, challenge for cardiovascular research and clinical practice. It seems clear that the distribution and composition of atherosclerotic plaque constitutes an important determinant of the prognosis and natural history of coronary artery disease. However, until recently, atherosclerotic coronary lesions could not be directly visualized by any available imaging modality. Accordingly, characterization of coronary disease has traditionally depended upon indirect methods that either depict the vessel lumen (angiography) or unmask the ischemic effect of coronary obstructions (functional studies). However, both methods are insensitive to the early, minimally obstructive disease associated with the dramatic and often lethal consequences of coronary atherosclerosis–acute coronary syndromes.

In the absence of a direct method for visualizing atherosclerotic plaques, angiography, following its introduction by Sones et al. in 1958, has constituted the principal modality used by clinicians and investigators to determine the anatomic severity of coronary artery disease. Indeed, for more than 35 years, coronary angiography has represented the "gold standard" for diagnosis of coronary disease, growing in frequency to more than 1 million procedures annually in the United States. Now, in the 1990s, for the first time, an alternative imaging modality, intravascular ultrasound, is challenging the dominance of coronary angiography in identification, characterization,, and quantification of coronary atherosclerosis. As a means to investigate atherosclerotic vessels, coronary ultrasound represents a radically different approach to the imaging of abnormal vascular anatomy.

The incremental value of intravascular ultrasound originates principally from two key features: the cross-sectional, tomographic perspective of the images and the ability of this imaging modality to visualize intramural coronary anatomy. Whereas angiography depicts complex coronary cross-sectional anatomy as a planar silhouette, ultrasound *directly* examines the atherosclerotic lesion within the vessel wall, allowing the operator to measure precisely atheroma size, distribution, and composition. Accordingly, coronary ultrasound is yielding important insights into diverse atherosclerotic phenomena, ranging from the pathophysiology of coronary syndromes to the patterns of disease associated with coronary risk factors.

II. RATIONALE FOR INTRAVASCULAR ULTRASOUND

A. Limitations of Coronary Angiography

The rationale for intracoronary ultrasound arises from extensively described limitations of coronary angiography. Clinical investigations have documented the limited accuracy and poor reproducibility of the coronary angiogram (1,2). Studies have established that visual interpretation of angiograms exhibits significant observer variability (1). Other reports demonstrate a large discrepancy between the apparent lesion severity by visual examination of angiography and postmortem examination (2). More recently, investigators have documented major differences between the apparent angiographic severity of lesions and measurements of the physiologic effects of stenoses (3). Although quantitative coronary angiography has improved the reproducibility of coronary luminal measurements, this technique is limited by magnification errors, inability to detect disease at the reference segment, and the limited number of projections available (4).

In the setting of percutaneous intervention, the theoretical limitations of angiography in classifying coronary disease are particularly relevant. Radiographic imaging depicts complex coronary cross-sectional anatomy from a planar silhouette of the contrast-filled lumen. Most mechanical interventions exaggerate the extent of luminal eccentricity by fracturing or dissecting the atheroma (5). This disruption of the atherosclerotic plaque permits extravasation of contrast media into (or beneath) the atheroma. The silhouette (angiographic appearance) of the complex postintervention vessel often consists of an enlarged, although frequently "hazy" lumen. In the setting of extensive plaque fracture, the hazy, broadened angiographic silhouette may overestimate the vessel cross-section and misrepresent the actual gain in lumen size.

The angiographic percentage stenosis represents an indirect and relative measure of luminal narrowing. To evaluate the severity of any specific lesion, the angiographer must identify and measure the diameter of an adjacent "reference site," which is presumed to be completely free of disease. However, necropsy studies have consistently demonstrated that coronary atherosclerosis is typically diffuse, not focal. Accordingly, in most patients, no truly normal reference segment exists from which to calculate the percentage narrowing. In this setting, the calculated percentage diameter stenosis will underestimate the actual lesion severity by comparing the stenosis diameter to a diffusely narrowed reference segment. Atherosclerotic involvement of the reference segment also has important implications for interventional practice, because reference segment disease can influence device selection and sizing.

Angiography is also significantly confounded by the phenomenon of coronary "remodeling" (Glagov phenomenon), originally observed by histology as the outward displacement of the external vessel wall in segments with atherosclerosis (6). The adventitial enlargement prevents an accumulating atheroma from encroaching on the lumen, thereby concealing the presence of atherosclerotic disease on angiography. Although remodeled lesions do not restrict blood flow, clinical studies have demonstrated that minimal, nonobstructive angiographic lesions represent the predominant atherosclerotic substrate underlying many acute coronary syndromes, including myocardial infarction (7). Angiographically unrecognized disease virtually always underlies an ergonovine-positive response in symptomatic patients with a "normal" coronary angiogram (8).

B. Advantages of Ultrasound

Intravascular ultrasound represents the first and only diagnostic technique that provides direct visualization of atherosclerotic coronary plaques in vivo. Coronary ultrasound has several unique properties of theoretical value in the detection and quantitation of atherosclerotic disease (4,9–11). The cross-sectional perspective of ultrasound permits visualization of the full 360° circumference of the vessel wall, not just two surfaces. This capability permits direct measurements of lumen dimensions, including minimum and maximum diameter and cross-sectional area. Luminal measurements are not dependent on the radiographic projection and can be determined by direct planimetry of the image. Because the velocity of sound in soft tissue represents a well-established constant, ultrasound scanners overlay an inherently accurate distance scale, which is electronically generated and superimposed on the image. This feature eliminates the troublesome requirement of traditional angiographic methods to correct for radiographic magnification (4). The tomographic perspective of ultrasound enables characterization of disease in vessels that are difficult to assess by conventional angiographic techniques, including diffusely diseased segments, bifurcation or ostial lesions and eccentric plaques.

C. Intravascular Ultrasound Artifacts

All current intravascular ultrasound devices generate artifacts that may adversely affect image quality, alter interpretation, or reduce quantitative accuracy (12). Studying lesions within small coronary arteries or stenoses requires imaging in close proximity to the transducer surface. However, near-field imaging is impaired by *ring-down artifact*, an imaging flaw that appears in most medical ultrasound devices. Ring-down artifacts arise from high-amplitude acoustic oscillations in the piezoelectric transducer material that precludes imaging within a few tenths of a millimeter of the transducer surface. Inability to image structures immediately adjacent to the transducer results in an "acoustic" catheter size slightly larger than its physical size. The most recent designs use carefully chosen transducer and backing materials, specialized coatings, and electronic filtering to suppress ring-down artifacts. In the nonmechanical electronic arrays, the transducer elements are surface mounted and ring-down must be reduced by digital subtraction, a process that is often incompletely effective.

The major branches of human epicardial coronaries typically range from 1.0 to 5.0 mm, while atherosclerotic lumina can reach 0.1 mm. Since the minimum size of current ultrasound catheters is approximately 1.0 mm, these devices cannot fully image severe stenoses prior to intervention. Further reductions in transducer size may be difficult because transducer miniaturization reduces the effective aperture of the device, which limits available acoustic power, reduces lateral resolution, and impairs the signal-to-noise ratio. Therefore, characterization of atherosclerotic coronary plaques by ultrasound is most effective for moderate lesions in large vessels. In the future, the resolution limits observed at small apertures (smaller catheter size) may be overcome using transducers operating at higher frequencies (40–50 MHz), an approach under active investigation.

All tomographic imaging techniques, including intravascular ultrasound, are vulnerable to distortion produced by imaging in oblique planes not perpendicular to the long axis of the vessel. This phenomenon increases the maximum, but not minimum, luminal dimensions, and can represent a significant confounding variable in quantitative plaque measurements. Under some circumstances, it is possible to recognize a nonorthogonal catheter position and manipulate the device to a more orthogonal position. Fortunately, the extent of this artifact is self-limiting, because the small size of the coronary vasculature geometrically limits the degree of obliquity possible during ultrasound examinations. However, obliquity-related distortion can be more troublesome when imaging larger vessels such as the aorta or the peripheral vasculature.

Mechanical transducers may exhibit cyclical oscillations in rotational speed, *nonuniform rotational distortion* (NURD), which arise from differential mechanical drag on the catheter drive–shaft producing visible distortion. NURD is most evident when the drive–shaft is bent into a small radius of curvature by a tortuous vessel and is recognized as circumferential "stretching" of a portion of the image with compression of the contralateral vessel wall. Improvements in the mechanical precision of ultrasound devices have reduced the impact of the artifact, but it still remains a troublesome problem during some examinations. NURD can distort measurements of atherosclerotic plaque by exaggerating or underestimating the circumferential extent of a lesion.

III. INTERPRETATION OF CORONARY ULTRASOUND

A. Normal Arterial Morphology

Studies performed in normal subjects or using excised, pressure-distended vessels have characterized the appearance of normal coronaries by intravascular ultrasound (13–17) (Fig. 1). Determinants of the vessel wall morphology include both the normal arterial structure and the inherent properties of ultrasound. A change in acoustic impedance between adjacent tissue layers is the most important factor responsible for the ultrasound appearance of the vessel wall (18). The leading edge of the intima (interface between the blood and endothelium) and the outer border of the media (the external elastic membrane) are two particularly strong acoustic interfaces. As a result, these two boundaries are typically well visualized by ultrasound.

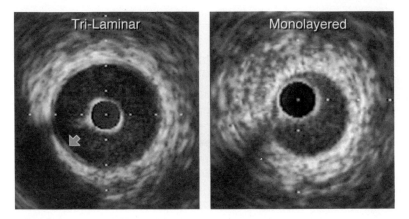

Figure 1   Two variants of normal anatomy. In the left frame, the vessel wall shows a tri-laminar pattern (outlined arrow), while in the right frame, the arterial wall is mono-layered.

However, these two classical interfaces are not well visualized in all normal subjects. At 30 MHz, theoretically, the theoretical axial resolution of intra-vascular ultrasound devices is approximately 80 μm, although actual perfor-mance is usually less, typically about 120–150 μm. The acoustic impedance shift at the blood–intima interface is highly dependent on patient-related factors, particularly the composition of the wall. In normals, the intima consists of a superficial layer of endothelial cells and connective tissue, resulting in a relatively small impedance difference between blood and vessel leading-edge. Accordingly, in young subjects, ultrasound frequently cannot distinguish in-tima from the subintimal layers, resulting in a monolayered appearance. This finding has led some observers to propose that any vessel with a trilaminar appearance represents evidence of coronary atherosclerosis (16). Others have studied young subjects and report a range of normal values for the intimal thickness, typically about 0.15 ± 0.07 millimeters (13). Most investigators use 0.25 to 0.30 mm as an upper limit of normal (2 standard deviations > normal).

In most adult patients, progressive intimal thickening or the development of pathologic intimal changes results in an ultrasound pattern consisting of two distinct echogenic layers sandwiching a sonolucent intermediate layer (three-layered appearance). A clear delineation of the inner border of the media (internal elastic membrane) is frequently difficult or impossible, so that only two layers are normally distinguished with ultrasound. The inner layer, often described as atherosclerotic plaque, should be more correctly described as "intima–media complex." Thus, the ultrasound definition of atheroma includes the media, whereas the histological definition does not.

Whether the artery is trilaminar or monolayered, the deepest layers representing the adventitia and periadventitial tissues, exhibit a characteristic "onionskin" pattern. The outer border of the vessel is usually indistinct, primarily because there are no acoustic differences between the adventitia and other encasing tissues. Accordingly, total wall thickness cannot be measured using ultrasound, except in vessels with a distinct outer border such as aorto-coronary saphenous vein grafts.

The blood within the vessel lumen exhibits a characteristic pattern of echogenicity in intravascular ultrasound examinations. At frequencies greater than 25 MHz, the lumen is characterized by subtle, finely textured, specular echoes that move in a characteristic swirling pattern during blood flow. The echogenicity arises from reflection of acoustic energy by circulating blood elements, although the precise anatomic origin of this effect remains uncertain. The presence of blood "speckle" can assist image interpretation by confirming the communication between a dissection plane and the lumen. The pattern of blood speckle is dependent upon the velocity of flow with increased intensity and a more coarse texture when flow is reduced. This latter property can represent a confounding variable in some examinations because the increased echogenicity of blood may interfere with identification of the blood tissue interface.

B. Classification of Atheromata

Vessels with classical atherosclerosis exhibit a diversity of abnormal features that reflect the severity, composition and distribution of the atheromata (10,11,14,15,18,19). Sites with low-grade disease exhibit circumferential or focal thickening of the intimal leading-edge, while advanced lesions appear as large echogenic masses protruding into the lumen. Three basic types of lesions are distinguished: 1. *Soft* cellular lesions with lipid infiltration, which have a low echogenicity (Fig. 2); 2. Dense *fibrous* lesions with a more echogenic pattern (Fig. 2); 3. *Calcified* lesions which generate the greatest degree of echogenicity with shadowing of underlying structures (Fig. 3).

There exists no uniformly accepted and standardized method for analysis of atheromata composition. Most classification approaches differentiate the predominant atheromata into one of the three general categories described previously according to plaque echogenicity (soft, fibrous, or calcified). However, the echogenicity of the atheroma is dependent, not only on the acoustic proper-

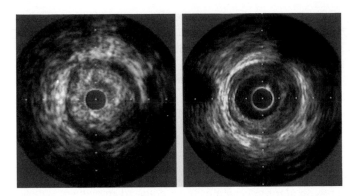

Figure 2   Soft and fibrous plaque variants. In the left panel, the atheroma is primarily sonolucent, while in the right panel, the echogenicity of the plaque approaches the brightness of the adventitia.

ties of tissue, but also the acquisition technique (gain, compression, etc.) of the ultrasound system. Accordingly, most classification methods compare the echointensity of the plaque to the adventitia as a means to correct for differences in ultrasound settings (14). Atheromata are termed "soft" if they are less echogenic than the adventitia and "fibrous" or "hard" if echodensity is similar

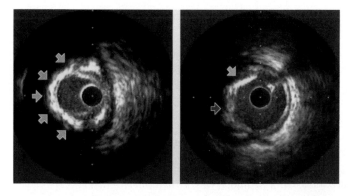

Figure 3   Calcified coronary atheroma. In the left panel, extensive calcification subtends approximately 180 degrees of the vessel circumference (solid arrows). In the right panel, more limited calcification is evident (outlined arrow). Although less echogenic than the adjacent arrow, the plaque indicated by the solid arrow also produces acoustic shadowing, probably representing microcalcification.

to the adventitia. Studies performed using excised vessels have confirmed that increasing tissue echogenicity correlates closely with a higher fibrous tissue content.

Calcified atheromata exhibit a characteristic morphology by intravascular ultrasound. Calcium attenuates transmission of high frequency ultrasound, thereby obscuring deeper layers of the vessel wall, a phenomenon known as "acoustic shadowing" (20). Obstruction of ultrasound transmission, not merely a high degree of echogenicity, is a requisite for identification of calcium. With the exception of multiple scattered microcalcification, ultrasound can be considered highly specific and sensitive for the detection of calcified plaque. Because of the importance of calcium for the selection of coronary interventional devices, most interpretation schemes further classify calcified atheroma. Additional descriptors include whether deposits are single or multiple, the circumferential extent of calcium expressed in degrees of arc, and the length in millimeters. Most approaches also determine the "depth" of the calcification, described as "superficial" or "deep" depending upon whether there exists tissue between the calcium deposit and lumen.

Few studies have examined unstable or degenerating atheromata using intravascular ultrasound. Some plaques contain a zone of reduced echogenicity within the central core of the atheroma, often covered by a distinct "cap" of greater echogenicity, presumably representing the classical fibrous cap described by histology. Current methods cannot distinguish whether these sonolucent zones represent areas of lipid deposition and necrotic degeneration, both of which can appear as areas of low density. Spontaneous plaque rupture associated with an unstable coronary syndrome is sometimes evident in ultrasound examination of the culprit lesions hours to days following the event. These lesions may show single or multiple flow channels within the plaque that appear to communicate with the lumen, most likely due to extrusion of the lipid-rich or necrotic core of the atheroma (Fig. 4). The presence of mobile intraluminal masses suggests the presence of thrombi, but, at 30 MHz, organizing thrombus appears visually indistinguishable from soft lipid-rich atheroma.

Although current devices produce highly detailed images of the vessel wall, determination of plaque composition must rely upon simple visual inspection of acoustic reflections. Validated methods do not yet exist for objective or automated classification of atheromatous lesions. Accordingly, some caution is warranted in interpretation of images. The echogenicity and texture of different atheroma features may overlap, making it difficult to arrive at definitive conclusions about plaque morphology. A sonolucent plaque may represent intracoronary thrombus, while a nearly identical appearance may result from an atheroma with a high lipid content. Thus, intravascular ultrasound can deter-

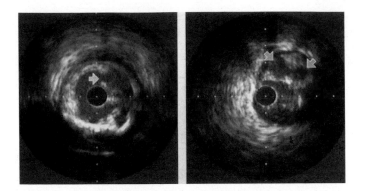

Figure 4   Unstable coronary lesions. The left panel shows a fracture of the fibrous cap with extrusion of the underlying lipid core. In the right panel, a large remodeled plaque contains two flow channels (arrows), which indicate recannulization through a previously necrotic or lipid laden core.

mine the thickness and echogenicity of intramural structures, but does not provide actual histology.

Despite these limitations, the classification of coronary plaques into the simple categories of soft, fibrous, or calcified has significant clinical implications. Initial experience suggests that the three different plaque subtypes may respond differently to interventional devices (21). For example, very dense fibrotic or calcified plaques typically resist removal with the current generation of directional atherectomy devices (22). Armed with this information, the practitioner may choose an alternative revascularization device, such as rotational atherectomy, for such lesions. Further refinement of interventional strategies based upon ultrasound lesion morphology are likely and may permit improved results or reduction in complications.

C.   Quantitation of Atherosclerosis

In addition to the aforementioned qualitative features, analysis of intravascular ultrasound images permits quantitative measurements of the extent and severity of coronary atherosclerosis (23). However, the physical properties of ultrasound require utilization of different anatomic landmarks than classical histology. In ultrasound imaging, reflections at the leading edge of any interface are located at the boundary where acoustic impedance abruptly changes. However, the precise location of the trailing edge of anatomic structures is determined by multiple nonanatomic factors, such as the properties of the ultrasound beam, particularly imaging frequency. Thus, leading-edge measurements accurately describe the precise location of a boundary, whereas trailing-edge measurements are ambiguous.

As previously noted, strong reflections occur at two locations, the interface between the lumen and the intimal leading-edge and the junction between the media and the external elastic membrane. In quantitative measurement of atherosclerotic lesions, the boundary at the trailing-edge of the intima is not accurately localized in intravascular ultrasound images. Accordingly, quantitative measurements must calculate atheroma cross-sectional area by subtracting the area bounded by the intimal leading-edge from the area enclosed by the external elastic lamina (Fig. 5). This approach results in an overestimation of plaque volume by including the area of the media within the atheroma calculation. Fortunately, in all but the most limited disease, the area of the media is small in comparison to atheroma area, thus limiting the impact of this overestimation.

The cross-sectional orientation of intravascular ultrasound represents an additional problem in quantifying atherosclerosis. Since each image contains information from only a thin "slice" of the vessel, measures of total atheroma burden require integration of multiple cross-sections. To facilitate measurements of multiple tomographic cross-sections, some studies employ a motorized device to slowly withdraw the ultrasound catheter through the vessel, typically at 0.5 to 1.0 mm per second. Since motor speed is kept constant, cross-

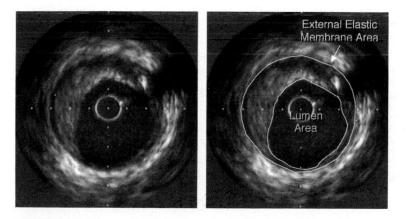

Figure 5   Boundaries for intravascular ultrasound measurements. The tracings in the right panel indicate the interface at the leading edges of the blood–lumen and the external elastic membrane.

sections obtained at any fixed time interval will be equally spaced longitudinally. This approach yields a series of tomograms, which are individually measured, and then summated to approximate total atheroma burden. A second approach to atheroma quantitation employs 3-dimensional (3-D) reconstruction of the vessel from the 2-dimensional ultrasound tomograms (24). Unfortunately, 3-D methods are exceedingly complex, have many unresolved confounding variables, and remain largely unvalidated.

D. Ultrasound Measurements

The lumen area is determined by manually tracing the circumference of the leading-edge of the blood–intima interface. Because of the speckled nature of ultrasound images, any individual frame of the video recording may not contain a continuous intimal leading-edge. Accordingly, review of the videotape with the vessel in motion may assist in accurate edge-detection by allowing the moving display of images to "fill-in" discontinuous portions of the vessel circumference. This process is also facilitated by differentiating the dynamic speckle pattern characteristic of flowing blood from the more static pattern of adjacent tissue. The injection of contrast dye or saline into the vessel temporarily clears the echogenic blood signals and may facilitate border delineation.

The cross-sectional area of the "normal" portion of the vessel wall is defined as the area enclosed by the interface between the media and adventitia—the leading edge of the external elastic membrane. The terms "total vessel area," "external elastic membrane area (EEM)," and "external elastic lamina area (EEL)" are used interchangeably. As previously discussed, measurement of the area within the external elastic lamina does not allow calculation of true plaque or intimal area because the *internal* elastic membrane is not well delineated with ultrasound. Calcium-induced acoustic shadowing can obscure a large portion of the vessel wall, requiring interpolation of missing portions of the vessel circumference.

The percentage of the vessel area occupied by atheroma is calculated using the formula:

$$\frac{\text{Total Vessel Area } - \text{ Lumen Area}}{\text{Total Vessel Area}} \times 100$$

This parameter has been referred to as "percentage vessel area stenosis," "plaque area stenosis," or, simply, "percent stenosis." It should be realized, however, that this measurement is not equivalent to angiographic percentage stenosis, which represents an expression of luminal narrowing at the stenosis relative to the reference segment.

In addition to cross-sectional area measurements, most laboratories also routinely measure atheroma thickness. Typically, maximal plaque thickness is defined as the longest distance between the intimal and adventitial leading-edges whereas the minimum thickness is the shortest distance between these two interfaces. The difference between maximum and minimum atheroma thickness represents a useful measure of plaque eccentricity, usually expressed by the following calculation:

$$\frac{\text{Maximum Plaque Thickness } - \text{ Minimum Plaque Thickness}}{\text{Maximum Plaque Thickness}} \times 100$$

The circumferential extent of disease is also commonly classified by determining whether abnormal intimal thickening involves the full $360°$ circumference of the vessel. The longitudinal extent of atherosclerosis is also sometimes reported and defined as diffuse if intimal thickness exceeds normal values at every site within an anatomic segment.

E. Discrepancies with Angiography

In general, the percentage of stenosis determined by ultrasound is greater than the extent of narrowing by angiography. This phenomenon is a consequence of two major factors: 1. The diffuse nature of coronary atherosclerosis, which frequently affects the angiographically normal "reference" vessel (Fig. 6) and 2. The presence of adaptive enlargement of the vessel, which opposes luminal encroachment, thereby keeping the lumen constant during the early phases of atherosclerosis (6) (Fig. 7). As previously discussed, angiography, a planar technique, has major limitations in measuring the size of vessels with complex luminal geometry (25). Accordingly, studies comparing angiographic and ultrasound assessment of luminal narrowing show close correlation for arteries with a nearly circular cross-section and progressively lower correlation with increasing luminal eccentricity (13,25).

A second frequent area of discrepancy concerns the eccentricity of the atheromata. In patients with coronary disease, the circumferential distribution of the atheroma varies from symmetrical, circumferential plaques to highly eccentric lesions in which the entire atheroma is located on only one side of the artery. The majority of plaques are eccentric by intravascular ultrasound with a maximum atheroma thickness more than twice the minimum plaque thickness (26). Comparative studies have demonstrated a poor correlation between the

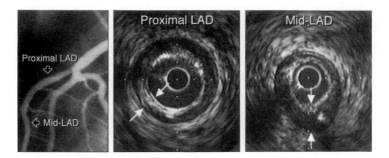

Figure 6   Underestimation of diffuse disease by angiography. In the angiogram, the two sites of ultrasound examination are indicated. In both the proximal and mid-LAD, diffuse atherosclerosis is present, which is not evident on the angiogram because of the concentric and symmetrical pattern of disease.

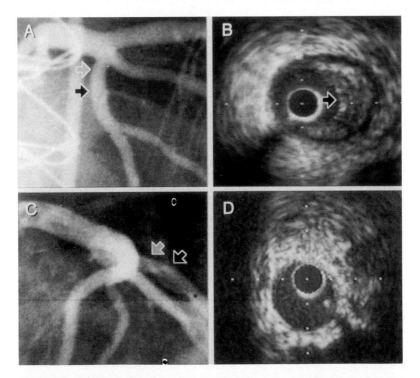

Figure 7   Coronary remodeling. Ultrasound at the site indicated by the black arrow in panel A is shown in panel D. Panel B shows the ultrasound image at the site of the gray arrow in panel A. Note that the lumen sizes in panels B and D are similar, despite the presence of a large atheroma in panel B (black arrow).

apparent plaque distribution by angiography and the actual circumferential pattern revealed by ultrasound examination (26). Such studies demonstrate the inaccuracy inherent in determining plaque distribution from the projected 2-dimensional silhouette of the lumen (angiography). This observation has important implications for guidance of coronary interventions, particularly techniques for selective plaque removal such as directional atherectomy.

Atheroma calcification represents an important sequela of coronary atherosclerosis, generally associated with disease of long duration. The traditional approach to identification of calcification employs cinefluoroscopy to visualize moving opacities in proximity to the vessel silhouette. However, this approach is limited by many factors, including the moderate spatial and contrast resolution of angiography and the confounding effects produced by the overlap of other calcium-containing structures. Studies comparing ultrasound and angiography studies demonstrate poor sensitivity for angiography in detection of coronary calcification (20,27). At interventional target lesions, Tuzcu et al. reported that angiography identified less than half (45%) of patients with calcification by ultrasound (20). Even in the presence of more extensive calcification, the sensitivity of angiography remains poor, correctly identifying only 52% of patients with calcium subtending more than 90° of vessel circumference and only 63% of lesions with >180° of involvement.

IV. CLINICAL APPLICATIONS

A. Angiographically Occult Disease

In patients with clinical symptoms of coronary disease, intravascular ultrasound commonly detects atherosclerotic abnormalities at angiographically normal sites (13,28,29). In the presence of any luminal irregularity by angiography, intravascular ultrasound typically demonstrates disease at all other examined coronary sites. The extent of disease in angiographically normal vessels confirms the finding, previously reported from necropsy studies, that coronary disease is frequently more diffuse than apparent by angiography (2).

There are 4 principal mechanisms by which angiography may underestimate the presence, extent or severity of atherosclerotic disease (4). First, to detect focal narrowing, angiography relies upon comparison of the interrogated site to an adjacent uninvolved segment. However, atherosclerosis is frequently a diffuse process. The diseased vessel may be reduced in caliber along its entire length, containing no truly normal segment for comparison (Fig. 6). In the absence of a focal stenosis, the angiographer could erroneously conclude that the vessel is simply "small in caliber."

Eccentric lesions, plaques that occupy only a portion of the vessel circumference, represent a second important source of false negative angiography. To detect eccentric disease, optimal angiographic projection angles are essential. However, in many clinical settings, physical limitations prevent the angiographer from obtaining optimal radiographic projections. For example, at certain angles, overlapping structures such as adjacent vessels can obscure some segments of the coronary. Mechanical constraints in positioning of the x-ray gantry preclude other potentially useful views. Therefore, an eccentric lesion may not be visualized by angiography, because the operator cannot obtain an appropriate projection orthogonal to the lesion. A third important mechanism underlying false-negative angiography results from the phenomenon of coronary remodeling, original described by Glagov from histology (6). As previously described, compensatory enlargement ("remodeling") of the vessel wall at atherosclerotic sites often preserves lumen diameter, resulting in an angiographic lumen size identical to adjacent, uninvolved segments (Fig. 7). A fourth mechanism of false negative angiography, vessel foreshortening, can conceal short "napkin-ring" lesions (usually less than 1–2 mm in length).

For each of these mechanisms of false negative angiography, ultrasound can confirm the presence and estimate the extent of atherosclerosis. There are important clinical implications for the higher sensitivity of ultrasound in detecting atherosclerosis. Patients who present with symptoms suggestive of coronary disease, but who have "normal" angiograms represent a common and perplexing group. In our experience, ultrasound will demonstrate coronary atherosclerosis in the many of these patients, a finding that may impact on the choice of therapy. The long-term implications of angiographically occult disease remain uncertain, since no outcome-based research has demonstrated a worse prognosis for patients with disease detected only by ultrasound. However, Little and others have demonstrated that plaques with minimal to moderate angiographic narrowing are the most likely to lead to myocardial infarction (7). Accordingly, the presence of angiographically-occult coronary disease may have important prognostic significance. Studies are currently underway to determine the predictive value of ultrasound in determining the prognosis in patients with angiographically-unrecognized coronary disease.

B. Ambiguous Lesions

Despite thorough radiographic examination using multiple projections, angiographers commonly encounter lesions that elude accurate characterization. Lesions of uncertain severity often include ostial lesions and moderate stenoses (angiographic severity ranging from 40% to 75%) in patients whose symptomatic status is difficult to evaluate. For these "ambiguous" coronary lesions, ultrasound provides precise tomographic measurements, enabling quantitation of the stenosis independent of the radiographic projection (30). Bifurcation lesions are particularly difficult to assess by angiography. Examination of bifurcation lesions by ultrasound involves specialized techniques, requiring subselective placement of the transducer in the main trunk and each of the daughter branches.

C. Cardiac Allograft Disease

Identification of atherosclerotic lesions in cardiac allograft recipients represents a particularly important and challenging task for diagnostic intravascular ultrasound (28). Transplant coronary artery disease is the leading cause of death beyond the first year after cardiac transplantation with a reported incidence of 15% to 20% per year. Although most transplant centers perform coronary arteriograms annually for screening, these surveillance studies often fail to detect atherosclerosis prior to a clinical event (31). These patients may have diffuse vessel involvement which, for reasons already enumerated, conceals the atherosclerosis from the angiographer. Necropsy studies have demonstrated that angiography systematically underestimates coronary atherosclerosis in transplant recipients (32). Many large centers now routinely perform intravascular ultrasound at the time of annual catheterization in all cardiac transplant recipients. Recent investigations using ultrasound to detect transplant vasculopathy report a very high incidence of this disease (33). Overall, abnormal intimal thickening is evident in 80% of patients at one year and in more than 92% of patients studied 4 or more years after transplantation (33).

Clinical investigations using intravascular ultrasound have revealed 2 pathways for development of transplant associated atherosclerosis. Some patients receive atherosclerotic plaques inadvertently transmitted via the donor heart, while others develop an immune-mediated vasculopathy (28,33). Thorough examination of the coronaries using ultrasound reveals a distinctly heterogeneous pattern of longitudinal and circumferential involvement (33). The evidence from clinical studies supports the hypothesis that the atherosclerotic pattern is related to the origins of the disease. Traditional atherosclerosis (usually donor-transmitted) has an eccentric plaque distribution with patchy longitudinal involvement, whereas immune-mediated (acquired) disease is more circumferential and diffuse (Fig. 8).

D. Risk Stratification of Atherosclerotic Lesions

In the early 1980s, Little et al. confirmed that plaques of minimal to moderate angiographic severity were the most likely to rupture and cause acute myocar-

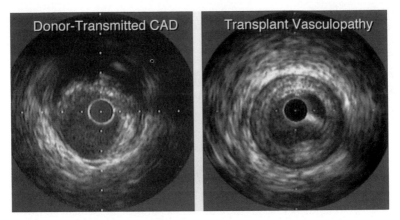

Figure 8 Patterns of atherosclerosis in transplant recipients. In the left panel, an eccentric lesion (donor transmitted disease) is evident. In the right panel, a diffuse and concentric pattern is consistent with immune-mediated transplant vasculopathy.

dial infarction. When intracoronary ultrasound interrogates lesions associated with acute coronary syndromes, most of these plaques contain a relatively echolucent material, consistent with a high lipid content. If a fibrous cap is present, this thick layer is most often ruptured and overlies a large, echolucent, lipid-laden area. Recent research indicates that lipids are the most thrombogenic component of atherosclerotic plaque. The ability of intravascular ultrasound to differentiate predominantly fibrous or calcified plaques from atheromata with a high lipid content offers the potential to determine which plaques are most susceptible to progression to acute coronary syndromes. However, clinical applications will require well-controlled prospective trials to determine if ultrasound-derived plaque morphology can predict the risk of unstable syndromes.

E. Vascular Responses to Intervention

A more complete understanding of restenosis has evolved from serial ultrasound measurements of plaque and lumen areas at follow-up studies after balloon angioplasty and directional atherectomy (34). In some studies, repeated ultrasound examinations have shown, that a late reduction in total vessel area (chronic negative remodeling) is an important mechanism of restenosis after mechanical revascularization procedures (nonstent) (34). These observations suggest that interventions to prevent chronic recoil (such as stenting) may be important in preventing restenosis and reduce the attractiveness of pharmacological treatment to prevent intimal hyperplasia. If further validated, this concept would explain the lower restenosis rate observed in randomized multicenter studies comparing balloon angioplasty and stent implantation. Although some strong evidence of "negative remodeling" exists, this concept remains controversial. In particular, there is uncertainty regarding the proportion of lumen loss produced by vessel versus neointimal proliferation.

F. Plaque Morphology and Directional Atherectomy

By determining both the location and composition of the target atheroma, ultrasound intravascular ultrasound has proven particularly valuable in guiding directional coronary atherectomy (22,23). As noted previously, lesions that appear concentric by angiography are often eccentric by ultrasound and conversely, angiographically eccentric lesions are often concentric by ultrasound. The improved spatial perspective provided by ultrasound can assist in the proper orientation of atherectomy cuts. However, successful application of this approach requires considerable skill, because precise orientation of the intravascular image remains difficult. Many interventional operators examine the target vessel prior to atherectomy to locate anatomic landmarks, especially side branches adjacent to the lesion. Using these landmarks to orient the ultrasound image, the operator can direct atherectomy cuts toward the appropriate side of the vessel. Some practitioners repeat ultrasound examinations between successive passes of the atherectomy device to assess the extent of plaque removal and the need for additional cuts.

With currently available directional atherectomy devices, the presence and extent of vessel calcification can dramatically affect the efficiency of plaque removal. As noted previously, ultrasound is more sensitive than angiography in detection of calcification, permitting identification of calcified atheromata despite the absence of any apparent calcification of fluoroscopy. However, ultrasound can determine not only the presence of calcification, but also its depth in relation to the lumen. Calcification at the luminal surface usually precludes successful tissue removal, whereas target lesions with extensive calcification deep within the atheroma can still undergo successful atherectomy.

Ultrasound studies before and after directional atherectomy confirm that plaque removal is the primary mechanism of luminal enlargement. Nevertheless, ultrasound also reveals that despite a successful angiographic result (<15% residual stenosis), 40–60% or more of the target site is still occupied by atheroma (22). Some investigators have proposed that a larger lumen after atherectomy would result in a lower restenosis rate (compared to balloon angioplasty). However, it remains untested whether a larger postprocedure lumen can be achieved using ultrasound guidance without a concomitant increase in dissection, perforation, or other complications. A promising approach under development will combine atherectomy and ultrasound devices to permit direct observation during atheroma debulking.

G. Plaque Morphology and Rotational Ablation

Rotational ablation (Rotablator™, Scimed Life Systems, Maple Grove, MN) employs a high-speed diamond-coated burr to debulk atheromata within coronary stenoses. This approach has been proven particularly effective at removing superficial calcium from stenotic vessels. As previously discussed, there is a poor correlation between ultrasound and fluoroscopy in assessment of the presence and amount of calcification (35). Vessels revascularized using rotational ablation are frequently diffusely diseased and the "normal" dimension can be difficult to determine angiographically. Ultrasound-guided vessel sizing can facilitate the selection of the largest burr. Observational ultrasound studies to date have confirmed that ablation of plaque constitutes the primary mechanism of rotational atherectomy, particularly the more fibrotic or calcified components of the lesion. In certain lesions, rotational atherectomy may be the only device capable of removing a hard, superficial layer of calcium, yet even

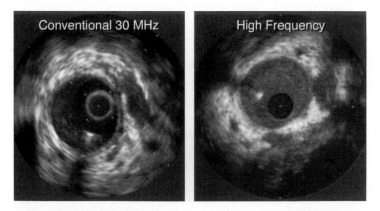

Figure 9 High-frequency intravascular ultrasound imaging. In the left panel, the coronary is shown using a conventional 30 MHz intravascular ultrasound system. In the right panel, a higher frequency transducer was employed and shows much improved axial and lateral resolution.

after this layer is removed, a large volume of plaque may remain. Post-Rotablator™ ultrasound can quantitate the size of the neo-lumen, characterize the morphology of the remaining plaque, and guide the technique and size of device used for further luminal enlargement.

H. Future Directions of Intravascular Ultrasound

During the next several years, technological advances in intravascular imaging will likely expand the utility of this procedure in assessing the atherosclerotic process. Further reduction in the size of imaging catheters is anticipated with the likely development of a guidewire-sized ultrasound probe. Very small devices would enable imaging of virtually any coronary stenosis prior to treatment. An ultrasound system operating at a higher frequency (40–50 MHz) is currently undergoing animal testing and, when released, will significantly increase spatial resolution (Fig. 9). As a consequence of refinements in equipment and expanded knowledge of clinical applications, we anticipate an increasing role for intravascular ultrasound in the assessment of the atherosclerotic lesions over the next decade.

REFERENCES

1. Zir LM, Miller SW, Dinsmore RE, Gilber JP, Harthorne JW. Interobserver variability in coronary angiography. Circulation 1976; 53:627–632.
2. Vlodaver Z, Frech R, van Tassel RA, Edwards JE. Correlation of the antemortem coronary angiogram and the postmortem specimen. Circulation 1973; 47:162–168.
3. White CW, Wright CB, Doty DB, Hirtza LF, Eastham CL, Harrison DG, Marcus ML. Does visual interpretation of the coronary arteriogram predict the physiologic importance of a coronary stenosis? N Engl J Med 1984; 310:819–824.
4. Topol EJ, Nissen SE. Our preoccupation with coronary luminology: The dissociation between clinical and angiographic findings in ischemic heart disease. Circulation 1995; 92:2333–2342.
5. Waller BF. "Crackers, breakers, stretchers, drillers, scrapers, shavers, burners, welders, and melters": the future treatment of atherosclerotic coronary artery disease? A clinical-morphologic assessment. J Am Coll Cardiol 1989; 13: 969–987.
6. Glagov S, Weisenberg E, Zarins CK, et al. Compensatory enlargement of human coronary arteries. N Engl J Med 1987; 316:1371–1375.
7. Little WC, Constantinescu M, Applegate RJ, et al. Can arteriography predict the site of a subsequent myocardial infarction in patients with mild-to-moderate coronary artery disease? Circulation 1988; 78:1157–1166.
8. Yamagishi M, Miyatake K, Tamai J, Nakatani S, Koyama J, Nissen SE. Detection of atherosclerosis at the site of focal vasospasm in angiographically normal or

minimally narrowed coronary segments by intravascular ultrasound. J Am Coll Cardiol 1994; 23:352–357.

9. Nissen SE, Gurley JC. Application of intravascular ultrasound to detection and quantitation of coronary atherosclerosis. Int J of Cardiac Imaging 1991; 6: 165–177.

10. Nissen SE, Gurley JC. Quantitative assessment of coronary dimensions, lumen shape and wall morphology by intravascular ultrasound. In: Tobis P, Yock P, eds., Intravascular Ultrasound. Churchill Livingstone, Inc., New York, 1992; pp. 71–83.

11. Nissen SE, DeFranco A, Tuzcu EM. Detection and quantification of atherosclerosis: the emerging role for intravascular ultrasound. In: Fuster V, ed., Syndromes of Atherosclerosis: Correlations of Clinical Imaging and Pathology. Futura Publishing Company, Inc., Armonk NY, 1996; pp. 291–312.

12. TenHoff H, Korbijn A, Smit ThH, Klinkhamer JFF, Borm N. Image artifacts in mechanically driven ultrasound catheters. Int J Cardiac Imag 1989; 4:195–199.

13. Nissen SE, Gurley JC, Grines CL, Booth DC, McClure R, Berk M, Fischer C, DeMaria AN. Intravascular ultrasound assessment of lumen size and wall morphology in normal subjects and coronary artery disease patients. Circulation 1991; 84(3):1087–1099.

14. Gussenhoven EJ, Essed CE, Lancee CT, Mastik F, Frietman P, Van Egmond FC, et al. Arterial wall characteristics determined by intravascular ultrasound imaging: an in vitro study. J Am Coll Cardiol 1989; 4:947–952.

15. Nishimura RA, Edwards WD, Warnes CA, Reeder GS, Holmes DR, Tajik AJ, et al. Intravascular ultrasound imaging: in vitro validation and pathologic correlation. J Am Coll Cardiol 1990; 16:145–154.

16. Fitzgerald PJ, St. Goar FG, Connolly AJ, Pinto FJ, Billingham ME, Popp RL, Yock PG. Intravascular ultrasound imaging of coronary arteries: is three layers the norm? Circulation 1992; 86:154–158.

17. St. Foar FG, Pinto FJ, Alderman EL, Fitzgerald PJ, Stadius ML, Popp RL. Intravascular ultrasound imaging of angiographically normal coronary arteries: an in vivo comparison with quantitative angiography. J Am Coll Cardiol 1991; 18: 952–958.

18. Siegel RJ, Chae JS, Maurer G, Berlin M, Fishbein MC. Histopathologic correlation of the layered intravascular ultrasound appearance of normal adult human muscular arteries. Am Heart J 1993; 126:872–878.

19. Tobis JM, Mallery J, Mahon D, Lehmann K, Zalesky P, Griffith J, Gessert J, Moriuchi M, McRae M, Dwyer ML, et al. Intravascular ultrasound imaging of human coronary arteries in vivo. Analysis of tissue characterizations with comparison to in vitro histological specimens. Circulation 1991; 83(3):913–926.

20. Tuzcu EM, Berkalp B, DeFranco AC, Ellis SG, Whitlow PL, Nissen SE. The dilemma of diagnosing coronary calcification: angiography versus intravascular ultrasound. J Am Coll Cardiol 1996; 27:832–838.

21. Mintz GS, Pichard AD, Kovach JA, et al. Impact of preintervention intravascular

ultrasound imaging on transcatheter treatment strategies in coronary artery disease. Am J Cardiol 1994; 73:423–430.

22. Matar FA, Mintz GS, Pinnow E, et al. Multivariate predictors of intravascular ultrasound end points after directional coronary atherectomy. J Am Coll Cardiol 1995; 25:318–324.

23. Nissen SE, Tuzcu EM, De Franco AC. Coronary intravascular ultrasound: diagnostic and interventional applications. In: Topol EJ, ed., Update to Textbook of Interventional Cardiology. WB Saunders, Philadelphia, PA 1994; pp. 207–222.

24. Gil R, von Birgelen C, Prati F, Di Mario C, Ligthart J, Serruys PW. Usefulness of three-dimensional reconstruction for interpretation and quantitative analysis of intracoronary ultrasound during stent deployment. Am J Cardiol 1996; 77: 761–764.

25. Nissen SE, Grines CL, Gurley JC, Sublett K, Haynie D, Diaz C, Booth DC, DeMaria AN. Application of a new phased-array ultrasound imaging catheter in the assessment of vascular dimensions: in vivo comparison to cineangiography. Circulation 1990; 81(2):660–666.

26. Mintz GS, Popma JJ, Pichard AD, et al. Limitations of angiography in the assessment of plaque distribution in coronary artery disease: a systematic study of target lesion eccentricity in 1446 lesions. Circulation 1996; 93:924–931.

27. Mintz GS, Popma JJ, Pichard AD, et al. Patterns of calcification in coronary artery disease: a statistical analysis of intravascular ultrasound and coronary angiography in 1,155 lesions. Circulation 1995; 91:1959–1965.

28. Tuzcu EM, Hobbs H, Rincon G, Bott-Silverman C, De Franco AC, Nissen SE. Occult and frequent transmission of atherosclerosis coronary disease with cardiac transplantation. Circulation 1995; 91:1706–1713.

29. Mintz GS. Painter JA, Pichard AD, et al. Atherosclerosis in angiographically "normal" coronary artery reference segments: an intravascular ultrasound study with clinical correlations. J Am Coll Cardiol 1995; 25:1479–1485.

30. White CJ, Ramee SR, Collin TJ, Jain A, Mesa JE. Ambiguous coronary angiography: clinical utility of intravascular ultrasound. Cathet Cardiovasc Diagn 1992; 26(3):200–203.

31. Uretsky BF, Kormos RL, Zerbe TR, Lee A, Tokarcyzk TR, Murah S, Reddy S, Dennys BG, Griffin BP, Hardesty RL, Armitage JM, Arena VC. Cardiac events after heart transplantation: incidence and predictive value of coronary arteriography. J Heart Transplant 1992; 11:S45–S50.

32. Johnson DE, Alderman EL, Schroeder JS, et al. Transplant coronary artery disease: histopathological correlations with angiographic morphology. J Am Coll Cardiol 1991; 17:449–457.

33. Tuzcu EM, DeFranco AC, Goormastic M, Hobbs RE, Bott-Silverman C, Nissen SE, et al. Dichotomous pattern of coronary atherosclerosis 1 to 9 years after transplantation: insights from systematic intravascular ultrasound imaging. J Am Coll Card 1996; 27:839–846.

34. Mintz GS, Popma JJ, Pichard AD, Kent KM, Satler LF, Wong SC, Hong MK,

Kovach JA, Leon MB. Arterial remodeling after coronary angioplasty. A serial intravascular ultrasound study. Circulation 1996; 94:35–43.
35. Kovach JA, Mintz GS, Pichard AD, Kent KM, Popma JJ, Satler LF, Leon MB. Sequential intravascular ultrasound characterization of the mechanism of rotational atherectomy and adjunct balloon angioplasty. J Am Coll Cardiol 1993; 22: 1024–1032.

9

Comparative Utility of Intravascular Ultrasound Versus the Doppler Flowire

Jerome Segal and Eduardo Moreyra *George Washington University, Washington, D.C.*

I. INTRODUCTION

For the past 40 years coronary angiography has been the method of choice for quantitative assessment of atherosclerotic vascular disease. Cardiologists have relied on this imaging method not only to determine the severity of coronary artery disease, but also to guide revascularization and interventions. Several well-performed studies, however, have questioned the accuracy and reproducibility of angiography, showing a significant intra- and interobserver variability (1–4). In addition, quantitative studies of necropsy specimens have shown a poor correlation with angiography in determining lesion severity (5–7). These findings can be explained by the fact that angiography provides a simple two-dimensional projection of the lumen, which is a poor representation of the three-dimensional coronary anatomy. This limitation is accentuated in vessels with distorted or eccentric luminal shapes and following interventional procedures, when angiography tends to overestimate the actual lumen gain as a result of plaque fracture and intimal dissections (8). Recently the development of new imaging techniques such as intravascular ultrasound and angioscopy have provided increased information regarding luminal and plaque characterization, as well as more precise dimensional measurements of vessel size. These new techniques, however, provide little information regarding the functional significance of a coronary stenosis. An easy-to-use and highly reliable method for measuring coronary flow (velocity, volume, and pattern) has long been the goal of investigators and clinicians alike. Clearly, a means of accurately measuring coronary flow would provide additional information concerning the physiological impact of a coronary stenosis and the results of pharmacological or mechanical interventions such as balloon angioplasty, laser angioplasty, atherectomy, and stent placement. This chapter reviews the basic principles, technique, and validation of Doppler flow velocity using wire-guided catheters and guidewires in assessing coronary blood flow in patients. It also compares its clinical applications to that of intravascular ultrasound.

II. CORONARY FLOW MEASUREMENT WITH DOPPLER CATHETERS AND FLOWIRE

Commonly utilized methods of measuring coronary artery blood flow have included coronary sinus thermodilution, indicator dilution including impedance measurement, digital substraction angiography, angiographic contrast transit time measurement, xenon 133 scintigraphy, and positron emission tomography. None of these methods have gained widespread acceptance due to problems with accuracy or reproducibility and because of the cumbersome nature of the measurements. Catheter-based Doppler ultrasound systems have been extensively investigated as a method for obtaining subselective coronary artery flow measurements during cardiac catheterization. Problems with the use of these Doppler catheters include the ability to measure flow velocity only in the proximal coronary artery and sensitivity to changes in vessel cross-sectional area, flow profile, angulation and position. Recently, a low-profile Doppler angioplasty guidewire with a spectral analysis flow velocimeter (Cardiometrics, Inc., Mountain View, CA), which overcomes many of the limitations observed with the Doppler catheter, has been extensively used in the clinical setting. The Doppler guidewire is constructed of a 175-cm-long, 0.018- or 0.014-in.-diameter, flexible, steerable guidewire with a 12-MHz piezoelectric ultrasound transducer integrated onto its tip (Fig. 1). The transducer produces a broad-beam ultrasound signal, which provides more uniform insonification of the vessel lumen and more accurate assessment of spatial mean velocity. In distinction to the existing Doppler catheters, velocity signals are processed by a real-time spectral analyzer using an on-line fast Fourier transform, providing a scrolling gray-scale display (Fig. 2). The Doppler system has the capacity to compute a variety of on-line spectral parameters including peak velocity, time-average peak velocity, proximal-to-distal velocity ratios, and diastolic-to-systolic velocity ratios. The profile of the Doppler Flowire (only

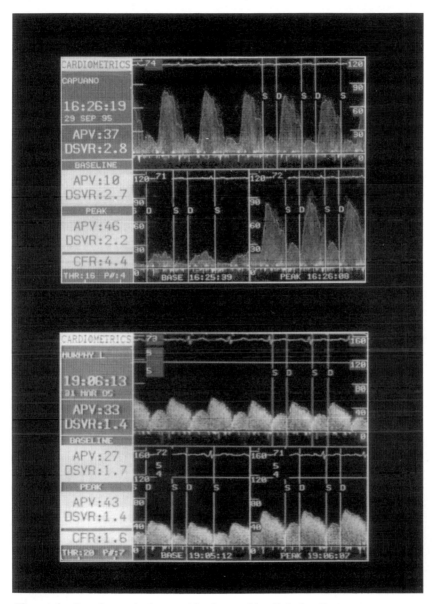

Figure 1 Doppler angioplasty guidewire used in clinical setting.

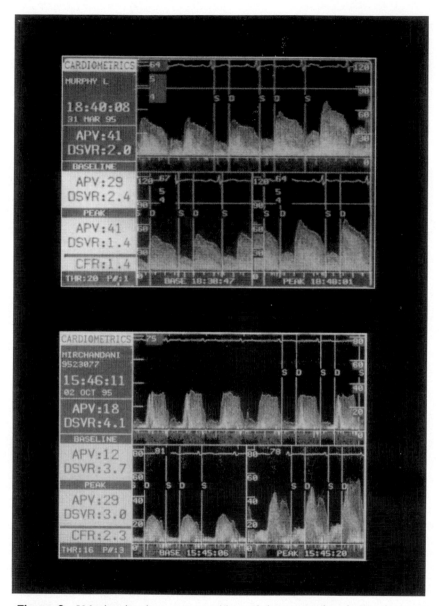

Figure 2   Velocity signals are processed by real-time spectral analyzer using an on-line fast Fourier transform, providing a scrolling gray-scale display.

one-fifth the cross-sectional area of the conventional Doppler catheter) allows the device to be advanced into small arteries and to areas distal to moderately severe stenoses for velocity sampling. The disturbance of flow distal to the tip of the wire is negligible. The Doppler guidewire system has been extensively validated in both in vitro and in vivo models of coronary artery flow (9), and Doppler-derived volume flow has been shown to be highly correlated with electromagnetic flow. Coronary flow reserve measured using the Doppler guidewire has also been validated and shown to be highly correlative with flow reserve measured using Doppler catheters in an animal model (10).

III. CORONARY FLOW VELOCITY PATTERNS IN NORMAL CORONARY ARTERIES

Doppler flow velocity patterns in normal human coronary arteries have been well characterized by Ofili et al. (11). Simultaneous flow velocity measurements in proximal and distal coronary segments were performed on 55 angiographically normal patients (11). Intracoronary adenosine was administered to induce coronary hyperemia. Flow velocity patterns were unchanged when measured in the proximal and distal segments in all three coronary arteries at baseline and during hyperemia. All arteries had predominant diastolic waveforms paired with a smaller systolic waveform. The diastolic-to-systolic flow velocity ratio was 1.5 or greater, and remained stable whether the measurements were performed in the proximal or distal segments. This patterns was more pronounced in the left anterior descending and circumflex coronary arteries than in the right coronary artery, probably due to the lower contractile force of the right ventricle during systole causing less resistance to the systolic flow. The average mean diastolic velocity in the left anterior descending and circumflex arteries was 30 cm/sec. The average peak diastolic velocity ranged between 40 and 80 cm/sec. The average peak systolic velocity was 10–20 cm/sec. When measurements were obtained in the right coronary artery or in distal segments, a reduction of up to 15% could be observed.

IV. CORONARY FLOW VELOCITY IN SIGNIFICANTLY STENOSED CORONARY ARTERIES

In animals, studies of phasic coronary artery flow have revealed changes in the normal diastolic predominant pattern to a less diastolic predominant pattern, with greater systolic flow contribution occurring with increasing severity of the epicardial coronary artery stenosis (12–14). Two multicenter trials evaluating alterations of phasic coronary artery flow velocity in patients with stenosed arteries have confirmed these results (15,16). In both trials a Doppler Flowire was used to measure blood flow velocity, flow reserve, and diastolic-to-systolic velocity ratio both proximal and distal to significant stenoses in the left anterior descending (LAD) or left circumflex (LCX) coronary arteries in patients undergoing angioplasty. Flow patterns distal to the stenoses were noted to be abnormal showing a significant decrease in mean diastolic-to-systolic velocity ratio as result of a decrease in the diastolic flow velocity with a relatively preserved systolic flow velocity (Fig. 2). This decrease in the diastolic-to-systolic flow ratio (DSVR) with increasing epicardial stenosis may be explained by the increased influence of an epicardial stenosis on flow during periods of low vascular resistance (diastole) as compared with periods of high vascular resistance (systole) (17). Phasic velocity patterns and mean diastolic-to-systolic velocity ratios measured proximal to a coronary stenosis were not statistically different from values in normal vessels. There was an important increase of proximal-to-distal mean velocity ratio in patients with coronary stenoses most likely due to blood runoff into branch vessels proximal to a significant coronary artery stenosis.

V. CORONARY FLOW RESERVE

For decades physiologists have recognized the capacity of normal coronary arteries to increase their flow nearly fourfold as a result of resistance vessel dilatation induced by maximal metabolic demands (18). This phenomenon is called coronary flow reserve (CFR) and can be reproduced in the catheterization laboratory by the intracoronary administration of vasodilators such as papaverine or adenosine, as long as the epicardial coronaries and the downstream myocardium are normal (19). The CFR is calculated as the ratio of hyperemic to basal mean flow velocity and can be normalized for blood pressure by dividing each flow value by its corresponding mean arterial pressure producing the reserve ratio (20). In flow-limiting lesions, the downstream coronaries vasodilate in an attempt to compensate for the decreased flow, blunting the hyperemic response when a vasodilator is administered. Thus, in the presence of significant epicardial coronary stenosis, the CFR is attenuated. These observations have been confirmed in studies comparing the hyperemic response between patients with significant coronary disease and patients with normal coronaries (15,16). The CFR was significantly blunted in patients with CAD when measured in the proximal or distal segments compared to patients with normal coronaries. However, distal measurements of CFR appear to be more reliable in assessing the significance of coronary artery disease than do proximal measurements, which remain near normal in the presence of significant runoff vessels proximal to the stenosis. In addition to assessing CAD significance, CFR is also useful in diagnosing microvascular disease (syndrome X) and following cardiac transplant patients especially during episodes of rejection (20–22). When using CFR to make clinical decisions, one must take into consideration that some factors may lead to erroneous conclusions. Hemodynamic factors including tachycardia and increased preload may decrease the CFR. Patients with previous infarctions, hypertrophy, microvascular disease, or rheological abnormalities such as anemia or hyperviscocity syndromes may present misleading flow reserve values. To exclude this confounding factor when assessing the severity of a lesion, it is sometimes useful to measure the CFR in a normal coronary from the same patient. Finally, flow reserve measurements are vessel- but not lesion-specific, because these measurements reflect all flow-limiting lesions in the vessel studied (19).

VI. ASSESSMENT OF ANGIOGRAPHICALLY INTERMEDIATE CORONARY ARTERY STENOSES

Often physicians are faced with the presence of coronary lesions of intermediate angiographic severity. Angiography has clearly been shown to be an unreliable method to determine physiological significance of these stenoses, even when performing quantitative analysis which is designed to minimize interobserver variability (23–25). The decision whether to intervene in these situations should rely on objective evidence of lesion significance utilizing perfusion or 2D echo stress testing (26) or documenting abnormal lesional hemodynamics (27,28). Several studies have shown coronary flow reserve to be a reliable marker of physiological significance for a given coronary obstruction (27,29,30). The development of the Doppler Flowire has facilitated the routine measurement of coronary flow both proximal and distal to stenoses. Donohue et al. (25) examined the relationship between angiography, coronary flow velocity, and translesional pressure gradients in patients with angiographic stenosis ranging from 50% to 70%. Nuclear imaging was not performed. They found that angiography was a poor predictor of translesional gradients ($r = 0.2$, $p = NS$) and distal flow velocity variables. Flow velocity ratio, however, correlated with translesional pressure gradients ($r = 0.8$, $p < 0.001$). This trial confirmed the close relationship between translesional pressure gradients and distal coronary flow velocity and their superiority over angiography in determining the hemodynamic significance of coronary artery stenoses. Several studies have evaluated the correlation between distal flow velocity variables and nuclear imaging in patients with angiographically intermediate lesions. Miller and co-workers (31) reported a strong correlation between hyperemic distal flow-velocity ratio measurements and TC-sestamibi perfusion imaging (89%; k = .78). Joye et al. (32) showed that the sensitivity, specificity, and overall predictive accuracy of Doppler-determined coronary flow reserve for stress SPECT thallium 201 results were 94%, 95%, and 94%, respectively. Distal measures of diastolic/systolic velocity ratio were 85% concordant with stress SPECT thallium-201 results in the left coronary system but were of limited utility in the right coronary artery. More recently, Deychak et al. (33), reported that a flow reserve < 1.8 and a diastolic/systolic flow velocity < 1.7 predicted a reversible thallium perfusion scintigram (concordance 96% and 88%, respectively).

The outcome of patients in whom revascularization procedures were not performed based on the presence of normal flow reserve measurements and/or translesional pressure gradients has also been reported. Lasser et al. (34) found that at 2 years, symptoms in nearly all patients greatly diminished without any interventional procedure. Subsequently, Kern et al. (35) demonstrated that in patients with lesions of intermediate angiographic severity and normal translesional hemodynamic data, in whom angioplasty was deferred, 92% of target arteries evaluated remained stable without the requirement for intervention at 10-month follow-up. No patient died or developed acute myocardial infarction or unstable angina as a result of progression of a target artery lesion.

In summary, these studies show that when faced with angiographically intermediate lesions, distal flow reserve measurements may accurately determine their physiological significance and are highly correlated with nuclear imaging results. The Doppler Flowire measurements available during the angiographic procedure may thus lead to improved clinical decision making.

VII. ALTERATION OF CORONARY FLOW AFTER BALLOON ANGIOPLASTY

The limitations of angiography in assessing severity of coronary disease are further compounded in cases of coronary interventions, where the architecture of the coronary vessel is distorted as a result of the intervention. Additional means of assessing the physiological significance of the residual stenosis after angioplasty is required. Segal et al. (16) reported the results of a multicenter trial in which the Doppler Flowire was used to measure coronary blood flow velocity, coronary flow reserve, and the diastolic-to-systolic flow ratio in 38 patients undergoing balloon angioplasty. Twelve patients without significant coronary artery disease served as a control group. Measurements performed in the distal coronary artery appeared to be more predictive of a successful angiographic outcome of balloon angioplasty than did measurements performed proximally to the stenosis. Average peak velocity (mean velocity) increased significantly from 19 ± 12 to 35 ± 16 cm/sec ($p < 0.01$) in the distal vessel following angioplasty, whereas changes in proximal average peak velocity were increased but to a lesser degree (preangioplasty, 34 ± 18 cm/sec, vs. postangioplasty, 41 ± 14 cm/sec, $p = 0.04$). Coronary flow reserve was unchanged after angioplasty, whether measured in the distal or proximal coronary artery ($p < 0.10$). When measured distal to significant stenosis ($> 70\%$), the diastolic/systolic flow patterns were noted to be abnormal, with low diastolic-to-systolic flow ratios (1.3 ± 0.5) when compared with coronary arteries in patients without significant stenoses (diastolic-to-systolic flow ratio of 1.8 ± 0.5, $p < 0.10$). Phasic velocity patterns were noted to normalize, with significant increases in diastolic-to-systolic flow ratios (1.9 ± 0.6, $p < 0.10$), within 10–15 min following successful balloon angioplasty.

Similar findings have been reported by Ofili et al. (15), who examined flow dynamics with the Doppler Flowire before and after angioplasty in 39 patients, 17 with angiographic normal arteries and 29 with significantly stenosed arteries before and after angioplasty. The mean and peak diastolic velocity, diastolic and total flow integral (flow-time area), and first one-third (portion of flow integral) flow fraction were compared. In addition to improvement in the phasic pattern, the total velocity integral, as well as the peak diastolic velocity distal to the lesion, was significantly improved after angioplasty. The mean and peak diastolic velocity during hyperemia was significantly higher proximal and distal to the stenotic regions following successful angioplasty compared with the preangioplasty values. The improvement in the ratio of proximal-to-distal mean velocity also correlated with the angiographic success of the procedure. These data suggest that measurement of the proximal-to-distal average velocity ratios and diastolic-to-systolic flow ratios in the distal vessel, after coronary interventions such as balloon angioplasty, may provide important information concerning the immediate physiological outcome of the procedure.

VIII. ALTERATION IN CORONARY FLOW FOLLOWING OTHER CORONARY INTERVENTIONAL PROCEDURES

Segal (36) reported the effects of excimer laser angioplasty, before and after adjunctive balloon angioplasty, on the distal coronary flow in 10 patients with significant ($> 70\%$) coronary artery stenoses. The mean diameter stenosis decreased from 95% to 55% ($p < 0.01$) following laser angioplasty alone, with a further decrease to 27% ($p < 0.01$) following adjunctive balloon angioplasty. The average peak velocity increased from 6.3 to 13.0 cm/sec following laser angioplasty ($p < 0.01$) to 20.6 cm/sec following adjunctive balloon angioplasty ($p < 0.01$). Diastolic-to-systolic velocity ratios increased from a prelaser angioplasty mean value of 1.1 to 2.0 following laser recanalization ($p < 0.01$), with a further increase to 2.9 following adjunctive balloon angioplasty ($p < 0.01$). Mean coronary flow remained unchanged following either laser or balloon angioplasty ($p < 0.10$). These data show that after excimer laser angioplasty, flow velocity in the distal vessel often remains abnormally low and phasic velocity patterns do not normalize. An increase in distal flow velocity and normalization in phasic flow patterns with an increase in diastolic-to-systolic flow ratio occurs following the use of adjunctive angioplasty following laser.

Deychak et al. (37) reported the coronary flow changes in 18 patients undergoing directional coronary atherectomy. Despite a significant angiographic improvement following directional atherectomy (76% pre- vs. 24% postdiameter stenosis, $p < 0.001$), mean average peak velocity increased modestly from 24.7 to 31.2 cm/sec ($p < 0.05$). Mean diastolic-to-systolic flow ratio did not increase significantly (1.78 vs. 2.04, $p = 0.18$). The improvements observed in average peak velocity and mean diastolic-to-systolic flow ratio following directional atherectomy are not as consistent as those following balloon angioplasty. The reason for this is unclear. It is possible that the eccentric channel with significant residual plaque burden and thrombus formation observed in necropsy and intravascular studies following directional atherectomy may explain it (38,39). Platelet adhesion following exposure of the media, and occasionally adventitia, may lead to the release of local vasoactive factors limiting the flow response. In addition, the normalization of phasic diastolic/systolic flow ratio may take longer following directional atherectomy than following balloon angioplasty.

Ge et al. (40) evaluated the coronary flow changes in eight patients who underwent balloon angioplasty and subsequent stent placement. Intravascular imaging was performed in each case. The lumen diameter was 2.42 ± 0.55 mm after angioplasty and increased to 2.74 ± 0.49 mm following stent placement. The CFR increased from 2.05 ± 1.01 to 2.99 ± 1.14 after angioplasty ($p = 0.015$). Following stent implantation the CFR further increased to 4.51 ± 1.33 ($p = 0.001$). Several case reports have described similar improvements in coronary flow parameters following stent deployment (41,42). In one report the coronary flow remained abnormal after stent implantation despite an excellent angiographic result. The patient presented 4 months later with restenosis raising the question of whether postprocedure coronary flow parameters may predict restenosis (43). Percutaneous transluminal coronary rotational atherectomy (PTCRA) has a unique mechanisms of action using a diamond-coated elliptical burr that rotates at high-speed ablating plaques. This results in the release of microparticulate debris into the circulation. Because the burr-to-artery ratio is always less than 1, the minimal luminal diameter (MLD) obtained is often suboptimal requiring adjunctive angioplasty. Nunez et al. (44) reported the coronary flow changes following PTCRA with adjunctive PTCA. The MLD increased from 1.3 ± 0.1 mm to 2.6 ± 0.2 mm and was associated with an increase in APC (20 ± 3 cm/sec to 36 ± 5 cm/sec; $p < 0.05$) and coronary flow (81 ± 14 ml/min to 154 ± 18 ml/min; $p < 0.05$), but no change in CFR (1.24 ± 0.1 to 1.6 ± 0.1, NS). Similar results were obtained by Khoury et al. (45), who evaluated the serial changes of coronary flow in 13 patients at baseline, following PTCRA and after adjunctive PTCA. The MLD increased from 0.7 ± 0.4 mm at baseline, to 1.9 ± 0.4 mm after PTCRA ($p < 0.01$), and increased to 2.4 ± 0.5 mm after PTCA ($p < 0.01$ vs. baseline and PTCRA). Poststenotic coronary flow at baseline was 47 ± 23 ml/min and 57 ± 38 ml/min during hyperemia. After PTCRA, coronary blood flow increased to 104 ± 59 ml/min and to 132 ± 73 ml/min with hyperemia. Following adjunctive PTCA, coronary blood flow showed no significant change. The poststenotic CFR increased from an initial value of 1.1 ± 0.2 ml/min to 1.3 ± 0.3 ml/min after PTCRA (p = NS vs. baseline) and to 1.6 ± 0.3 ml/min after adjunctive PTCA ($p < 0.01$ vs. baseline; p = NS vs. PTCRA). As demonstrated by these two studies, PTCRA improves basal and hyperemic coronary blood flow, but despite an adequate MLD gain, coronary flow remains physiologically compromised as suggested by the persistently impaired CFR. This may result from stunning and occlusion of the microcirculation as a result of showering of microparticulate debris into the distal vascular bed induced by PTCRA (45). The recovery time of the microcirculation and CFR remain to be determined.

IX. CORONARY FLOW MONITORING DURING INTERVENTIONS

The development of the Doppler Flowire has made possible monitoring blood flow distal to the target lesion not only at the time of balloon inflation, but also during the period immediately following the intervention, allowing the evaluation of important features of coronary behavior. Anderson et al. (46) demonstrated that occlusion of the coronary artery by an angioplasty balloon produces ischemia, inducing a transient posthyperemic phase similar to that produced by agents such as papaverine, dipyridamole, and adenosine. Sequential brief balloon inflations enlarge the lumen, enhancing the hyperemic response each time. Following coronary interventions most patients demonstrate higher coronary flows, which tend to remain stable (46). Several unstable or unsatisfactory flow patterns have been identified. Abrupt decrease of blood flow has been described with spasm or vasovagal hypotension (46). Diffuse spasm has also been associated with an acceleration in flow velocity (47,48). A gradual decline of blood flow has been observed in patients developing elastic recoil or impending vessel occlusion (46,47). The presence of cyclic flow variations may reflect thrombus formation. This phenomenon was first described by Folts et al. (49) and has further been characterized in animal models (50–52). This abnormal flow pattern results from the accumulation of platelets at sites of injury postintervention. As the accumulation of platelet aggregates increases, the flow declines. A pressure gradient develops across the mass of platelet causing it to dislodge with a sudden increase in flow. Angiographically this phenomenon correlates with the presence of thrombus (46). Following PTCA, cyclic alterations in coronary flow have been detected in approximately 20% of cases (53). Whether this flow pattern is a marker for abrupt closure in humans is unknown, but animal studies suggest it may be, since it often precedes complete thrombotic occlusion in animal models. The identification of these abnormal flow patterns is important because they may allow the interventionalist to alter therapy to prevent catastrophic complications. In cases of spasm, IC nitroglycerin may be given. Impending closure or recoil may require stent placement. Abnormal coronary phasic flow has also been reverted or abolished with the administration of glycoprotein receptor IIb/IIIa (53,54).

X. ASSESSMENT OF COLLATERAL FLOW WITH DOPPLER FLOWIRE

Until recently collateral channels have been evaluated mainly by angiographic grading systems, which are qualitative and subjective (55,56). The development of the Doppler Flowire has permitted the quantitative assessment of both antegrade and retrograde flow distal to totally or subtotally occluded vessels supplied by mature collateral vessels or acutely recruitable conduits. Kern et al. (57) studied 21 patients undergoing routine angioplasty. Collateral flow was defined as retrograde or persistent antegrade flow during balloon occlusion. Retrograde flow was observed in 17 patients. The collateral flow had a phasic pattern that was highly variable. Mean collateral flow velocity was approximately 30% of normal postangioplasty antegrade flow velocity. The mean time of appearance or retrograde collateral flow velocity was 18 ± 7 sec. The collateral data demonstrated no differences between left-to-right collateral flow patterns with respect to mean velocity, diastolic, or systolic velocity integrals or the ratio of the diastolic-to-systolic flow integrals. Two patients had persistent antegrade flow during balloon occlusion. Both patients had right-to-septal-to-left anterior descending communications. Absolute flow velocity values were similar to retrograde flow velocity data. There was poor correlation (r = 0.4) between the magnitude of collateral flow velocity and angiographic score because 11 patients had only acutely recruitable collaterals. The largest epicardial communicating branches had the highest retrograde diastolic flow. At the conclusion of the angioplasty, restoration of the normal coronary flow velocity was evident.

Doppler Flowire has also been helpful to quantitate the influence of different pharmacological agents on the enhancement of collateral flow. Donohue et al. (58) reported that the effect of intracoronary nitroglycerine and adenosine on retrograde collateral flow during balloon angioplasty was negligible, whereas significant enhancement of collateral flow was produced by repeated balloon occlusions in the recipient artery.

The plausible applications of accurately measuring collateral flow include identifying patients who may have an increased margin of safety undergoing coronary angioplasty, or identifying patients in whom collateral flow may obviate more invasive and potentially complicating hemodynamic support measures, such as intra-aortic balloon pump or cardiopulmonary bypass in the catheterization laboratory. It will also permit the assessment of new pharmacological agents that may potentially enhance collateral flow (57).

XI. COMPARATIVE UTILITY OF DOPPLER FLOWIRE AND INTRAVASCULAR ULTRASOUND (IVUS)

IVUS and Doppler Flowire are new intravascular imaging modalities that have contributed to overcome the deficiencies of angiography in assessing coronary artery disease. IVUS has supplemented the morphological information provided by angiography and the Doppler Flowire has added physiological data. Both intravascular tools have important diagnostic and interventional applications.

A. Diagnostic Applications

The tomographic images of the coronary vessels provided by IVUS enable direct and accurate measurements of the lumen dimensions including diameter and cross-sectional area. The superiority of IVUS examination over quantitative angiography for assessment of anatomical features is well established (59). IVUS has made possible the diagnosis of angiographically unrecognized atherosclerosis including diffuse concentric lesions (60), and is emerging as the gold standard for the detection of coronary vasculopathy in cardiac transplant patients (61). Problem lesions such as ostial stenosis and disease at bifurcations or left main coronary arteries are precisely defined by IVUS. In addition, angiographic stenoses of intermediate significance may be quantitated more accurately (62). The unique and detailed cross-sectional images of the arterial wall have allowed IVUS to characterize plaques, making it an important research tool for the understanding of coronary artery disease pathophysiology and for quantitating atherosclerosis in regression trials. IVUS, however, provides no information concerning the physiological significance of the lesions noted. The Doppler guidewire provides significant physiological measurements which detail flow dynamics and myocardial perfusion. The Doppler Flowire, however, provides no anatomical detail concerning the characteristics or severity of a coronary stenosis as provided by IVUS and angiography. The combination of these modalities to precisely determine both the anatomy and physiological significance of coronary lesions appears preferable.

B. Interventional Applications

By providing precise measurements of the coronary reference segments, and being able to characterize plaques, IVUS has become critical in choosing the type and size of mechanical devices for different interventions. IVUS may identify the presence of calcium missed by fluoroscopy. If extensive superficial calcification is identified, the lesion should be approached with rotational atherectomy. Directional atherectomy can be utilized when calcification is present deep within the lesion. IVUS is also useful in assessing the length of the vessel affected by atherosclerotic plaque that needs to be covered by stents.

Following an intervention, IVUS permits the evaluation of the mechanism and extent of luminal enlargement poorly defined by angiography. In cases of stent implantation it determines whether the stent has been well deployed and whether significant plaques or dissections have been left uncovered. This important postprocedural information provided by IVUS can be complemented by physiological data acquired with the Doppler Flowire. Restoration of normal flow confirms that the luminal enlargement obtained with the procedure has been sufficient. In addition, monitoring flow velocity immediately after an intervention may identify the development of abnormal flow patterns. These patterns are usually due to specific clinical situations that can be treated preventing poor outcomes. Isner et al. (63) investigated the feasibility of combining IVUS and Doppler Flowire for evaluation of patients undergoing percutaneous revascularization of stenotic or occluded coronary and peripheral arteries. A total of 76 patients were evaluated using the Flowire to guide an IVUS catheter. Revascularization was achieved by balloon angioplasty, direction atherectomy, excimer laser angioplasty, and thrombolytic therapy, alone or in combination. The study showed that the physiological findings obtained with the Flowire reinforced conclusions regarding morphological severity of candidate stenoses and anatomical adequacy of revascularization following IVUS examination. In certain ambiguous cases, information gained by one modality clarified information obtained with the other.

Several studies are underway to determine whether IVUS or coronary flow data may predict restenosis. Mintz et al. (64) recently showed that IVUS variables are more powerful and consistent predictors of angiographic stenosis than currently accepted clinical or angiographic risk factors. Serruys and Mario have recently completed the Debate Trial that evaluated postprocedural flow data as potential predictor of angiographic restenosis. They found that if the residual angiographic stenosis was $\leq$ 35% and the coronary flow reserve by Doppler Flowire was >2.5, there was a low angiographic restenosis rate as well as a reduced need for coronary intervention. This combination of angiographic and Doppler coronary flow reserve parameters allowed the identification of a group of patients immediately postangioplasty with a low restenosis rate of 16% compared to the patients who did not meet this criterion and who had a restenosis rate of 41% (p = 0.002) (65).

It is also clear that the physiological data provided by the Doppler Flowire and the anatomical information obtained with IVUS are complementary. Combining this data may provide a more sensitive and possibly more accurate analysis of significance and adequacy of revascularization than has been previously obtained with angiography alone. Whether such a detailed investigation on a routine basis will improve clinical outcome warrants further investigation.

REFERENCES

1. Detre KM, Wright E, Murphy MC, Takaro T. Observer agreement in evaluating coronary angiograms. Circulation 1975; 52:979–986.
2. Zir LM, Miller SW, Dinsmore RE, Gilbert JP, Harthorne JW. Interobserver variability in coronary angiography. Circulation 1976; 53:627–632.
3. DeRouen TA, Murray JA, Owen W. Variability analysis of coronary arteriograms. Circulation 1977; 55:324–328.
4. Galbraith JE, Murphy ML, DeSoyza N. Coronary angiogram interpretation: interobserver variability. JAMA 1978; 240:2053–2056.
5. Hutchins GM, Bulkley BH, Ridolfi RL, Griffith LSC, Lohr FT, Piasio MA. Correlation of coronary arteriograms and left ventriculograms with postmortem studies. Circulation 1977; 56:32–37.
6. Grondin CM, Dyrda I, Pasternac A, Campeau L, Bourassa MG, Lesperance J. Discrepancies between cineangiographic and postmortem findings in patients with

coronary artery disease and recent myocardial revascularization. Circulation 1974; 49:703–708.

7. Arnett EN, Isner JM, Redwood DR, Kent KM, Baker WP, Ackerstein H, Roberts WC. Coronary artery narrowing in coronary heart disease: comparison of cine-angiographic and necropsy findings. Ann Intern Med 1979; 91:350–356.

8. Waller BF. "Crackers, breakers, stretchers, drillers, scrapers, shavers, burners, welders, and melters": the future treatment of atherosclerotic coronary artery disease? A clinical-morphological assessment. J Am Coll Cardiol 1989; 13: 969–987.

9. Doucette JW, Corl PD, Payne HM, Flynn AE, Goto M, Nassi M, Segal J. Validation of a Doppler gadder for intravascular measurement of coronary artery flow velocity. Circulation 1992; 85:1899–1911.

10. Vanyi J, Bowers T, Jarvis G, White CW. Can an intracoronary Doppler wire accurately measure changes in coronary blood flow velocity? Cathet Card Diagnosis 1993; 29:240–246.

11. Ofili EO, Labovitz AJ, Kern MJ. Coronary flow velocity dynamics in normal and diseased arteries. Am J Cardiol 1993; 71:3D–9D.

12. Gould KL, Lipscomb K, Hamilton GW. Physiologic basis for assessing critical coronary stenosis. Am J Cardiol 1974; 33:87.

13. Furuse A, Klopp EH, Brawley RK, Gott VL. Hemodynamic determinations in the assessment of distal coronary artery disease. J Surg Res 1975; 19:25–33.

14. Wiesner TF, Levesque MJ, Rooz E, et al. Epicardial coronary blood flow including the presence of stenoses and aortocoronary bypasses. II. Experimental comparison and parametric investigations. Trans Am Soc Mech Eng 1988; 110:144.

15. Ofili EO, Kern MJ, Labovitz AJ, St. Vrain JA, Segal J, Aguirre FV, Castello R. Analysis of coronary blood flow velocity dynamics in angiographically normal and stenoses arteries before and after endolumen by angioplasty. J Am Coll Cardiol 1993; 21:308–316.

16. Segal J, Kern MJ, Scott NA, King SB, Doucette JW, Heuser RR, Ofili E, Siegel R. Alterations of phasic coronary artery flow velocity in humans during percutaneous angioplasty. J Am Coll Cardiol 1992; 20:276–286.

17. Logan SE. On the fluid mechanics of human coronary artery stenosis. IEEE Trans Biomed Eng 1975; 22:327.

18. Katz LN, Linder E. Quantitative relation between reactive hyperemia and the myocardial ischemia which it follows. Am J Physiol 1939; 126:283–288.

19. White CW. Clinical applications of Doppler coronary flow reserve measurements. Am J Cardiol 1993; 71:10D–16D.

20. Kern MJ. Interpretation and application of intracoronary Doppler flow velocity for coronary interventions. In: Current Review of Interventional Cardiology. 1994: 14.1–14.30.

21. Nitenberg A, Tavolaro O, Benvenuti C, Loisance D, Foult J-M, Hittinger L, Castigne A, Cachera J-P, Vernant P. Recovery of a normal coronary vascular reserve after rejection therapy in acute human cardiac allograft rejection. Circulation 1990; 81:1312–1318.

22. Cannon RO, Epstein SE. Chest pain and "normal" coronary arteries: role of small coronary arteries. Am J Cardiol 1985; 55:508.

23. White CW, Wright CB, Doty DB, Hiratza LF, Eastham CL, Harrison DG, Marcus ML. Does visual interpretation of the coronary arteriogram predict the physiologic importance of a coronary stenosis? N Engl J Med 1984; 310:819–824.

24. Vogel RA. Assessing stenosis significance by coronary arteriography. Are the best variables good enough? J Am Coll Cardiol 1988; 12:692–693.

25. Donohue TJ, Kern MJ, Aguirre FV, Bach RG, Wolford T, Bell CA, Segal J. Assessing the hemodynamic significance of coronary artery stenoses: analysis of translesional pressure-flow velocity relations in patients. J Am Coll Cardiol 1993; 22:449–458.

26. American College of Physicians. Efficacy of exercise thallium-201 scintigraphy in the diagnosis and prognosis of coronary artery disease. Ann Intern Med 1990; 113: 703–704.

27. Gould KL, Lipscomb K, Hamilton GW. Physiologic basis for assessing critical coronary stenosis: instantaneous flow response and regional distribution during coronary hyperemia as measures of coronary flow reserve. Am J Cardiol 1974; 33: 87–94.

28. Kern MJ, Donohue TJ, Aguirre FV, Bach RG, Caracciolo EA, Ofili E, Labovitz AJ. Assessment of angiographically intermediate coronary artery stenosis using the Doppler Flowire. Am J Cardiol 1993; 71:26D–33D.

29. Gould KL, Lipscomb K. Effects of coronary stenoses on coronary flow reserve and resistance. Am J Cardiol 1974; 34:48–55.

30. Marcus ML, Wright CB, Doty DB, Eastham C, Laughlin D, Krum P, Fastenow C, Brody M. Measurements of coronary velocity and reactive hyperemia in the coronary circulation of humans. Circ Res 1981; 49:877–891.

31. Miller DD, Donohue TJ, Younis LT, Bach RG, Aguirre FV, Wittry MD, Goodgold HM, Chaitman BR, Kern MJ. Correlation of pharmacological 99mTC-Sestamibi myocardial perfusion imaging with poststenotic coronary flow reserve in patients with angiographically intermediate coronary artery stenoses. Circulation 1994; 89: 2150–2160.

32. Joye FD, Schulman DS, Lasorda D, Farah T, Donohue BC, Reichek N. Intracoronary Doppler guide wire stress single-photon emission computed tomographic thallium-201 imaging in assessment of intermediate coronary stenoses. J Am Coll Cardiol 1994; 24:940–947.

33. Deychak YA, Segal J, Reiner JS, Rohrbeck SC, Thompson MA, Lundergan CF, Ross AM, Wasserman AG. Doppler guide wire flow-velocity indexes measured distal to coronary stenoses associated with reversible thallium perfusion defects. Am Heart J 1995; 129:219–227.

34. Lesser JR, Wilson RF, White CW. Physiologic assessment of coronary stenoses of intermediate severity can facilitate patient selection for coronary angioplasty. Coronary Artery Dis 1990; 1:697–705.

35. Kern MJ, Donohue TJ, Aguirre FV, Bach RG, Caracciolo EA, Wolford T, Mechem CJ, Flynn MS, Chaitman B. Clinical outcome of deferring angioplasty in patients

with normal translesional pressure-flow velocity measurements. J Am Coll Cardiol 1995; 1:178–187.

36. Segal J. Applications of coronary flow velocity during angioplasty and other coronary intervention procedures. Am J Cardiol 1993; 71:17D–25D.

37. Deychak Y, Segal J, Thompson MA, Lundergan CL. Changes in coronary artery flow velocity in humans following directional coronary atherectomy. Circulation 1992 (abstract).

38. Yock PG, Fitzgerald PJ, Linker DT, Angelsen BAJ. Intravascular guidance for catheter based interventions. Circulation 1991; 17:39B–45B.

39. Yock PG, Fitzgerald PJ, Sudhir K, Linker DT, White W, Ports A. Intravascular ultrasound imaging for guidance of atherectomy and other plaque removal techniques. Int J Cardiac Imaging 1991; 6:179–189.

40. Ge J, Erbel R, Zamorano J, Haude M, Kearney P, Gorge G, Meyer J. Improvement of coronary morphology and blood after stenting. Assessment by intravascular ultrasound and intracoronary Doppler. Int J Cardiac Imaging 1995; 11:81–87.

41. Bach RG, Kern MJ, Bell C, Donohue TJ, Aguirre F. Clinical application of coronary flow velocity for stent placement during coronary angioplasty. Am Heart J 1993; 125:873–876.

42. Kern MJ, Donohue T, Bach R, Aguirre F, Bell C. Monitoring cyclical coronary blood flow alterations after coronary angioplasty for stent restenosis with a Doppler guide wire. Am Heart J 1993; 125:1159–1161.

43. Hong MK, Wong C, Mintz G, Popma JJ, Kent KM, Pichard AD, Satler L, Leon MB. Can coronary flow parameters after stent placement predict restenosis? Cath Cardiov Diag 1995; 36:278–280.

44. Nunez BD, Keelan ET, Lerman A, Higano ST, Garratt KN, Nishimura RA, Holmes DR Jr. Coronary hemodynamics after rotational atherectomy. JACC 1995; 95A (Suppl) (abstract).

45. Khoury AF, Aguirre FV, Bach RG, Caracciolo EA, Donohue TJ, Wolford TH, Mechem C, Herrmann SC, Kern MJ. Influence of percutaneous transluminal coronary rotational atherectomy with adjunctive percutaneous transluminal coronary angioplasty on coronary blood flow. Am Heart J 1996; 131:631–638.

46. Anderson HV, Kirkeeide RL, Stuart Y, Smalling RW, Heibig J, Willerson JT. Coronary artery flow monitoring following coronary interventions. Am J Cardiol 1993; 71:62D–69D.

47. Kern MJ, Bach RG, Donohue TJ, Caracciolo EA, Aguirre FV, Mechem C, Cauley M, Abbott L. Clinical utility of continuous coronary flow velocity monitoring during interventional studies. Cathet Cardiovasc Diagn 1993; 29:81 (abstract).

48. Kern MJ, Aguirre FV, Donohue TJ, Bach RG, Caracciolo EA, Flynn MS, Wolford T, Moore JA. Continuous coronary flow velocity monitoring during coronary interventions: velocity trend patterns associated with adverse events. Am Heart J 1994; 128:426–434.

49. Folts JD, Crowell EB, Rowe GG. Platelet aggregation in partially obstructed vessels and its elimination with aspirin. Circulation 1976; 54:365–370.

50. Eidt JF, Ashton J, Golino P, McNatt J, Buja LM, Willerson JT. Thomboxane A2 and serotonin mediated coronary blood flow reductions in unsedated dogs. Am J Physiol 1989; 257:H873–H882.

51. Yao SK, Rosolowski M, Anderson HV, Golino P, McNatt, DeClerck F, Buja LM, Willerson JT. Combined thromboxane A2 synthetase inhibition and receptor blockade are effective in preventing spontaneous and epinephrine-induced canine coronary cyclic flow variations. J Am Coll Cardiol 1990; 16:705–713.

52. Yao SK, Ober JC, McNatt J, Benedict CR, Rosolowski M, Anderson HV, Cui K, Maffrand JP, Campbell WP, Buja LM, Willerson JT. ADP plays an important role in mediating platelet aggregation and cyclic flow variations in vivo in stenosed and endothelium-injured canine arteries. Circ Res 1992; 70:39–48.

53. Anderson HV, Kireeide RL, Krishnaswami A, Weigelt LA, Revana M, Weisman HF, Willerson JT. Cyclic variations after coronary angioplasty in humans: clinical and angiographic characteristics and elimination with 7E3 monoclonal antiplatelet antibody. J Am Coll Cardiol 1994; 23:1031–1037.

54. Anderson HV, Revana M, Rosales O, Brannigan L, Stuart Y, Weisman H, Willerson JT. Intravenous administration of monoclonal antibody to the platelet GPIIb/IIIa receptor to treat abrupt closure during coronary angioplasty. Am J Cardiol 1992; 69:1373–1376.

55. Cohen M, Rentrop KP. Limitation of myocardial ischemia by collateral circulation during sudden controlled coronary artery occlusion in human subjects: a prospective study. Circulation 1986; 74:469–476.

56. Rentrop KP, Thornton JC, Feit F, VanBuskirk M. Determinants and protective potential of coronary arterial collateral as assessed by an angioplasty mode. Am J Cardiol 1988; 61:677–684.

57. Kern MJ, Donohue TJ, Bach RG, Aguirre FV, Caracciolo EA, Ofili EO. Quantitating coronary collateral flow velocity in patients during coronary angioplasty using a Doppler guidewire. Am J Cardiol 1993; 71:34D–40D.

58. Donohue T, Kern MJ, Bach R, Aguirre F, Wolford T. An examination of the effects of hemodynamic and pharmacologic interventions on coronary collateral flow in a patient during cardiac catheterization. Cathet Cardiovasc Diagn 1993; 28:155–161.

59. Topol EJ, Nissen SE. Our preoccupation with coronary luminology. The dissociation between clinical and angiographic findings in ischemic heart disease. Circulation 1995; 92:2333–2342.

60. Sheikh KH, Harrison JK, Harding MB, et al. Detection of angiographically silent coronary atherosclerosis by intracoronary ultrasonography. Am Heart J 1991; 121: 1803–1807.

61. Valantine H, Pinto FJ, St. Goar FG. Intracoronary ultrasound imaging in heart transplant recipients: the Stanford experience. J Heart Lung Transplant 1992; 11: S60–S64.

62. Nissen SE, Tuzcu EM, De Franco AC. Coronary intravascular ultrasound: diagnostic and interventional applications. In: Textbook of Interventional Cardiology.

63. Isner JM, Kaufman J, Rosenfield K, Pieczek A, Schainfeld R, Ramaswamy K, Kosowsky BD. Combined physiologic and anatomic assessment of percutaneous revascularization using a Doppler guidewire and ultrasound catheter. Am J Cardiol 1993; 71:70D–86D.

64. Mintz GS, Popma JJ, Pichard AD, Kent DM, Satler LF, Chuang YC, Griffin J, Leon MB. Intravascular ultrasound predictors of restenosis after percutaneous transcatheter coronary revascularization. J Am Coll Cardiol 1996; 27:1678–1687.

65. Serruys PW, Mario CD. Prognostic value of coronary flow velocity and diameter stenosis in assessing the short and long term outcome of balloon angioplasty: the Debate Study (Doppler endpoints balloon angioplasty trial Europe). Am Heart Assoc 1996; 94:1847.

10

Three-Dimensional Intravascular Ultrasound Reconstruction and Quantification: A Valuable Approach for Clinical Decision-Making

Clemens von Birgelen, Maria Teresa Mallus, and Patrick W. Serruys *Thorax Center, University Hospital Rotterdam-Dijkzigt, Erasmus University, Rotterdam, The Netherlands*

I. INTRODUCTION

Intravascular ultrasound (IVUS) permits the examination of the extent, distribution, and result of therapy of the atherosclerotic plaque as it provides a unique tomographic visualization of both the lumen and vessel wall (1–8). However, in conventional IVUS there is a lack of "angiography-like" longitudinal visualization of the examined coronary segment which is provided only by three-dimensional (3D) IVUS approaches (9–16). This ability to visualize the plaque in an entire coronary segment helps to avoid the difficult mental conceptualization process required when using 2D IVUS, provides a more detailed insight into the complex plaque architecture, and facilitates serial IVUS studies (14, 17–20). Moreover, in parallel with the progress in quantitative angiography techniques that started with manual caliper assessment and finally reached computer-assisted methods (21, 22), automated methods of quantitative 3D IVUS analysis have been developed (14,15,19,23–27) to reduce the analysis time and the subjectivity of manual tracing (28). These

177

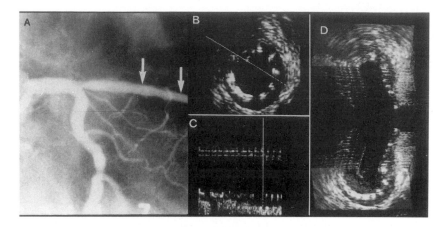

Figure 1 Left anterior descending coronary artery with a Wallstent (A, arrows) implanted. The IVUS revealed proximally an incomplete stent deployment, shown as a zone of low echogenicy between the bright stent struts and the vessel wall. The black area is displayed in cross-sectional (B; between 1 and 6 o'clock), longitudinal (C, lower right-hand side), and spatial cylindrical views (D; anterior right-hand side), suggesting additional balloon dilatations at this site. There are image artifacts (B, at 11 o'clock; C, upper part; D, left-hand side), resulting from the strut of the 4.3 F IVUS catheter. The new sheath-based IVUS catheters do not show such artifacts as they operate with a flexible rotating imaging core inside an echo-transparent sheath.

techniques permit the careful evaluation of coronary segments of interest before and/or after interventional procedures (10–13,16,29–31) (Fig. 1) and allow online measurements of the target lesion and the reference segments (16,25,26), which may facilitate the selection of the optimal type and size of interventional device and the evaluation of potential complications.

II. METHODS AND TECHNICAL NOTES

Before any 3D feature can be used in clinical practice, data processing has to be performed that follows similar basic steps for all 3D systems currently available. Nevertheless, there are significant differences in the manner of image acquisition, the method of image segmentation, and the features provided for 3D visualization and measurement of the vascular segment examined.

A. Image Acquisition

After the IVUS machine settings have been optimized (e.g., time-gain compensation and zoom factor), image acquisition is started distal to the stenosis while the imaging catheter is withdrawn through the arterial segment to be reconstructed.

1. IVUS Catheter Design

Sheath-based IVUS catheters are frequently used, as they are designed for repeated pullbacks and have the advantage that the imaging core has no direct contact with the vessel wall. Such catheters are equipped with a long transparent distal sheath which houses the transducer. There are two catheter designs: a short monorail, and a common distal lumen catheter. The distal lumen of the latter alternatively houses the guidewire (during catheter introduction) or the transducer (during imaging when the guidewire has been pulled back). These IVUS catheter designs reduce the risks of nonuniformity of speed in continuous pullbacks. However, during the first 5 to 10 sec of a continuous pullback the imaging core may straighten out inside the catheter before a constant withdrawal speed is achieved.

2. Continuous Transducer Pullback

There are different pullback methods that can be applied. A continuous uniform-speed pullback, resulting in an equidistant spacing of adjacent images (32) is still the most common approach (Fig. 2). Sidebranches or spots of calcium are used as topographic landmarks to ensure a reliable comparison of the same arterial segment in serial studies. However, systolic-diastolic artifacts can hamper the reconstruction of IVUS images acquired during such pullbacks (Fig. 3).

3. ECG-Gated Image Acquisition

Combined use of an ECG-gated image acquisition station and a dedicated pullback device (stepping motor) is the most sophisticated and accurate way to overcome the problem of cyclic motion artifacts (Fig. 4). However, the time required for the image acquisition is still somewhat longer than for a conventional acquisition. Using a dynamic 3D reconstruction system, initially designed for 3D reconstruction of echocardiographic images (EchoScan, TomTec, Munich, Germany), the arterial segment can be displayed in 3D and vascular dimensions may be measured at any time of the cardiac cycle. Before image acquisition starts, the upper and lower limits of the R-R interval are defined. Up to 25 IVUS images per cardiac cycle can be sampled (if the length of the

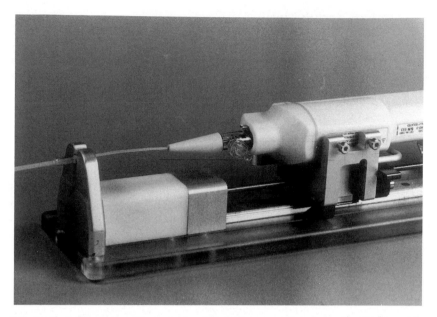

Figure 2 Motorized pullback device for continuous uniform-speed pullbacks of the IVUS transducer. A sheath-based IVUS catheter is connected to the handle of the IVUS machine, which is attached on the sledge (right-hand side) of the pullback device. As the proximal end of the external sheath is fixed, the motion of the telescopic IVUS imaging core with the transducer at its tip corresponds to the motion of the handle on the sledge of the pull-back device.

R-R interval meets the preset range) which permits various transverse or longitudinal reconstructions of the arterial segment and allows to show its motion (dynamic visualization) during an entire cardiac cycle (33,34).

B. Digitization and Segmentation

Digitization of the IVUS images can be performed on line or off-line by sampling the IVUS frames with a frame grabber at a defined rate. The segmentation of the IVUS images, a processing step which identifies structures of interest according to a certain gray-scale scheme, can be achieved by the application of dedicated algorithms which discriminate between the blood-pool inside the lumen and structures of the vessel wall (35). The quality of the reconstruction and the accuracy of the quantitative analysis are highly influenced by the characteristics of the chosen segmentation algorithm (Table 1).

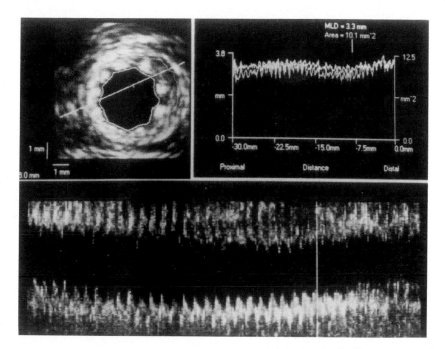

Figure 3 Cyclic artifacts in a venous bypass graft. The longitudinally reconstructed image of a stented bypass graft shows enormous saw-shaped artifacts, resulting from the cyclic vessel pulsation and the movement of the IVUS catheter inside ("catheter fluttering"). The artifacts are visible in both the longitudinal display and the graph, showing the measurements of the luminal cross-sectional area and the minimum diameter (right upper panel). (Reprinted from Ref. 31, with permission.)

The applicability of thresholding, which is based on the definition of a threshold value in the grayscale (9), depends significantly upon the basic IVUS image quality. Nevertheless, in instances with optimal IVUS image quality, remarkable 3D reconstructions can be obtained. Segmentation can also be achieved by the application of more sophisticated algorithms such as acoustic quantification (24,25) or contour detection algorithms (14,15,36).

The acoustic quantification method (Fig. 1) distinguishes between the blood pool and the vessel wall by use of an algorithm for statistical pattern recognition (16,24–26) (EchoQuant, Indec, Capitola, CA). The algorithm is able to distinguish between these two patterns and to detect the interface between blood and vessel wall.

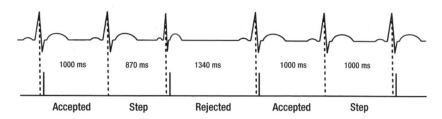

Figure 4 Combined use of an ECG-gated 3D image acquisition station (EchoScan, TomTec, Munich, Germany) and a dedicated pullback device allows to overcome the problem of cyclic image artifacts. The range of the R-R interval is defined (here: 1000 ± 100 msec), before the image acquisition starts. Images for each scanning site are digitized and sampled in the computer memory, unless the length of the R-R interval fails to meet the preset range (here: third cardiac cycle). Each time a cycle has been stored, the following heart beat is required to perform a pullback step to reach the adjacent scanning site.

A contour detection system, developed at the Thoraxcenter Rotterdam, applies a minimum cost algorithm to detect not only the intimal leading edge but also the external vascular boundary, which corresponds to the external elastic lamina (14,15,19,36) (Fig. 5). Another contour detection system, developed by Sonka and colleagues, detects the luminal contour and the contours of the internal and external elastic laminae; initial studies show a good correlation with lumen and plaque area measurements obtained by manual tracing (27,37).

Table 1 Characteristics of Selected 3D IVUS Systems

	Acoustic quantification	Contour detection
Applicability	• No geometric assumption on lumen shape required • Depends much on image quality	• User interaction is required in irregular lumen shape • Depends less on image quality
On-line use	• Feasible	• Feasible with ECG-gated image acquisition
Automated detection	• Only detection of intimal leading edge is possible	• Detection of both intimal leading edge and external vessel contour is possible

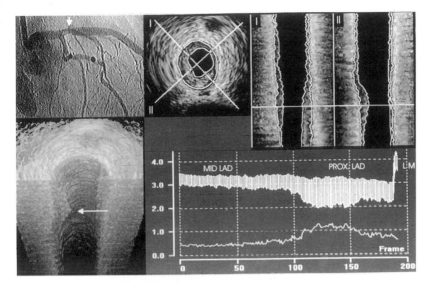

Figure 5 Primary lesion in a proximal left anterior descending coronary artery (LAD), assessed by 3D IVUS and the Thoraxcenter contour detection system. An arrowhead indicates the target stenosis in the cylindrical reconstruction (left lower panel). The mean diameter measurements are shown in the right lower panel. The white zone represents the plaque; the absolute values of the plaque diameter are also shown as a single line. The plaque burden at the site of the mid-LAD was 20%. According to the mechanism described by Glagov, an enlargement of the total vessel partly compensating the plaque burden may be expected at the site of relatively focal plaque formation. In this case, however, a paradoxical reduction of the total vessel dimensions from the distal reference in the mid LAD to the target stenosis in the proximal segment was observed. (Reprinted from Ref. 41, with permission.)

C. Three-Dimensional Reconstruction and Display

Specific shading and rendering techniques are used to give the 3D-reconstructed views a spatial aspect when displayed on the 2D computer screen. Different display formats can be used to present the 3D data sets (Fig. 5). A longitudinal and a cylindrical format are most commonly generated. General programs for 3D presentation display the reconstructed vascular segment in various views including oblique and tangential sections, comparable to display options available in magnetic resonance imaging systems. A dynamic visualization of the artery after ECG-gated image acquisition is also possible (33).

D. 3D IVUS Systems: The Thoraxcenter Experience

Different 3D IVUS systems are available which are based on different techni-cal approaches with specific advantages and disadvantages in applicability, imaging, and quantification. At the Thoraxcenter the largest experience was gained with an acoustic quantification system and the Thoraxcenter contour detection system; the latter can be used in combination with an ECG-gated IVUS image acquisition station (EchoScan).

1. Acoustic Quantification System

This 3D IVUS system (EchoQuant) samples images with a digitization frame rate of 8.5 frames per second. The length of the reconstructed coronary seg-ment is determined by the pullback speed, since the image acquisition and digitization rates are fixed (e.g., 80 mm at a pullback speed of 1.0 mm/sec). Segmentation and reconstruction of a vascular segment of 30 mm length can be performed within 3 min.

The pattern recognition algorithm which detects the bloodpool inside the lumen does not require a geometric assumption of the lumen shape (24) and may therefore provide accurate detection of an irregularly shaped lumen. However, application of the algorithm may be hampered by the quality of the basic IVUS images (24,25). It is not capable of detecting the external vascular boundary, but as the reconstruction is performed within a few minutes, it can be used online in the catheterization laboratory (25) (Fig. 6). A selected cross-sectional image, a longitudinally reconstructed image, and a cylindrical 3D view (presenting the segment opened longitudinally) are displayed by the system.

2. Thoraxcenter Contour Detection System

This 3D analysis system allows for the analysis of a 3D set of IVUS images, digitized off-line from videotape or online by an ECG-gated image acquisition station (EchoScan). A maximum of 200 IVUS images can be examined, permitting the reliable analysis of approximately 25 mm long (uniform pull-back) or 40 mm long (ECG-gated pullback) segments. This method depends less on the image quality than the acoustic quantification method does, and reliable segmentation and 3D reconstruction remain possible even when the image quality is not optimal; however, a certain degree of user interaction is required in the presence of very irregular lumen shapes. On-line application of this system has recently been introduced, using the ECG-gated image acquisi-tion approach.

The contour detection procedure consists of three steps (14,15,36) (Fig. 7). First, the IVUS images are modeled in a voxel space (38), and two perpendicu-

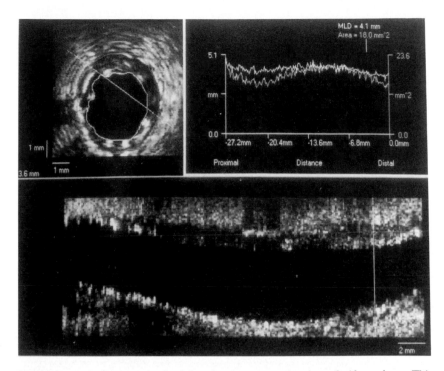

Figure 6   Stented segment of a right coronary artery, showing a fusiform shape. This luminal silhouette results from the use of a short balloon of low compliance, which was chosen to optimize the result of stenting without the risk of an injury of the nonstented references proximal and distal to the stent. The maximum instent lumen diameter is in the midportion and the minimal lumen diameter is at the distal ending (vertical cursor in the lower panel) of the stent. Note the lack of difference between the size of the lumen at the smallest in-stent site and the distal vessel segment. (Reprinted from Ref. 26, with permission.)

lar longitudinal sections of the vascular segment are reconstructed. In a second step an automated detection of the longitudinal contours of the luminal and external vascular boundaries (external elastic lamina) is performed, based on the application of a minimum cost algorithm (39). In each individual cross-sectional image the contours of the longitudinal sections (Fig. 8) are depicted as points that guide the automated contour detection in the cross-sectional IVUS images (third step) and permit area and volume measurements of both lumen and plaque (14,15,19,36) (Fig. 9).

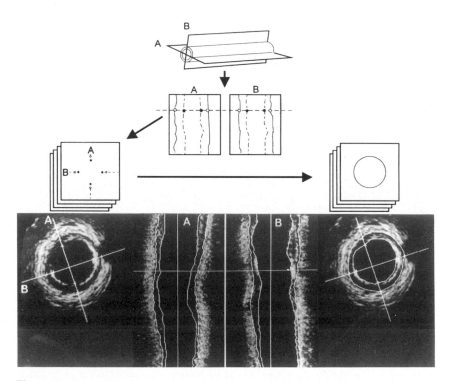

Figure 7 Principle of the 3D contour detection system. The IVUS images, obtained during a motorized pullback, are stored in the computer memory as a "voxel space." The method has the concept that edge points, derived from longitudinal contours which were previously detected on two longitudinally reconstructed images (A,B), guide and facilitate the final contour detection on the transverse IVUS images. The position of an individual transverse plane in the longitudinal sections is indicated by a horizontal cursor line, which can be used to scroll through the whole series of transverse IVUS images. (Reprinted from Ref. 14, with permission.)

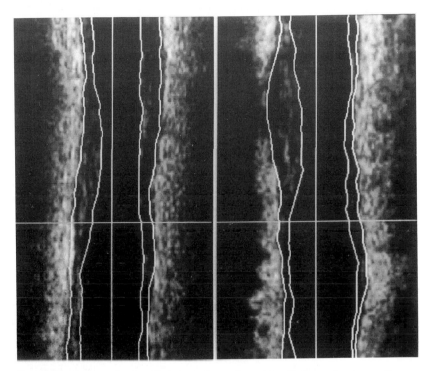

Figure 8 Two longitudinal IVUS sections of a proximal left anterior descending coronary artery at 6-months follow-up after directional coronary atherectomy; the longitudinal views were obtained from the Thoraxcenter contour detection system (reprinted from Ref. 14, with permission).

III. CLINICAL VALIDATION AND APPLICATION

A. Automated Measurement of Vascular Dimensions

The 3D systems extend the measurement features of IVUS by longitudinal and volumetric measurements and provide an automated quantitation of the plaque and/or the vascular lumen (19,40). These measurements are used to plan interventional strategies, appropriately size devices, and guide the procedures. Therefore it is very important to determine the reliability of these automated measurement tools and to perform a decent validation. Such a comprehensive validation has been performed only for a few 3D IVUS systems such as, for in-

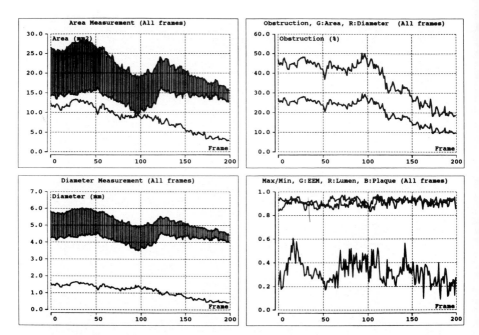

Figure 9   Display of 3D IVUS measurement results corresponding to the coronary segment displayed in Figure 8. The left panels show area and mean diameter measurements of lumen, total vessel, and plaque, provided by the Thoraxcenter contour detection method. The gray areas represent the coronary plaque, and the upper and lower boundaries of these gray zones correspond with the dimensions of the coronary lumen and the total vessel. Absolute plaque measurements are shown as a single-line function for both area and diameter measurements (left panels). Functions of the diameter-stenosis (%) and area-obstruction (%) are displayed in the right upper panel. The right lower panel shows the symmetry of lumen and total vessel and the eccentricity of the plaque. (Reprinted from Ref. 14, with permission.)

stance, the binary threshold-based system validated by Matar et al. (23) or the contour detection-based approach of Sonka and colleagues (27,37).

1. Acoustic Quantification System

The pattern recognition algorithm of the acoustic quantification system which is able to distinguish between the blood pool inside the lumen and the vessel wall has been validated by Hausmann et al. in 29 aortal segments of New Zealand rabbits (24). Lumen area measurements by repeated automated analyses, and automated and manual analyses showed high correlations ($r = .97$ for both) and differences of $1 \pm 10\%$ and $-2 \pm 10\%$, respectively. The correlation between quantitative angiographic measurements and automated 3D IVUS measurements was also high ($r = .93$); the between-measurement difference was $7 \pm 14\%$ (24).

The acoustic quantification system permits the on-line quantification of the coronary lumen and has frequently been used at the Thoraxcenter Rotterdam during stent procedures (Fig. 4). To evaluate the reliability of the automated measurement of the minimal luminal cross-sectional area, we performed a clinical validation by comparing the 3D IVUS measurements in 38 coronary stents with results obtained by conventional 2D IVUS, and both geometric and videodensitometric quantitative coronary angiography (25). The results by 3D IVUS were slightly (NS) smaller than the results by 2D IVUS (8.1 ± 2.7 mm^2 vs. 8.3 ± 2.5 mm^2). The correlation between the measurements by 3D and 2D IVUS ($r = .81$) was almost as high as the correlation between the two standard techniques of quantitative coronary angiography ($r = .84$) (25), which is known to be high in relatively circular lumen shapes (21). Measurements by 3D IVUS showed a higher correlation with videodensitometry ($r = .70$) than with geometric quantitative coronary angiography ($r = .58$) (35), most likely because measurement of the luminal area is the basic quantification approach of both IVUS and videodensitometry whereas the geometric angiographic approach depends on the angiographic projection used, which is especially important in eccentric stent configurations.

2. Thoraxcenter Contour Detection System

This has been carefully validated both in vitro and in vivo. We used the 3D IVUS approach in a tubular phantom, consisting of four segments with luminal diameters between 2 and 5 mm, and found excellent correlations ($r = .99$) between the 3D lumen area and volume measurements and the true values (14). Deviation between the 3D measurements and the true values were small (-0.7 to 3.9%, areas; 0.3 to 1.7%, volumes) (14). A histomorphometric validation study was performed in vitro in 13 atherosclerotic human coronary segments with area stenoses of at least 40%, demonstrating the reliability of the contour detection system (15). Measurements of lumen, total vessel, and plaque, obtained by the 3D contour detection system, showed a good correlation with morphometric measurements on histologic sections ($r = .80$ to $.94$, areas; $.83$ to $.98$, volumes). A good agreement (mean difference $\leq 3.7\%$ with SD $\leq 6.2\%$) and high correlation ($r = .97$ to $.99$) was found between area measurements provided by this 3D analysis system and manual tracing on single IVUS images (15).

The intraobserver and interobserver measurements by the contour detection system that were performed in atherosclerotic coronary arteries of 20 patients in vivo showed high correlations ($r = .95$ to 0.98, areas; .99, volumes) and small between-measurement differences (-0.87 to 1.1%) (14). The standard deviations of the between-measurement differences of the lumen, total vessel, and plaque measurements did not exceed 2.7%, 0.7%, and 2.8% for the volume (Fig. 10), and 7.3%, 4.4%, and 10.8% for the area measurements (14) (Fig. 11). By use of ECG-gated 3D IVUS (33), the variability of the cross-sectional area measurements can be further reduced to standard deviations of the between-measurement differences, not exceeding 5.2%, 2.7%, and 7.2% (own unpublished data), respectively.

B. Diagnostic Value Before and During Angioplasty and Atherectomy

Visualization and measurement with 3D IVUS prior to coronary interventions facilitates perception of plaque distribution and provides valuable information about target lesion, reference, and potential "tapering" of the vessel segment which may influence the interventional strategy. The benefit of 3D IVUS should be most significant in long, complex, or unclear lesions. In our experience, on-line 3D reconstruction prior to atherectomy is feasible for the examination of plaque eccentricity along an entire coronary segment.

We recently reported a case of deferred angioplasty, based on information obtained from 3D IVUS and intracoronary Doppler in an intermediate LAD lesion (41) (Fig. 5). In this patient, referred for balloon angioplasty, no compensatory enlargement of the coronary arterial wall, but a "reverse Glagovian modeling" was found, recently described in peripheral vessels (42). Based on the information provided by 3D IVUS imaging and the normal coronary flow reserve, as demonstrated by intracoronary Doppler, no coronary intervention was performed and the absence of inducible ischemia in the myocardial territory subtended by the LAD was confirmed by dobutamine stress-echocardiography. Nevertheless, the question whether coronary lesions with reverse Glagovian modeling have a specific prognosis or a different response to treatment requires further clinical investigation.

Guidance of atherectomy can be facilitated by 3D reconstruction of IVUS images, as the spatial relation between side branches and the orientation of the plaque may help to correctly direct the atherectomy cutter, reduce the frequency of deep cuts, and minimize the procedure-related damage to the non-diseased vessel wall. Volumetric IVUS evaluation before and after atherectomy allows reliable quantification of both plaque ablation and luminal enlargement

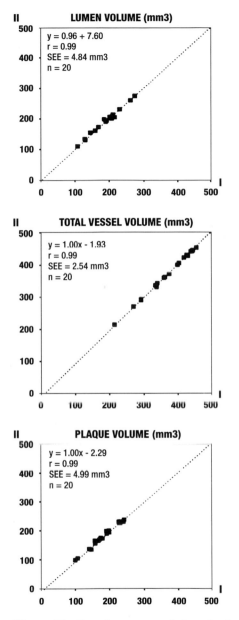

Figure 10 Interobserver correlation of volumetric IVUS measurements by the Thoraxcenter analysis system. The lumen, total vessel, and plaque volume measurements in 20 coronary segments by two independent observers (I, II) showed a high correlation in vivo; dotted lines mark the lines of identity. (Reprinted from Ref. 14, with permission.).

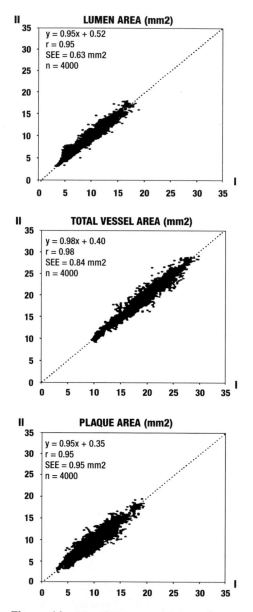

Figure 11 Interobserver correlation of cross-sectional IVUS measurements in vivo, obtained with the Thoraxcenter analysis system. The lumen, total vessel, and plaque area measurements in 4000 IVUS cross sections (20 coronary segments) by two observers (I, II) correlated well; dotted lines mark the lines of identity. (Reprinted from Ref. 14, with permission.)

and thus the understanding of the mechanism and efficacy of the device; however, to date only volumetric approaches based on 2D analysis of images acquired at 1 mm increments have been applied to evaluate this issue (43,44).

After balloon angioplasty the most significant benefit can be expected in the evaluation of postprocedural complications such as severe dissections, which may require the implantation of coronary stents (45). A comprehensive in vitro validation of both the sensitivity of 3D IVUS in the detection of dissections ($\geq$ 92% in noncalcified arteries) and in the accuracy of length and depth measurements of dissections in 3D ($\kappa \geq 0.72$ in noncalcified arteries) has been reported by Coy et al., who studied 41 peripheral arterial specimen with a threshold-based 3D IVUS system (10). The clinical feasibility of 3D IVUS (threshold-based approach) for the assessent of postinterventional dissections and plaque fractures has been evaluated by Rosenfield et al. in 12 coronary and 40 peripheral or renal arteries in vivo (9).

C. Guidance and Optimization of Stenting

Preintervention 3D IVUS examination of the coronary segment to be treated provides insight into the relation between plaque and sidebranches, permits appropriate sizing of the stent (diameter and length), and may help to reduce the frequency of procedural complications of high-pressure stenting (46). The spatial geometry of coronary stents can accurately be reconstructed (13). Automated measurement of lumen area by 3D IVUS facilitates the detection of stent underexpansion (Fig. 12), as changes of the instent cross-sectional lumen area during motorized pullbacks are frequently smooth and gradual and often difficult to recognize by conventional 2D IVUS (26). The advantages and feasibility of online 3D IVUS (acoustic quantification) for the guidance of stent implantation have recently been demonstrated. In a series of 49 stents (33 pts.) we could show that 3D IVUS is more sensitive than 2D IVUS in assessing optimal stent expansion and requires less time for analysis (2.6 ± 0.4 mm (3D) vs. 4.4 ± 1.5 min (2D); $P > .05$) (26).

We then performed 2D and 3D IVUS (acoustic quantification) examinations in 20 Wallstents and 20 Palmaz-Schatz stents (34 pts.) to study the approach of optimized angiography-guided stenting (16). The rationale for performing this study was that the strategy of optimized stent expansion by high-pressure inflations of oversized balloons had been derived from experience obtained with the Palmaz-Schatz stent, while there was little experience with such a strategy in longer stents such as the Wallstent (Fig. 13). Ultrasound criteria of adequate stent expansion were defined as 1) complete apposition of the stent to the vessel wall, 2) stent symmetry index (= minimum/maximum lumen diameter) ≥ 0.7, and 3) stent-reference lumen area ratio (= minimum instent lumen area/average of proximal and distal reference lumen area) ≥ 0.8.

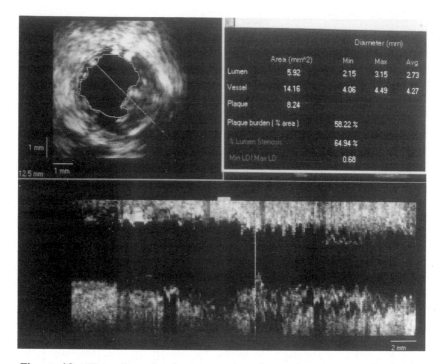

The following table appears within the figure:

	Area (mm^2)	Diameter (mm)		
		Min	Max	Avg
Lumen	5.92	2.15	3.15	2.73
Vessel	14.16	4.06	4.49	4.27
Plaque	8.24			
Plaque burden (% area)	58.22 %			
% Lumen Stenosis	64.94 %			
Min LD / Max LD	0.68			

Figure 12 Three-dimensional reconstruction of a coronary segment after implantation of three AVE Microstents (Applied Vascular Engineering, Edmonton, Canada). Asymmetric stent expansion and protrusion of stent struts of the midstent into the vessel lumen (at the site of the cursor in the lower panel) are shown. The longitudinal view (lower panel) reveals an adequate deployment of the rest of the stent. The table (right upper panel) provides measurements of the transverse IVUS image displayed (left upper panel). Avg, Max, and Min = average, minimum, and maximum, respectively; Min LD/Max LD: ratio of minimal to maximal lumen diameters. (Reprinted from Ref. 26, with permission.).

In all cases a smooth angiographic lumen and a negative diameter stenosis, based on a distal reference, was achieved. Ninety percent of failure in meeting these IVUS criteria resulted from a low stent-reference lumen area ratio. The Wallstents met the IVUS-criteria less often (2D: 10% vs. 50%, $P < .01$; 3D: 15% vs. 45%, $P < .05$), were significantly longer, and demonstrated a trend toward a larger vessel tapering (Fig. 13), measured as proximal minus distal IVUS reference lumen area (1.33 ± 2.91 mm^2 vs. 0.44 ± 1.97 mm^2; not

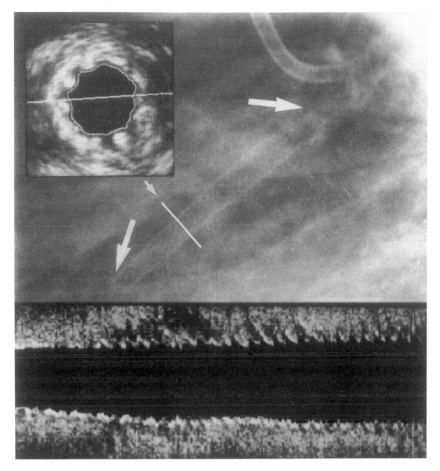

Figure 13 Long Wallstent implanted in left anterior descending coronary artery. Arrowheads indicate the proximal and distal ends of the stent on the radiographic image (upper panel). The location of the transverse IVUS image (insert) is indicated by a small arrowhead. A longitudinal view (lower panel) is reconstructed, showing a smooth tapering of the luminal dimensions from proximal (right) to distal (left). (Reprinted from Ref. 16, with permission.)

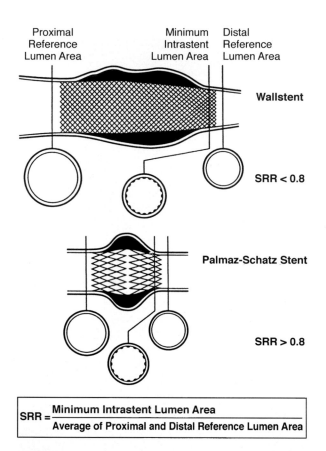

Figure 14 Possible explanation for the difficulty in achieving a stent/reference lumen area ratio (SRR) $\geq$ 0.8 following Wallstent implantation. In this scheme the Wallstent clearly tapers and does not fulfill the SRR criterion, as the minimal lumen area is located near the distal reference site, with lumen dimensions significantly smaller than the proximal reference. The example of the Palmaz-Schatz stent, however, shows little vessel tapering and is much more likely to fulfill the SRR criterion. (Reprinted from Ref. 16, with permission.)

significant); Wallstents meeting the IVUS criteria, however, showed less vessel tapering (0.18 $\pm$ 1.64 mm^2). Thus, although angiographic results and visual assessment of the IVUS examination suggested a good outcome for both Palmaz-Schatz and Wallstent, few Wallstents met the IVUS criteria in contrast to the Palmaz-Schatz stents. This is most likely due to vessel tapering, which suggests that the stent-reference lumen area ratio may be unsuitable for the assessment of the adequacy of relatively long stents such as the Wallstent (16) (Fig. 14).

A display of the lumen symmetry measurements, as provided by the Thoraxcenter contour detection system, allows to review the stent symmetry along the entire stented segment at a quick glance. Moreover, the algorithm of the Thoraxcenter contour detection system (14,15) has been modified for the computerized assessment of instent neointima at follow-up; it allows the detection of both neointimal leading edge and stent struts, and thus the quantification of instent neointimal volume, which is evaluated in both the ERASER trial (studying the effect of ReoPro in Palmaz-Schatz stents) and the TRAPIST trial (studying the effect of Trapidil in Wallstents).

IV. LIMITATIONS, CHALLENGES, AND FUTURE DIRECTIONS

Several factors, including general problems related to IVUS (47,48) as well as specific limitations of the 3D reconstruction (49), influence the quality of the reconstruction. Measurement of both lumen and plaque volumes showed minimal short-term biologic variability upon repeated pullbacks of the same coronary artery segment (50). The quality of the basic IVUS images is crucial, as poor or incomplete visualization of the lumen-plaque and plaque-adventitia boundaries in the presence of calcification is a problem that hampers both reconstruction and quantification. Currently available transducers have limited lateral resolution (51), and image distortion by nonuniform rotation or a noncoaxial position of the IVUS catheter in the lumen may create complex artifacts in 3D reconstructions (49). Moreover, motorized pullback devices cannot always assure an equal distance between adjacent images, as bends of the ultrasound catheter may induce a difference between the movement of the distal transducer and the proximal part of the IVUS catheter. ECG-gated image acquisition and pullback have the potential to minimize the typical cyclic saw tooth-shaped artifacts (48,52) (Fig. 3) and optimize image acquisition, permitting reliable volumetric measurement (49,53). However, compared with continuous pullback, image acquisition by the ECG-gated approach requires a longer acquisition time which may cause problems in patients with very severe coronary stenoses.

Vessel curvatures with a radius of less than 5 cm cause a significant distortion of the 3D reconstructed image (54). Overestimation and underestimation of certain portions of the plaque may be caused by a curved transducer pullback trajectory (49,55). The current 3D systems do not show the real curvatures and spatial orientation of the reconstructed vascular segment. The combined use of data obtained from biplane angiography and IVUS may help to overcome this limitation (56,57) as demonstrated by the ANGUS approach (57), which was shown to be highly accurate in both a vessel phantom and in the first human applications (Fig. 15). These findings have been confirmed by another group using a similar technical approach (58).

Many of the current limitations may soon be overcome by the use of these combined techniques, ECG-gated image acquisition (59,60), advanced segmentation algorithms based on radio frequency data (61) and forward-looking transducers (62); however, the value of the latter is still limited by the low image resolution and the large dimensions of the transducer. Miniaturization of the imaging catheters and improvement of the computer technology will help

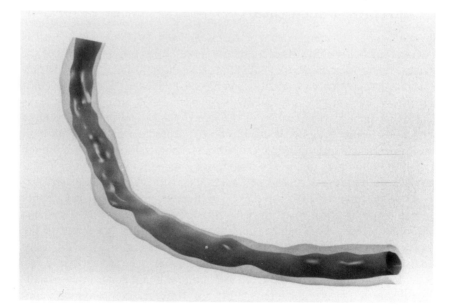

Figure 15 Combined use of biplane angiography and 3D IVUS by ANGUS. This novel method allows investigation of the true geometry of the coronary lumen and plaque, taking arterial curvatures and catheter bends into account. A reconstruction of an atherosclerotic right coronary artery is displayed in a frontal projection. IVUS data provided by the contour detection method were spatially arranged and interpolated, using biplane data on both the pullback trajectory and the angiogram. (Reprinted from Ref. 19, with permission.)

to increase the future applications of 3D IVUS and permit a volumetric quantification (14,19) without need of laborious manual tracing (43).

Thus, 3D IVUS is not restricted to research applications but a valuable clinical approach, which will gain further importance and become a routine technique if the interest of the clinicians and the effort of both the engineering and the clinical research groups is sustained.

REFERENCES

1. Yock PJ, Linker DT. Intravascular ultrasound: looking below the surface of vascular disease. Circulation 1990; 81:1715–1718.
2. Nissen SE, Gurley JC, Grines CL, et al. Intravascular ultrasound assessment of lumen size and wall morphology in normal subjects and patients with coronary artery disease. Circulation 1991; 84:1087–1099.
3. Ge J, Erbel R, Rupprecht H-J, Koch L, et al. Comparison of intravascular ultrasound and angiography in the assessment of myocardial bridging. Circulation 1994; 89:1725–1732.
4. Mintz GS, Painter JA, Pichard AD, et al. Atherosclerosis in angiographically "normal" coronary artery reference segments: an intravascular ultrasound study with clinical correlations. J Am Coll Cardiol 1995; 25:1479–1485.
5. Gerber TC, Erbel R, Görge G, Ge J, Rupprecht H-J, Meyer J. Extent of atherosclerosis and remodeling of the left main coronary artery determined by intravascular ultrasound. Am J Cardiol 1994; 73:666–671.
6. Yamagishi M, Miyatake K, Tamai J, Nakatani S, Kojama J, Nissen SE. Intravascular ultrasound detection of atherosclerosis at the site of focal vasospasm in angiographically normal or minimally narrowed coronary segments. J Am Coll Cardiol 1994; 23:352–357.
7. Görge G, Haude M, Ge J, et al. Intravascular ultrasound after low and high inflation pressure coronary artery stent implantation. J Am Coll Cardiol 1995; 26: 725–730.
8. Mintz GS, Popma JJ, Pichard AD, et al. Limitations of angiography in the assessment of plaque distribution in coronary artery disease: a systematic study of target lesion eccentricity in 1446 lesions. Circulation 1996; 93:924–931.
9. Rosenfield K, Losordo DW, Ramaswamy K, Isner JM. Three-dimensional reconstruction of human coronary and peripheral arteries from images recorded during two-dimensional intravascular ultrasound examination. Circulation 1991; 84: 1938–1956.
10. Coy KM, Park JC, Fishbein MC, et al. In vitro validation of three-dimensional intravascular ultrasound for the evaluation of arterial injury after balloon angioplasty. J Am Coll Cardiol 1992; 20:692–700.
11. Rosenfield K, Kaufman J, Pieczek AM, et al. Human coronary and peripheral arteries: on-line three-dimensional reconstruction from two-dimensional intravascular US scans. Radiology 1992; 184:823–832.

12. Schryver TE, Popma JJ, Kent KM, Leon MB, Eldredge S, Mintz GS. Use of intracoronary ultrasound to identify the true coronary lumen in chronic coronary dissection treated with intracoronary stenting. Am J Cardiol 1992; 69:1107–1108.

13. Mintz GS, Pichard AD, Satler LF, Popma JJ, Kent KM, Leon MB. Three-dimensional intravascular ultrasonography: reconstruction of endovascular stents in vitro and in vivo. J Clin Ultrasound 1993; 21:609–615.

14. von Birgelen C, Di Mario C, Li W, et al. Morphometric analysis in three-dimensional intracoronary ultrasound: an in-vitro and in-vivo study using a novel system for the contour detection of lumen and plaque. Am Heart J 1996; 132: 516–527.

15. von Birgelen C, van der Lugt A, Nicosia A, et al. Computerized assessment of coronary lumen and atherosclerotic plaque dimensions in three-dimensional intra-vascular ultrasound correlated with histomorphometry. Am J Cardiol 1996; 78: 1202–1209.

16. von Birgelen C, Gil R, Ruygrok P, et al. Optimized expansion of the Wallstent compared with the Palmaz-Schatz stent: online observations with two- and three-dimensional intracoronary ultrasound after angiographic guidance. Am Heart J 1996; 131:1067–1075.

17. Losordo DW, Rosenfield K, Pieczek A, Baker K, Harding M, Isner JM. How does angioplasty work? Serial analysis of human iliac arteries using intravascular ultrasound. Circulation 1992; 86:1845–1858.

18. Dhawale PJ, Rasheed Q, Mecca W, Nair R, Hodgson JM. Analysis of plaque volume during DCA using a volumetrically accurate three dimensional ultrasound technique. Circulation 1993; 88:I-550. Abstract.

19. von Birgelen C, Slager CJ, Di Mario C, de Feyter PJ, Serruys PW. Volumetric intracoronary ultrasound: a new maximum confidence approach for the quantitative assessment of progression/regression of atherosclerosis? Atherosclerosis 1995; 118(suppl):S103–S113.

20. Galli FC, Sudhir K, Kao AK, Fitgerald PJ, Yock PG. Direct measurement of plaque volume by three-dimensional ultrasound: potentials and pitfalls. J Am Coll Cardiol 1992; 19:115A. Abstract.

21. von Birgelen C, Umans V, Di Mario C, et al. Mechanism of high-speed rotational atherectomy and adjunctive balloon angioplasty revisited by quantitative coronary angiography: edge detection versus videodensitometry. Am Heart J 1995; 130: 4055–4012.

22. Keane D, Serruys PW. Quantitative coronary angiography: an integral component of interventional cardiology. In: Topol EJ, Serruys PW, eds. Current Review of Interventional Cardiology. (2nd ed). Philadelphia: Current Medicine, 1995: 205–233.

23. Matar FA, Mintz GS, Douck P, et al. Coronary artery lumen volume measurement using three-dimensional intravascular ultrasound: validation of a new technique. Cathet Cardiovasc Diagn 1994; 33:214–220.

24. Hausmann D, Friedrich G, Sudhir K, et al. 3D intravascular ultrasound imaging with automated border detection using 2.9 F catheters. J Am Coll Cardiol 1994; 23:174A. Abstract.
25. von Birgelen C, Kutryk MJB, Gil R, et al. Quantification of the minimal luminal cross-sectional area after coronary stenting: two- and three-dimensional intravascular ultrasound versus edge detection and videodensitometry. Am J Cardiol 1996; 78:520–525.
26. Gil R, von Birgelen C, Prati F, Di Mario C, Ligthart J, Serruys PW. Usefulness of three-dimensional reconstruction for interpretation and quantitative analysis of intracoronary ultrasound during stent deployment. Am J Cardiol 1996; 77:761–764.
27. Sonka M, Liang W, Zhang X, et al. Three-dimensional automated segmentation of coronary wall and plaque from intravascular ultrasound pullback sequences. In: Computers in Cardiology 1995. Los Alamitos, CA: IEEE Computer Society Press, 1995:637–640.
28. Hausmann D, Lundkvist AJS, Friedrich GJ, Mullen WL, Fitzgerald PJ, Yock PG. Intracoronary ultrasound imaging: intraobserver and interobserver variability of morphometric measurements. Am Heart J 1994; 128:674–680.
29. Rosenfield K, Kaufman J, Pieczek A, Langevin RE, Razvi S, Ilsner JM. Real-time three-dimensional reconstruction of intravascular ultrasound images of iliac arteries. Am J Cardiol 1992; 70:412–415.
30. Mintz GS, Leon MB, Satler LF, et al. Clinical experience using a new three-dimensional intravascular ultrasound system before and after transcatheter coronary therapics. J Am Coll Cardiol 1992, 19:292A. Abstract.
31. von Birgelen C, Di Mario C, Reimers B, et al. Three-dimensional intracoronary ultrasound imaging: methodology and clinical relevance for the assessment of coronary arteries and bypass grafts. J Cardiovasc Surg 1996; 37:129–139.
32. Mintz GS, Keller MB, Fay FG. Motorized ICUS transducer pull-back permits accurate quantitative axial measurements. Circulation 1992; 86:I-323. Abstract.
33. Bruining N, von Birgelen C, Di Mario C, et al. Dynamic three-dimensional reconstruction of ICUS images based on an ECG gated pull-back device. In: Computers in Cardiology 1995. Los Alamitos, CA: IEEE Computer Society Press, 1995:633–636.
34. Fehske W, Pizzulli, Hagendorff A, Lüderitz B. Real-time three-dimensional intracoronary ultrasonography: high resolution dynamic images of coronary artery lesions. J Am Coll Cardiol 1995; 25:180A. Abstract.
35. Chandrasekaran K, D'Adamo AJ, Sehgal CM. Three-dimensional reconstruction of intravascular ultrasound images. In: Yock PG, Tobis JM (eds). Intravascular Ultrasound Imaging. New York: Churchill-Livingston, 1992:141–147.
36. Li W, von Birgelen C, Di Mario C, et al. Semi-automatic contour detection for volumetric quantification of intracoronary ultrasound. In: Computers in Cardiology 1994. Los Alamitos, CA: IEEE Computer Society Press, 1994:277–280.
37. Sonka M, Zhang X, Siebes M, DeJong S, McKay CR, Collins SM. Automated segmentation of coronary wall and plaque from intravascular ultrasound image

sequences. In: Computers in Cardiology 1994. Los Alamitos, CA: IEEE Computer Society Press, 1994:281–284.

38. Kitney R, Moura L, Straughan K. 3-D visualization of arterial structures using ultrasound and voxel modelling. Int J Cardiac Imag 1989; 4:135–143.

39. Li W, Bosch JG. Zhong Y, et al. Image segmentation and 3D reconstruction of intravascular ultrasound images. In: Wei Y, Gu B, eds. Acoustical Imaging, Vol. 20. New York: Plenum Press, 1993:489–496.

40. von Birgelen C, Mintz GS, de Feyter PJ, et al. Reconstruction and quantification with three-dimensional intracoronary ultrasound: an update on techniques, challenges, and future directions. Eur Heart J 1997; 18:1056–1067.

41. von Birgelen C, Di Mario C, Serruys PW. Structural and functional characterization of an intermediate stenosis with intracoronary ultrasound and Doppler: a case of "reverse Glagovian modeling." Am Heart J 1996; 132:694–696.

42. Pasterkamp G, Wensing PJW, Post MJ, Hillen B, Mali WPTM, Borst C. Paradoxical arterial wall shrinkage may contribute to luminal narrowing of human atherosclerotic femoral arteries. Circulation 1995; 91:1444–1449.

43. Matar FA, Mintz GS, Farb A, et al. The contribution of tissue removal to lumen improvement after directional coronary atherectomy. Am J Cardiol 1994; 74: 647–650.

44. Weissman NJ, Palacios IF, Nidorf SM, Dinsmore RE, Weyman AE. Three-dimensional intravascular ultrasound assessment of plaque volume after successful atherectomy. Am Heart J 1995; 130:413–419.

45. Cavaye DM, White RA, Lerman RD, et al. Usefulness of intravascular ultrasound imaging for detecting experimentally induced aortic dissection in dogs and for determining the effectiveness of endoluminal stenting. Am J Cardiol 1992, 69: 705–707.

46. Reimers B, von Birgelen C, van der Giessen WJ, Serruys PW. A word of caution on optimizing stent deployment in calcified lesions: a case of acute coronary rupture with cardiac tamponade. Am Heart J 1996; 131:192–194.

47. Ge J, Erbel R, Seidel I, et al. Experimentelle Überprüfung der Genauigkeit und Sicherheit des intraluminalen Ultraschalls. Z Kardiol 1991; 80:595–601.

48. Di Mario C, Madretsma S, Linker D, et al. The angle of incidence of the ultrasonic beam: a critical factor for the image quality in intravascular ultrasonography. Am Heart J 1993; 125:442–448.

49. Roelandt, JRTC, Di Mario C, Pandian NG, et al. Three-dimensional reconstruction of intracoronary ultrasound images: rationale, approaches, problems and directions. Circulation 1994; 90:1044–1055.

50. Dhawale P, Rasheed Q, Berry J, Hodgson J McB. Quantification of lumen and plaque volume with ultrasound: accuracy and short term variability in patients. Circulation 1994; 90:I-164. Abstract.

51. Benkeser PJ, Churchwell AL, Lee C, Abouelnasr DM. Resolution limitations in intravascular ultrasound imaging. J Am Soc Echocardiogr 1993; 6:158–165.

52. Di Mario C, von Birgelen C, Prati F, et al. Three-dimensional reconstruction of

two-dimensional intracoronary ultrasound: clinical or research tool? Br Heart J 1995; 73(Suppl 2):26–32.

53. Dhawale PJ, Wilson DL, Hodgson JM. Optimal data acquisition for volumetric intracoronary ultrasound. Cathet Cardiovasc Diagn 1994; 32:288–299.

54. Waligora MJ, Vonesh MJ, Wiet SP, McPherson DD. Effect of vascular curvature on three-dimensional reconstruction of intravascular ultrasound images. Circulation 1994; 90:I-227. Abstract.

55. Klein HM, Günther RW, Verlande M, et al. 3D-surface reconstruction of intravascular ultrasound images using personal computer hardware and a motorized catheter control. Cardiovasc Intervent Radiol 1992; 15:97–101.

56. Koch L, Kearney P, Erbel R, et al. Three dimensional reconstruction of intracoronary ultrasound images: roadmapping with simultaneously digitised coronary angiograms. In: Computers in Cardiology 1993. Los Alamitos, CA: IEEE Computer Society Press, 1993:89–91.

57. Slager CJ, Laban M, von Birgelen C, et al. ANGUS: a new approach to three-dimensional reconstruction of geometry and orientation of coronary lumen and plaque by combined use of coronary angiography and ICUS. J Am Coll Cardiol 1995; 25:144A. Abstract.

58. Evans JL, Ng KH, Wiet SG, et al. Accurate three-dimensional reconstruction of intravascular ultrasound data: spatially correct three dimensional reconstructions. Circulation 1996; 93:567–576.

59. von Birgelen C, Mintz GS, Nicosia A, et al. Electrocardiogram-gated intravascular ultrasound image acquisition after coronary stent deployment facilitates on-line three-dimensional reconstruction and automated lumen quantification. J Am Coll Cardiol 1997. In press.

60. von Birgelen C, de Vrey EA, Mintz GS, et al. ECG-gated three-dimensional intravascular ultrasound: feasibility and reproducibility of an automated analysis of coronary lumen and atherosclerotic plaque dimensions in humans. Circulation. In press.

61. Bom N, Li W, van der Steen AFW, de Korte CL, Gussenhoven EJ, von Birgelen C, Lancee C. Intravascular ultrasound: possibilities of image enhancement by signal processing. In: van der Wall E, Marwick TH, Reiber JHC (eds). Advances in Imaging Techniques in Ischemic Heart Disease. Dordrecht, Netherlands: Kluwer Academic Publishers, 1995:113–125.

62. Ng K-H, Evans JL, Vonesh MJ, et al. Arterial imaging with a new forward-viewing intravascular ultrasound catheter. II. Three-dimensional reconstruction and display of data. Circulation 1994; 89:718–723.

11

Intravascular Ultrasound Assessment of PTCA Results: Mechanisms and Clinical Implications

Anthony C. De Franco *Moses H. Cone Memorial Hospital, Greensboro, and University of North Carolina at Chapel Hill, Chapel Hill, North Carolina*

E. Murat Tuzcu, Khaled Ziada, and Steven E. Nissen
Cleveland Clinic Foundation, Cleveland, Ohio

I. INTRODUCTION

During the 20 years since Greuntzig first described percutaneous transluminal coronary angioplasty, contrast angiography has been the primary method to guide the size and type of balloon, to determine the number and force of inflations, to triage lesions to different interventional devices, and to assess the adequacy of results. Unlike angiography, intravascular ultrasound (IVUS) allows direct observation of atherosclerotic plaque before and after mechanical interventions; the interventional cardiologist can use this information incrementally to confirm, to modify, or to extend the angiographic findings. It is evident even from the initial studies published to date that IVUS will continue to provide information on elastic recoil, pathologic dissection, abrupt closure, and restenosis.

In this chapter we first discuss the contributions of intravascular ultrasound in understanding the mechanisms of lumen enlargement after balloon angioplasty, which is followed by a discussion on the quantitative assessment of balloon angioplasty results. Among the studies reviewed is the recently completed Clinical Outcomes with Ultrasound Trial (CLOUT); the results of this study have important implications for balloon sizing during angioplasty procedures. We then discuss the contributions that ultrasound is making toward our understanding of restenosis after balloon procedures. Finally, we summarize other potential contributions of ultrasound during balloon angioplasty procedures, such as its potential to decrease acute complications, to improve long-term results, and to triage selected lesions to other transcatheter devices or surgical intervention.

II. MECHANISMS OF LUMINAL ENLARGEMENT FOLLOWING BALLOON ANGIOPLASTY

Intravascular ultrasound studies that have included both pre- and postinterventional imaging have identified three potential mechanisms of luminal enlargement after balloon angioplasty. Prior to the development of ultrasound, necropsy studies suggested that plaque fracturing or disruption were common after balloon PTCA and that plaque fracturing was the probable mechanism of lumen enlargement after successful balloon dilation (1–4). Although angiography can often detect this mechanism when it appears as a dissection, it is often insufficient to diagnose its extent and severity (5,6). For example, necropsy studies have demonstrated a relatively weak correlation between the angiographic extent of dissection and pathologic examination (6). Intravascular ultrasound studies (7–11) have confirmed these necropsy observations (Fig. 1). Taken as a group, these IVUS series suggest that dissection occurs in at least 50% to 80% of patients who have a successful angiographic result after balloon angioplasty. This relatively wide range is due to several factors, including the small numbers of patients in some series and, more importantly, the inclusion of patients studied with prototype IVUS devices, which are far inferior to the image quality obtainable from all manufacturers in 1997.

Ultrasound studies have also revealed that dissections after transcatheter interventions are not random events; rather, dissection tends to occur at particular anatomic locations. For example, localized calcium deposits are important determinants of fracture sites (8,11,12). Presumably, balloon expansion generates shear forces; because calcified plaque and adjacent, less dense tissue have different elastic properties, this zone is particularly susceptible to dissection

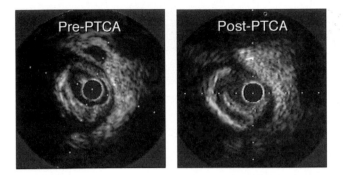

Figure 1 An example of typical plaque fracture after a balloon angoplasty. The mechanism of lumen enlargement is fracturing of the plaque, which occurs at a junction of the soft echolucent atheroma (which is more superficial) with a layer of more echo-dense atheroma with shadowing, which most likely represents a deep calcification.

(13). However, the interventionalist is more concerned with whether a post-balloon angioplasty dissection will become *angiographically* apparent, because these dissections are usually much larger and, presumably, more prone to acute vessel closure. (This is not to diminish the fact that some very large dissections are angiographically inapparent.) The juxtaposition of an echo dense or overtly calcified plaque to an echo-lucent area (which sonographers frequently describe as "soft," although the histologic accuracy of this term in a specific vessel is often questionable) is a risk factor for extensive (>5 mm), *angiographically* apparent dissection (14) (Fig. 2). Importantly, in a multiple logistic regression, this preprocedure ultrasound morphology was the strongest predictor of angiographic dissection among the clinical, angiographic, and ultrasonic variables tested.

In addition to localized calcium deposits, other lesion morphologies may also predispose to dissection. Ultrasound studies have shown that the majority (approximately 60%) of human atherosclerotic lesions are eccentric (when eccentricity is defined as the ratio of maximum to minimum plaque thickness ≥2.0). Thus, many lesions have a majority of the atheroma burden within one or two quadrants of the vessel wall with relative or complete sparing of the remaining two or three quadrants (15). After balloon angioplasty, fractures often originate at or near the juncture of an arc with a relatively large plaque burden with an arc that is less diseased or which is nearly normal (Fig. 3). Finite element analysis predicts that this region is often under the greatest circum-

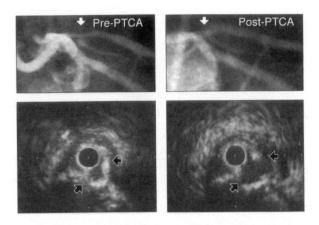

Figure 2   An example of an extensive plaque fracture after balloon angioplasty. In this patient, fluoroscopy did not reveal any calcification. However, the lesion was extensively calcified in more than two quadrants, as demonstrated in the pre-PTCA ultrasound image (lower left panel). When directional atherectomy failed to retrieve any tissue from this lesion, balloon angioplasty was attempted, but inflation pressures of 12 atm were required to achieve the modest improvement attained in the post-PTCA angiogram (upper right panel). The postangioplasty IVUS demonstrates extensive fracturing directly through the fibrocalcific layer and deep into the media (lower right panel, arrows).

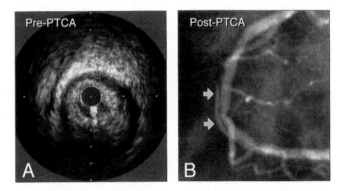

Figure 3   Although the juxtaposition of calcified and echolucent plaque is probably the most important risk factor for angiographic dissection (see Fig. 1), other atheroma morphologies may also be predisposed to extensive dissection. The pre-PTCA IVUS image (A) demonstrates an extensive and very eccentric atheroma. Balloon dilatation of this lesion resulted in extensive dissection (B, arrows). The postballoon IVUS image (not shown) demonstrated that the dissection originated at the junction of the heavily diseased and least diseased quadrants.

ference stress during balloon inflation (16). Although ultrasound may ultimately assist is stratifying dissection risk prior to angioplasty, additional research is needed to confirm the clinical utility of these observations. Honye and her colleagues (8) have proposed a classification scheme of post-angioplasty dissections based on ultrasonic characteristics (Table 1); such schemata can be useful in a research setting but are not commonly applied in daily clinical practice. Although some angiographic series from the 1980s suggested that the absence of dissection leads to a higher incidence of restenosis (17,18), few data regarding ultrasonically detected dissection (or lack of dissection) and subsequent restenosis are available. Honye et al. (8) noted that lesions without fracture on post-PTCA ultrasound imaging appeared to have a higher rate of restenosis (approximately 50%) than those with fracture (12%).

The second potential mechanism of lumen enlargement identified after balloon angioplasty is vessel stretching (Fig. 4). Vessel stretch is usually defined as an enlargement of the area subtended by the external elastic membrane (EEM); meticulous pre- and postintervention imaging at precisely the same site is necessary to document this mechanism. Several studies have suggested that vessel stretching is the predominant mechanism of lumen enlargement in perhaps 20% of lesions; the actual proportion of lesions that undergo stretching as a contributing factor to lumen enlargement is probably much larger (9,10,12). As with dissection, anecdotal experience suggests that some lesion morphologies are particularly susceptible to stretching as the predominant mechanism of balloon dilatation. For example, in extremely eccentric lesions, such as those with a heavy plaque burden in one or two quadrants with relative or complete sparing of the remaining arcs, balloon angioplasty often results in significant stretching of the normal wall opposite the atheroma. Although recoil is probably more prevalent in this situation, whether all such lesions should undergo some form of therapy other than

Table 1 Morphologic Patterns of Balloon
Angioplasty Dissections as Defined by Intravascular
Ultrasound, as Defined by Honye et al. (8)

Type	Pattern
A	Linear, partial tear of the plaque
B	Split in the plaque that extends to the media
C	Dissection behind the plaque, but < 180°
D	Extensive dissection ≥ 180°
E	No evidence of dissection

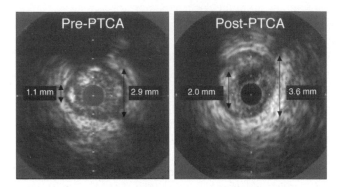

Figure 4   An example of a vessel stretching as the primary mechanism of lumen enlargement. In the pre-PTCA image on the left, the ultrasound catheter completely occupies the lumen; the luminal diameter is therefore 1.1 mm (the size of the catheter) at maximum dimension. The media-to-media diameter is 2.9 mm. After balloon dilatation, the lumen diameter has increased to approximately 2.0 mm, and the media-to-media diameter has increased to 3.6.

balloon angioplasty remains a matter of speculation. In the study by Honye et al. cited above (8), lesions with IVUS evidence of fracture after angioplasty presumably had a higher restenosis rate because vessel stretching was a predominant mechanism of lumen enlargement and this subset was more prone to elastic recoil. Another lesion type that may be predisposed to stretching is the focally constricted stenosis. Not all coronary stenoses are due predominantly to atheroma accumulation; some are due to focal contraction of the external elastic membrane ("scarring" or "negative remodeling") as well as plaque accumulation (19). Although some of these lesions (particularly those in vein grafts [20]) are very fibrotic and may completely resist balloon dilation, others are relatively easy to expand with average dilatation pressures (nominal balloon size) and result in a marked increase in lumen area with a low residual cross-sectional plaque burden (21) and minimal dissection. Although this situation is uncommon, in our experience, many of these lesions have a favorable long-term outcome with stand-alone balloon angioplasty.

The third potential mechanism of balloon angioplasty is redistribution of atheroma along the axial length of the vessel. To discern this mechanism, it is necessary to use an automatic pullback device, which withdraws the ultrasound transducer through the target site at a constant rate. Plaque volume is measured at regular intervals (usually every 0.5 mm), and the volume of atheroma pre-PTCA at each site is compared to the volume of atheroma at each site at the conclusion of the procedure. Prior to studies that routinely used automatic pullback devices, many reports described plaque "compression" as a mechanism of balloon angioplasty; however, this conclusion may have been a limitation of analyzing only the target site before and after intervention. A recent ultrasound study limited to stand-alone balloon angioplasty has confirmed that in axial redistribution, although there is a reduction of plaque-plus-media volume at the target site, there is a corresponding increase in sites proximal and distal to this site (22) (Fig. 5). As with dissection and vessel stretch, certain lesion morphologies may be more prone to axial redistribution. Kearney et al. (23) have reported that plaques in patients with unstable coronary syndromes are much more likely to undergo "compression" (or redistribution) than are lesions from patients with chronic stable angina, presumably because the former have a higher thrombus and soft plaque elements, which may be more amenable to dissolution, redistribution, or both. Cao at cl. have reported similar findings using computerized videodensitometry (24).

Of course, these potential mechanisms of luminal enlargement are not

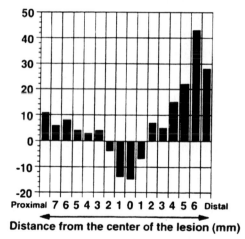

Distance from the center of the lesion (mm)

Figure 5   Mintz et al. (22) have demonstrated using an automatic pullback device that plaque redistribution along the axial length of the vessel is a third mechanism of lumen enlargement after balloon angioplasty. The Y axis represents the percent change in cross-sectional area; the X axis represents the distance in millimeters from the center of the lesion. Note that at the center of the lesion, plaque volume decreases from 10% to 15%; conversely, both proximally or distally to the precise target, plaque volume increases. Data from Mintz et al. (22), with permission.

mutually exclusive; all three mechanisms may occur to some degree within a single target lesion. This is an important contribution of intravascular ultrasound. Of the three potential mechanisms of balloon angioplasty, necropsy studies can discern only dissection; confirmation of vessel stretching and atheroma redistribution is impossible without preintervention measurements.

III. QUANTITATIVE ASSESSMENT OF PTCA RESULTS

Perhaps the most important contribution of IVUS to our understanding of vascular intervention has been the more accurate measurement of actual lumen gain from transcatheter therapies and the realization that angiography often significantly overestimates lumen gain. The tomographic perspective of ultrasound allows the investigator to planimeter lumen, vessel, and plaque areas directly, rather than indirectly from the angiographic silhouette (Figs. 6, 7). Even in atherosclerotic vessels that have not been treated with interventional devices, there is only a modest correlation between ultrasonic and angiographic dimensions, probably due to the inability of angiography to accurately represent the complex, irregular cross-sectional profiles of diseased arteries (25). The correlation between ultrasonic and angiographic dimensions is even worse following mechanical interventions (7, 8, 26–33), especially after balloon angioplasty (34). At the target site, angiography often *overestimates* actual luminal diameter, because contrast material penetrates into the complex cracks and fissures that follow balloon angioplasty, which creates a silhouette (the angiogram) that *appears* larger than it actually is. At the reference site, angiography often *underestimates* the actual vessel diameter, because angiographically occult atherosclerosis is often present. Then, to calculate a postprocedure percent diameter stenosis, the lumen diameter at the target site (an overestimate) is divided by the reference lumen diameter (an underestimate), which minimizes the percent diameter stenosis and exaggerates the magnitude of the gain in lumen area. This pitfall of angiography is inherent in applying a silhouette technique to a fractured and irregularly shaped lumen and is not overcome by the addition of "sophisticated" computerized edge-detection systems. Thus, when quantitative angiographic methods report a residual stenosis of only 10% to 15%, ultrasound commonly reports that 40% to 60% or more of the vessel is still occupied by plaque. For example, in one series after balloon angioplasty, the mean cross-sectional reduction by residual atheroma averaged 63% (35) although the quantitative angiographic percent stenosis was <20%. This large discrepancy has important implications for our understanding of restenosis and for the design of clinical trials that compare different devices, both of which we discuss below.

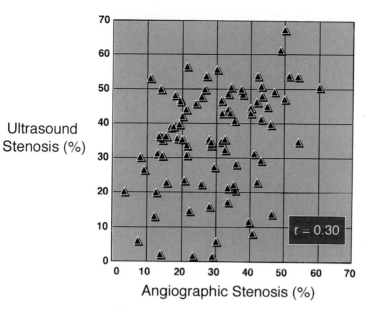

Figure 6 After balloon angioplasty, the ultrasound-determined percent stenosis (represented on the Y axis) has a poor correlation with the angiographically determined percent stenosis (represented on the X axis). See text for full details. Data from De Franco et al (33), with permission.

IV. QUANTITATIVE MEASUREMENTS AND BALLOON SIZING

Evaluation of the "normal" reference segment used for device sizing is an important potential application for intravascular imaging, because the diameter of the reference segment can affect the choice and the size of the interventional device and may affect clinical outcome (36). Ultrasound often reveals that "normal reference" segments may contain extensive, angiographically occult atherosclerosis or ectatic dilatation or be truly normal (37). As we have mentioned, angiographic and ultrasonic measurements of luminal diameter at these "normal reference" sites have only modest correlation (r^a .70) with a relatively large standard error, typically in the range of 0.50 mm (33,38,39). This phenomenon presents a complex dilemma for the operator who is selecting the type and size of the device for an interventional procedure. Is the "normal" reference segment diseased, ectatic, or truly normal?

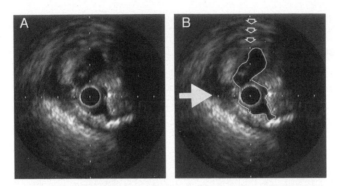

Figure 7   An example of a very irregular lumen shape after a balloon angioplasty. The postangioplasty image is in both frames, the irregular shape of the lumen is outlined in the right. Note that in one angiographic projection (B) (left to right, large arrow), the lumen would appear to be normal in diameter since the lumen extends from the media-to-media borders. However, in an orthogonal angiographic projection taken at 90° (small arrows), the lumen would appear to be only one-third as large. A planimetric method is more accurate than a silhouette technique when precise measurement of lumen areas is vital. (Modified after De Franco and Topol. Elective coronary intervention. In Sigwart, ed. Handbook of Cardiovascular Interventions. New York: Churchill Livingstone, 1996; with permission.)

   Although ultrasound can answer this question, its availability potentially makes device sizing more complex. Should device size be selected on the basis of lumen or vessel dimensions at the target site, at the reference site, or some combination of the two? If a particular method of device sizing does result in a larger postprocedure lumen areas, can this gain be accomplished without a corresponding increase in dissections or other acute complications? Although these questions may need to be addressed for each specific transcatheter therapy as discussed elsewhere in this text, the recently completed CLOUT pilot study addressed these issues with respect to balloon angioplasty (40). Because ultrasound frequently demonstrates angiographically occult atherosclerosis and extensive remodeling at the angiographic reference site, the CLOUT investigators hypothesized that in this circumstance the target lesions would safely accommodate a larger balloon size than what angiography would suggest, and that this larger balloon size would result in an increase in postprocedure target site lumen dimensions. Initially, all lesions were treated with a balloon judged to be 1.1:1 as estimated visually from the angiogram; balloon dilatation was then carried to angiographic completion. IVUS was then performed and the reference segments proximal and distal to the target lesions were analyzed. A second, IVUS-guided balloon size was calculated taking the average of the proximal and distal reference segment measurements as follows:

Proximal Reference (Media-to-Media Diameter − Lumen Diameter) −
Distal Reference (Media-to-Media Diameter − Lumen Diameter)

Regardless of the results of the angiographically guided initial balloon dilatation, the protocol called for additional inflations with the larger balloon in 76 of the 104 lesions (73%) using balloon : artery ratios that averaged 1.30 ± 17 as determined angiographically. After additional inflations with these larger balloons, the mean minimal lumen diameter for the entire cohort of 104 lesions increased from 1.78 to 2.04 mm and the mean post-PTCA residual stenosis decreased from 27% to 19% by quantitative angiography. Similarly, after inflations with the larger balloons, the IVUS determined lumen area increased from 3.31 to 4.34 mm². Thus, the authors concluded that when significant remodeling is present at the reference segment, the use of balloons larger than that considered safe by angiographic criteria can lead to larger postprocedure lumen dimensions by both angiographic and ultrasonic criteria.

Although this phase of CLOUT is only a pilot for a larger randomized trial, this preliminary study nevertheless has important implications for the practicing interventionalist. First, this is the only study to date that provides independent, core-lab analysis of a set of parameters for the selection of balloon sizing based on ultrasound measurement. This is an important issue, because when preintervention IVUS is performed and balloon angioplasty is selected as the primary device, the operator can use these data for sizing the balloon. Second, although this strategy of balloon sizing led to balloons that were considerably larger than conventionally accepted based on angiography alone, the investigators were able to achieve larger postprocedure lumen sizes without an increase in the rates of major complications. Finally, the larger postprocedure lumen sizes (as determined both angiographically and by ultrasound) may translate into a lower restenosis rate (41,42), although this awaits confirmation in the larger, randomized portion of the trial.

V. IVUS INSIGHTS INTO RESTENOSIS AFTER BALLOON ANGIOPLASTY

Restenosis remains the major limitation to percutaneous intervention techniques, particularly for balloon angioplasty. In the past, necropsy and animal studies suggested that restenosis was due to a characteristic neointimal hyperplasia that progressively narrowed the vessel lumen during the months that followed a successful intervention (2,43,44). However, during the past several years the paradigm of restenosis has changed. In the contemporary paradigm, all angioplasty procedures are considered to be a form of arterial injury; restenosis is considered to be a complex *set* of responses to this injury (45). Although this set of responses occurs to some degree in all patients during the months after transcatheter intervention, in some cases it is excessive and results in a recurrence of either the stenosis, clinical ischemia, or both.

For the purposes of discussion, we can divide this set of responses into three groups: recoil of the residual atheroma; thrombus deposition and organization; and vascular remodeling. As we have discussed, even when dissection or plaque redistribution is the predominant mechanism of luminal enlargement after balloon angioplasty, stretching of the vessel wall with displacement of atheroma is often present to some degree. *Recoil* refers to the rapid loss of the arterial cross-sectional area gained by the intervention occurring within minutes to hours after successful procedure. Thrombus is the second component of restenosis and its deposition may be directly related to the subsequent development of neointimal hyperplasia (46). Most percutaneous interventions expose subendothelial collagen and tissue factor, thereby stimulating platelet adhesion and accumulation within the first hours to days after the interventional procedure (47–50). The third component of restenosis is arterial remodeling, which refers to the process by which the injured arterial wall repairs itself over time. In the days following arterial injury, smooth muscle cells migrate to and proliferate in the injured arterial area and are transformed into cells that produce an extracellular matrix of connective tissue (45,46). If this process is robust, it can so encroach upon the lumen that recurrent stenosis of the lesion site occurs.

Although the division of the restenotic process into the three components of recoil, thrombus deposition, and remodeling is to some extent arbitrary and reflects our incomplete understanding, it serves as a convenient framework in which to discuss the contributions that IVUS studies have made to our concepts of this complex series of events. Although considerable data have been published using angiography to assess acute recoil (51–54), relatively few data are available using ultrasound to assess this phenomenon. In a small series of 43 patients who underwent IVUS imaging immediately and 20 min after balloon angioplasty, Koenig et al. (55) concluded that 35% of lesions experienced additional loss of lumen area attributable to recoil; importantly, in this subpopulation, mean lumen are decreased from 4.74 ± 1.19 to 3.87 ± 1.0 mm^2, a decline of nearly 20%.

After vessel recoil, thrombus deposition is the second major component of restenosis; unfortunately, currently available ultrasound systems are unreliable in identifying thrombus (29,56). With high-quality systems blood itself is seen as low-intensity, speckled reflections from within the vascular lumen; red thrombus usually has an echo density so similar to that of plaque that currently available ultrasound systems cannot reliably distinguish between them. Small series utilizing both angioscopy and intravascular ultrasound have confirmed that in an excellent ultrasound image, thrombus often has a characteristic scintillating appearance with brighter individual speckles than "fibrous" or fibrofatty plaque (57,58). Other qualitative features, such as the shape of an object (59) or an inner, demarcating "band" that separates a superficial layer (which is presumably thrombus) from the underlying atheroma (23), can sometimes "identify" thrombus with reasonable specificity. In clinical practice, angioscopy is the only available technology that can reliably differentiate thrombus from other material; ultrasound has contributed little in this area.

The most important contribution of intravascular ultrasound to our understanding of restenosis has been in the concept of arterial remodeling. In the old paradigm of restenosis, necropsy studies and animal models led to the concept that remodeling was due to proliferation of smooth muscle cells and the deposition of connective tissue matrix at the intervention site (Fig. 8). Thus, if this is true, serial ultrasound studies in restenotic sites should demonstrate that the decrease in lumen area occurred with a corresponding increase in plaque area (or, more accurately, plaque-plus-media area). However, recent data from intravascular ultrasound have challenged this notion. Mintz et al. (60) identified 360 native coronary lesions that were examined with IVUS at the end of the index procedure; all of these sites had follow-up angiographic data at a mean of 6.4 ± 3.6 months. The conventional, binary definition of restenosis (≥50% diameter stenosis) was the primary end point; follow-up diameter stenosis, late lumen loss, and follow-up minimum lumen diameter were also examined. Of all the clinical, angiographic, and ultrasound parameters tested, reference vessel size, preintervention lesion severity by quantitative coronary angiography, and the postintervention cross-sectional narrowing (plaque-plus media cross-sectional area divided by the area within the external elastic membrane, often abbreviated percent CSN) as measured by intravascular ultrasound predicted late angiographic results and the probability of restenosis. These investigators concluded that intravascular ultrasound was the most consistent predictor of restenosis, because it correlated most strongly with the primary end point of angiographic restenosis and also predicted two of the three secondary endpoints, late lumen loss, and follow-up diameter stenosis. The authors readily identify several important limitations of this study. First, interventional operators were not blinded to the ultrasound data; in many cases, ultrasound findings were monitored during the procedure to minimize the

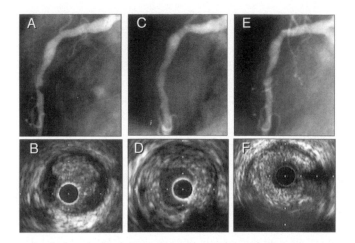

Figure 8   An example of restenosis both angiographically and ultrasonically, with the latter technique demonstrating a dramatic increase in plaque-plus-media areas as the mechanism. Preprocedure angiographc and ultrasound images are represented in A and B, respectively. After balloon angioplasty (C and D), the lumen area increases from 1.1 mm^2 to 4.3 mm^2, and the EEM area increases from approximately 13 mm^2 to 16.8 mm^2, indicating that the mechanism of lumen enlargement has been predominantly vessel stretch. Three months later the patient returned with clinical restenosis (E and F). Note that in the ultrasound image the EEM area has *increased* further to nearly 23 mm^2, concurrent with a significant decrease in lumen area and thus an increase in the plaque-plus-media area (from 12.3 mm^2 to 20.1 mm^2). Thus, the mechanism of restenosis is neointimal hyperplasia rather than negative remodeling.

residual cross-sectional narrowing and maximize lumen dimensions on the assumption that these goals would minimize restenosis and provide the best outcome for these patients. Second, the majority of patients underwent angiographic follow-up predominantly because of symptomatic recurrence; this selection bias is one factor that prevents one from the conclusion that IVUS parameters can be used routinely at the end of an interventional procedure to predict the probability of restenosis in an individual patient. Finally, the vast majority of patients were treated with new devices, and the results may or may not be applicable to patients treated with stand-alone balloon angioplasty. Nevertheless, if these results are confirmed in prospective series, the concept that an ultrasonic parameter such as percent cross-sectional narrowing can predict subsequent restenosis might have profound implications for the routine performance of balloon angioplasty. Patients whose treated lesions had a "favorable" final percent cross-sectional narrowing could be reassured of a low probability of restenosis; patients whose lesions failed to achieve an "acceptable" final percent cross-sectional narrowing could immediate undergo another adjunctive procedure (such as stenting or additional debulking) in an attempt to minimize the percent CSN.

If the observation that percent cross-sectional narrowing is the most important predictor of restenosis is in fact correct, why should this be so? Under the conventional paradigm of restenosis, animal models of arterial injury and necropsy studies on relatively small numbers of patients led to the concept that most late lumen loss after balloon angioplasty is due to neointimal hyperplasia. However, recent data from intravascular ultrasound suggest that restenosis after balloon angioplasty may be associated with a reduction in the total vessel cross-sectional area, or "circumferential coronary constriction" at the treated site rather than neointimal hyperplasia. Luo and his colleagues (61) interrogated 17 restenotic lesions with IVUS and compared vessel and lumen measurements at the target site with measurements at the proximal and distal reference sites. Importantly, vessel cross-sectional area (the area within the external elastic membrane) at the balloon angioplasty site averaged 10.1 ± 2.4 mm², significantly less than at the proximal and distal reference sites (14.8 ± 3.2 mm² and 13.8 + 3.1 mm², respectively). Thus, these investigators concluded that on average 83% of the late lumen loss at the angioplasty site was due to "constriction" of the total vessel cross-sectional area. In addition to "constriction," other investigators have used the terms "negative remodeling," "shrinkage," or "focal contraction" to refer to this phenomenon. An example of focal constriction as the predomant mechanism of restenosis is illustrated in Figure 9.

Although this series by Luo et al. is limited by its small number of patients and by the lack of ultrasonic data at the time of the initial intervention, the study is provocative for two reasons. First, as with data generated primarily from nonballoon angioplasty procedures reported by Mintz et al. (60) (above), this study challenges the conventional notion that restenosis after balloon angioplasty in humans is due to neointimal hyperplasia. Second, if the observation that "constriction" is the most important mechanism of restenosis after balloon angioplasty is correct, it suggests a potential mechanism for the observation that percent cross-sectional narrowing is the most important predictor of restenosis. Lesion sites with a small percent CSN after angioplasty could undergo some degree of constriction during the follow-up period and still maintain an adequate lumen size to prevent symptoms or myocardial ischemia; however, at a lesion site with the same absolute postprocedure lumen area but with a large

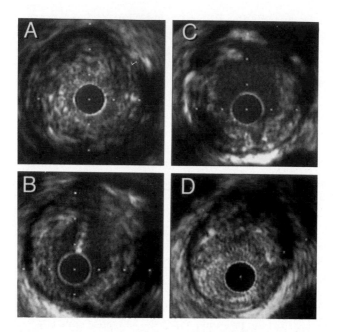

Figure 9   An example of vessel constriction (or negative remodeling) as the mechanism of restenosis. The predirectional atherectomy image is represented in A, the
postathrectomy image in B. Adjunct balloon angioplasty (C) enlarges the lumen further
by creating a moderate-size fracture at approximately 1 o'clock. When the patient
returns with clinical restenosis (D), the EEM area has decreased from 22.9 mm^2 to 16.1
mm^2; there is no difference in total plaque-plus-media area between the postprocedure
image (C) and the follow-up image (D) (15.6 mm^2 versus 13.9 mm^2, respectively).
Therefore, the mechanism of restenosis is purely negative remodeling.

percent CSN, the same degree of constriction would result in a much smaller
follow-up lumen area.

Another contribution of intravascular ultrasound to our understanding of
restenosis after angioplasty is the concept that vessel and lumen size can, in
some cases, enlarge in the months following interventional procedures. Under
the old paradigm of restenosis, remodeling after angioplasty was assumed to
result in a decrease in lumen size. Data from IVUS series suggest that some
coronary sites treated with angioplasty demonstrate luminal enlargement during the months after the procedure (62). An example of such a lesion from our
laboratory is illustrated in Figure 10. Remarkably, several investigators in the

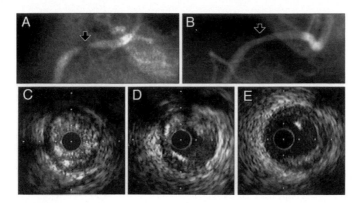

Figure 10   An example of positive remodeling (vessel expansion) after balloon angioplasty. The preangioplasty IVUS image is represented in C, the postangioplasty image in D. Lumen and vessel area have increased from 1.7 mm^2 to 5.2 mm^2 and from 11.9 mm^2 to 13.2 mm^2, respectively. At follow-up (E), the lumen area has increased further to 7.1 mm^2 and EEM area has increased to 14.0 mm^2. Therefore, favorable remodeling has occurred during the follow-up period, with an additional increase in lumen area.

field of nuclear cardiology speculated about the mechanism of improvement in flow as early as the mid-1980s. Manyari et al. (63) assessed thallium results after various intervals before and after successful angioplasty. Within 1 to 3 weeks after angioplasty, myocardial perfusion improved in the majority of patients; however, in approximately one-third of patients thallium results did not revert to normal until *1 month or more* after angioplasty. The authors speculated that this delay in thallium reperfusion may depend on progressive improvements in coronary flow, which, in retrospect, may have been due to progressive compensatory enlargement. As we will discuss, this concept has important implications for the timing and interpretation of functional testing and the design of clinical trials that compare interventional devices.

A.   Can Ultrasound Predict the Probability of Restenosis?

Several nonrandomized series have presented data to support the proposition that intravascular ultrasound analysis of the vessel following intervention can predict the probability of restenosis. This issue is of vital importance to interventional cardiology: If vessels treated with "plain old balloon angioplasty" could be stratified according to their risk of restenosis at the time of the initial procedure, these vessels could be triaged immediately to a different transcatheter intervention (such as atherectomy or stenting) that might reduce this risk and decrease the need for repeat revascularization. Conversely, if ultrasound could identify lesions with a low probability of restenosis after balloon angioplasty, these vessels could be effectively treated with this less expensive technology, obviating the need to stent the vast majority of coronary vessels.

Expanding on these concepts, Mintz and his colleagues (60) have developed a predictive model of restenosis based on their data that the percent cross-sectional narrowing is the most consistent predictor of angiographic restenosis. This model is supported by observations from other series, such as Phase II of the GUIDE trial (64). Although these reports may ultimately prove to be landmark studies in interventional cardiology, these results need to be validated in prospective series in which the operator is completely blinded to the ultrasound findings at the end of the intervention. Furthermore, these studies included patients who were treated with a variety of transcatheter therapies; the results may or may not be applicable to lesions treated with balloon angioplasty. The INSPIRE trial (intravascular predictors of Restenosis) is a multicenter study in which the operator is blinded to the pre- and postprocedure IVUS images; all patients undergo 6-month exercise nuclear studies as well as repeat angiography and follow-up intravascular ultrasound. This study has completed its pilot phase and is beginning enrollment in its final phase. This study should provide considerable data on whether IVUS criteria and the end of an intervention can predict the probability of restenosis after balloon angioplasty.

Until this issue is resolved conclusively in a research setting, from a practical standpoint, in clinical practice many experienced operators strive to achieve the lowest percent cross-sectional narrowing in the expectation that such a strategy will reduce the risk of restenosis. For example, after achieving a satisfactory angiographic result, IVUS is performed and the percent CSN is assessed. According to the model proposed by Mintz (60), lesions with a percent CSN of <40% have a favorable restenosis rate, lesions with a 50% to 60% have an intermediate restenosis rate (40% to 50%), and lesions with a high percent CSN (>60%) have a very unfavorable restenosis rate (>60%). Thus, in an individual patient, the operator determines the percent cross-sectional narrowing on line at the end of the procedure and, based on the morphology of the residual lesion by IVUS, estimates the feasibility, risk, and additional cost of attempting to reduce further the percent cross-sectional narrowing. For example, if a large residual flap is present and the precise position of this mass can be determined combining the information from angioplasty and IVUS, directional atherectomy might be attempted; if the position is less certain or the operator is inexperienced with DCA, a stent may be placed. Conversely, if the angiogram shows a satisfactory but "imperfect" result (for example, a residual 30% narrowing estimated visually in a 2.5-mm vessel) but the IVUS demonstrates an excellent result with a minimal percent CSN, this lesion may have a favorable restenosis rate with stand-alone balloon angioplasty, and additional attempts to improve the lumen further might be deferred.

B. Dissociation of Angiographic and Clinical Restenosis

In a research setting, clinical trials of drugs or devices designed to reduce restenosis usually use angiographic restenosis (usually defined as a binary end point, the presence or absence of a 50% diameter stenosis at a predetermined follow-up time point). However, from a practical standpoint, the most relevant definition of restenosis is a clinical one: whether or not the patient has symptoms, provokable ischemia, or both. Although many clinical trials report angiographic restenosis rates of 30% to 50%, the same trials frequently report evidence of ischemia; i.e., a need for repeat revascularization in only 20% to 30%. Although many authors have recognized the discrepancy between angiographic and clinical stenoses (65–70), many clinicians assume that this merely reflects the "inaccuracy" of functional testing. For example, some lesions that project a >50% diameter reduction by an angiographic silhouette may produce neither symptoms nor abnormalities on functional testing. This may occur in 25% or more of patients with angiographic restenosis (71). Conversely, other lesions that project "only" a 30% to 50% angiographic narrowing (and which would not qualify for the conventional angiographic definition of restenosis) nevertheless result in angina or provokable ischemia on functional testing. One study, by Duerr and Topol (71), has suggested that this may occur in 10% to 15% of patients without angiographic restenosis.

Recent information from IVUS has suggested the mechanism for the dissociation between angiographic and clinical stenosis. As we have discussed, the calculated luminal area from the angiographic silhouette has only a modest correlation with the actual lumen area as planimetered by intravascular ultrasound. Thus, it is not surprising that some patients with a clear-cut angiographic "stenosis" have an actual lumen area that is large enough to provide adequate blood flow, even at high rates of oxygen demand, whereas other patients, with an "intermediate" lesion angiographically, actually have a stenosis that is severe enough to produce ischemia (Fig. 11). This observation is simply another example of the limitations of a two-dimensional silhouette (the angiogram) of what is often a complex, three-dimensional structure (the coro-

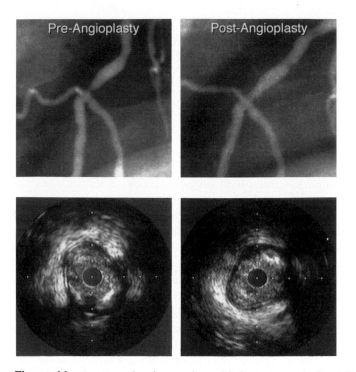

Figure 11   An example of an angiographic improvement after balloon angioplasty without any significant change in lumen area as measured by IVUS. Note that the lumen area in the pre-IVUS image is identical to the lumen area measured postballoon angioplasty. The catheter completely occupies the lumen in both images; since the size of the catheter is 1.1 mm^2, changes in lumen area that result in a lumen less than 1.1 mm cannot be discerned by current IVUS catheters.

nary lumen after balloon angioplasty). Thus, it is not surprising that the PICTURE study (72), which was a prospective series that attempted to determine whether IVUS data could predict the subsequent probability of angiographic restenosis, was negative. However, as Topol and Nissen have emphasized (73), from the standpoint of the individual patient, it is more important to determine whether a lesion produces *clinical ischemia* (either recurrent symptoms or a positive functional test) than an angiographic imperfection. Therefore, the more important issue for intravascular ultrasound studies will be not whether IVUS can predict subsequent angiographic restenosis, but the subsequent development of symptoms or provokable ischemia or the need for repeat revascularization.

The dissociation of angiographic and clinical restenosis underscores the fundamental difference of measuring the artery versus assessing the patient and has important implications for daily practice and clinical trials. On a practical level, the interventionalist should be guided by the functional significance of a lesion. On a research level, the use of an arbitrary, binary angiographic definition of restenosis will overestimate the clinical significance of a substantial portion of these recurrent angiographic lesions a priori. Although clinical trials of devices or drugs to reduce restenosis will continue to use different definitions to measure restenosis and different methods to determine its incidence, it is our opinion that the most relevant definition of restenosis is one that provides the most information about the patient's clinical outcome—specifically, the probability of survival free from recurrent angina, provokable ischemia, myocardial infarction, and death. Future clinical trials may adopt clinical end points (such as the persistence or recurrence of ischemia) because they are clinically more relevant than angiographic restenosis to judge the relative benefit of coronary revascularization procedures, although larger sample sizes will be required. Angiographic restenosis can still be measured in a predefined subset of patients in order to study procedural and technical aspects of the intervention.

C. "Pseudorestenosis"

Intravascular ultrasound has clearly demonstrated that a substantial minority of patients treated with balloon angioplasty have a dramatic improvement in the angiographic silhouette but a much less dramatic improvement in lumen area when the actual lumen is planimetered by ultrasound. Examples of such a patient is demonstrated in Figures 12 and 13. Topol has labeled this "pseudorestenosis" to signify that although this population may be at high risk for the recurrence of clinical ischemia, the initial gain in lumen area was minimal and, thus, a minimal amount of loss (whether by recoil, thrombus deposition, negative remodeling, or some combination of these) will completely negate the minimal initial gain. Balloon angioplasty is probably the interventional device most likely to generate this finding because, compared to other interventional devices, it is the most likely to produce dissections that will lead to an overestimation of lumen area by angiographic assessment (34). Interestingly, in the 1980s and early 1990s, a series of publications reported on the ability of early functional testing in asymptomatic patients to "predict" the subsequent development of restenosis (74–76). Although there is no published series that

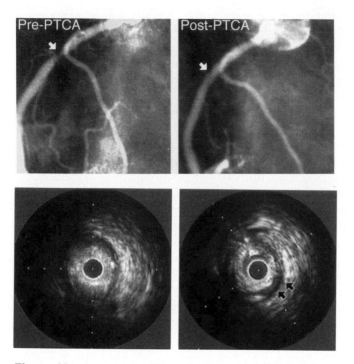

Figure 12 An example of "pseudorestenosis." Despite a dramatic improvement in the angiogram after balloon angioplasty, IVUS demonstrates that the mechanism of lumen enlargement is an extensive media fracture (black arrows, lower right panel); there has been little change in lumen area. This patient was studied as part of an IVUS protocol in which the operator was blinded to the IVUS image; the procedure was taken to angiographic completion. This patient had only modest improvement in his symptoms despite the successful angiographic result; when "restenosis" occurred 1.5 months after the procedure, penetration into the media was no longer present by IVUS. Thus, in some cases early restenosis may represent a failure of the initial procedure to enlarge the lumen by mechanisms that result in a high probability of a sustained favorable result.

correlates postprocedure ultrasound findings with the results of functional testing data soon (within 1 month) after balloon angioplasty, in our experience, many patients with a positive functional test soon after a "successful" intervention as defined angiographically probably have either a disproportionate amount of recoil, thrombus deposition, or "pseudorestenosis."

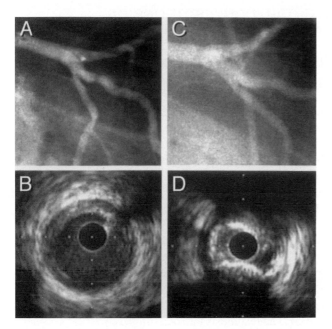

Figure 13 An example of an ambiguous angiogram in which IVUS establishes the correct diagnosis. This patient initially presented with new-onset angina, Canadian Functional Class III. Angiography revealed a 50%, slightly "hazy" area in a large obtuse marginal branch (A); the lesion was completely not apparent in other views (B). This was the only coronary lesion. Thus, intervention was deferred and the patient was referred for exercise testing, which provoked the patient's symptoms. Thallium scintigraphy demonstrated a large area of lateral wall ischemia. At repeat angiography, IVUS demonstrated only a minimal amount of atheroma at the reference site (C), but within the hazy area (D) a "napkin ring" of calcium nearly obliterated the lumen. Presumably, even a small amount of calcification placed strategically can impair the ability of angiography to measure a stenosis. After rotational ablation and adjunctive balloon angioplasty, ultrasound demonstrated a significant increase in lumen area (not shown), and the subsequent follow-up thallium exercise test was negative for ischemia. Thus, the angiogram can underestimate true lesion severity and its hemodynamic significance; in this circumstance, a functional test (or Doppler flow) may provide more reliable clinical information. (Modified after De Franco and Topol. Functional testing following percutaneous coronary intervention. In Marwick, ed. Stress Testing. New York: Churchill Livingstone, 1996; with permission.)

VI. OTHER POTENTIAL CONTRIBUTIONS OF ULTRASOUND

A. Determination of the End Points of Balloon Angioplasty

Although two multicenter, randomized clinical trials have demonstrated that stenting of specific lesion subsets reduces angiographic restenosis at 6 months, stenting every lesion in every patient is neither practical nor economically feasible. Thus, an important issue in interventional cardiology is whether some subsets of patients can achieve excellent long-term results from balloon angioplasty as a stand-alone device. Serruys and his colleagues, using data extracted from the Benestent-I trial, compared to the subset of patients who achieved a "stentlike" result following balloon angioplasty, defined as a QCA diameter stenosis of ≤30% (n = 213) with two groups of stent patients: the entire stent cohort in the study (n = 259), and the subset of stented patients who achieved a diameter stenosis ≤30% (n = 213). Procedural success was similar in all three groups (87%, 87%, and 93%, respectively). Importantly, there were no differences in minimum lumen diameter at follow up (1.84 ± 0.52 mm, 1.82 ± 0.64 mm, and 1.84 ± 0.62 mm). The restenosis rate determined by repeat coronary angiography in >95% of patients was 16% in those with a stentlike balloon angioplasty versus 22% in the total stent population and 18% in the patients who achieved a less than 30% residual with coronary stenting (P = NS). There were no statistical differences in major adverse clinical events across the three groups. Thus, in patients who were able to achieve an optimal postballoon result as rigorously defined by on-line QCA, the clinical event rate and angiographic restenosis rate were identical to those of patients treated with coronary stenting. These data suggest that the subset of patients treated with conventional balloon angioplasty who achieve an excellent acute angiographic result have the same angiographic restenosis rate as patients treated with coronary stent deployment. Serruys has also presented data that suggests that postangioplasty analysis by Doppler flow may add incremental information to on-line QCA to stratify the risk of restenosis at the end of the initial procedure.

During the past 2 years several trials have reported more favorable results for balloon angioplasty. Whereas multicenter, randomized trials of new devices that used conventional balloon angioplasty as a control group and that had independent, blinded core laboratory analysis frequently reported restenosis rates in the 30% to 45% range, more recent multicenter trials have reported restenosis rates for balloon angioplasty to be in the 20% to 30% range. Among the possible reasons for this improvement is that the availability of stents as a "bail-out" device allows a more "aggressive" initial balloon approach (e.g., a slightly larger balloon : artery ratio, etc.) which results in a lower postprocedure angiographic minimum lumen diameter (MLD) and, thus, a lower restenosis rate. Patients who dissect or who have a high residual MLD despite this approach are then treated with stent implantation. This approach has also been called "provisional" stenting; an example of such an approach from our laboratory is illustrated in Figures 14 and 15.

B. Distinguishing Therapeutic Results from Complications

In the early 1990s, many investigators speculated that IVUS would be particularly valuable in evaluating angioplasty complications, such as differentiating therapeutic plaque fractures from more severe dissections that increase the risk of acute closure or other adverse events. Although ultrasound clearly has a higher sensitivity for detecting dissections following balloon angioplasty, it

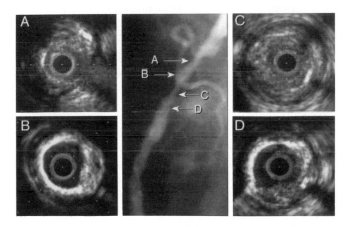

Figure 14 An example of a successful provisional stenting with IVUS guidance. By fluoroscopy, this vessel was diffusely and heavily calcified. The lesion was nearly 25 mm in length (from point A to point D). Prior to ultrasound, the planned procedure was rotational ablation followed by coronary stenting. However, the preprocedure ultrasound demonstrates that the calcification is present at segments with only moderate stenosis (points B and D). The most severely diseased portions (points A and C) have a very large plaque burden that consists of only soft plaque elements with minimal, if any, calcification. Thus, rotational ablation was not necessary based on preprocedural IVUS imaging, and redilatation was carried out, with the intent of placing two coronary stents.

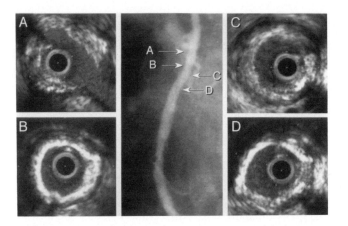

Figure 15 The same patient as in Figure 14 after balloon angioplasty; ultrasound images correspond to the same sites as in Figure 14. After predilatation, the angiogram is markedly improved with a <20% residual stenosis. Note that at the most severe stenoses (A and C) there has been a dramatic improvement in lumen area both angiographically and by IVUS. As expected, lumen area at B and D has improved only modestly. Despite the extensive superficial calcification at B and D, there is no evidence of plaque fracture. The excellent lumen areas and the relatively low residual cross-sectional narrowing throughout the entire length of this lesion balloon angioplasty alone obviated the need for the operator to defer placing two coronary stents.

can be difficult to distinguish therapeutic from pathologic dissection. Nevertheless, dissections identify patients at increased risk of subsequent adverse events (77), and the operator must decide whether or not to stent the lesion on the basis of the ultrasound findings (Fig. 15). On the basis of necropsy findings, Waller has proposed that dissections that encompass an arc of more than 180° (Table 1; type D) or those that are more than 1 cm in length are inherently unstable (78); therefore, we almost always recommend that dissections that occupy more than two quadrants (180°) or that have a relatively long false channel (>5 mm) or that are "bulky" (are >1 to 1.5 mm thick) are almost always stented (Fig. 16). Unfortunately, there are even fewer data on which to base recommendations for "less impressive" dissections. We often recommend stenting if the dissection flap occupies more than one quadrant or if it clearly prolapses across to the opposite vessel wall, especially if it is >5 mm in length or if it appears to be "stented" by the ultrasound catheter itself. This last feature is important to

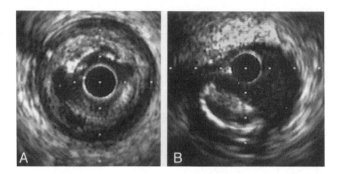

Figure 16 An example of two postballoon angioplasty plaque fractures that would not be stented in our laboratory. In (A), the ultrasound after balloon angioplasty revealed a significant increase in lumen area; the mechanism of lumen enlargement is multiple superficial fractures; none appear to have the potential to occlude the lumen completely. In (B), a more extensive dissection has occurred in the lower left portion of the image; however, this flap is less than one quadrant in size and the resulting lumen is large. Although there are no data yet to support this management strategy, these lesions would not be recommended for bailout stenting currently.

note. Since most ultrasound catheters are 1.1 mm in size, in small vessels (<3.0 mm) with a mere 50% cross-sectional plaque burden, it is possible for the IVUS catheter to compress even a large dissection flap against the vessel wall, making the dissection appear less severe than it actually is. On rare occasions, one occasionally sees a dissection angiographically that cannot be readily identified by ultrasound. In these last two situations, a combination of the ultrasound and angiographic appearances is used to determine the recommendation on a case-by-case basis. If a dissection is suspected but cannot be definitely diagnosed, contrast injection can help identify tissue planes (79). Long-term studies to establish the relationship between ultrasound appearance and clinical outcome may resolve these uncertainties.

Ultrasound can be particularly useful in assessing complications of balloon angioplasty procedures, such as abrupt vessel closure. Ultrasound can often be used to distinguish among dissection, thrombus, or vasospasm as the cause, particularly if a preintervention IVUS run is available for comparison. For example, if thrombus is the cause of the occlusion, ultrasound usually shows a significant increase in "plaque" mass with or without a clear dissection plane. On the other hand, if vasospasm is the cause, ultrasound usually demonstrates a

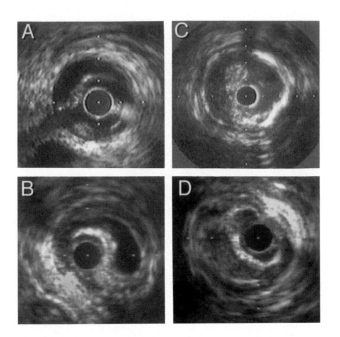

Figure 17 Examples of plaque disruptions that would be recommended for stenting in our laboratory. Image A demonstrates a large dissection extending from the side branch that extends more than two quadrants. This image was taken from a patient with a spontaneous coronary artery dissection that was angiographically inapparent; the image was obtained on routine preprocedural IVUS imaging. Because this dissection occupied two quadrants or more and was long (>10 mm), this lesion was recommended for stenting. In (B), a large dissection flap is seen in the center of the lumen, occupying two quadrants. Images (C) and (D) are taken more than 5 mm apart from the same patient—a long spiral dissection (arrows) is present that was completely inapparent angiographically.

marked reduction in vessel caliber (area within the EEM) without a significant increase in plaque mass. Another situation in which IVUS is particularly useful after balloon angioplasty is the angiographically improved but "hazy" lesion. In this situation, the operator must decide whether the haze is due to dissection, an irregular lumen shape (but one which is uncompromised), thrombus, an atheromatous filling defect, or some combination of these findings. As we have discussed, ultrasound can often be used to distinguish among these possibilities.

C.   Triage to Other Transcatheter Revascularization Strategies

In many patients undergoing interventional procedures, areas of severe ath-erosclerosis are detected at sites with little or no abnormality by angiography. For example, necropsy studies decades ago suggested that angiography under-estimates the extent of left main coronary atherosclerosis (80); recent ultra-sound studies have confirmed that the severity of left main disease is often underestimated in patients undergoing left coronary interventions (81,82). Rarely, ultrasound demonstrates a left main lesion so severe that the interven-tionalist decides that surgical revascularization is preferable to a transcatheter approach. In other cases, ultrasound may reveal specific details of plaque morphology that are thought to respond poorly to stand-alone balloon as the primary device. For example, angiography and fluoroscopy are very poor at identifying lesion calcification; many operators consider rotational ablation to be a preferable option for such lesions, especially when the calcium is super-ficial and extensive. Similarly, because angiography underestimates the amount of disease at the reference site, lesions that are much longer than they appear angiographically are occasionally triaged to rotational ablation. In other cases, large, extensively remodeled lesions, particularly those in large vessels, are sometimes triaged to directional atherectomy for "debulking" even if stent deployment is used as an adjunct. Although these triage strategies are common in centers that frequently use preinterventional IVUS imaging (83), clinical trials of such strategies are needed to confirm that they have a beneficial effect on long-term clinical outcome.

Occasionally, preprocedural IVUS imaging identifies a morphology that is probably best treated with a modality other than balloon angioplasty. For example, spontaneous coronary dissections (84) (particularly those that are >5 mm) and pseudoaneurysms (85–88) are often triaged to stent deployment because anecdotal evidence (such as imaging after balloon dilatation and before stent deployment) suggests that balloon dilatation alone often makes the ultrasonic appearance of these lesions considerably worse. Before the approval of stents, angiographic filling defects (which may be thrombi or atheromatous material) or overt dissections were often treated with balloon angioplasty to "tack up" the defect against the vessel wall (89). In our experience, despite occasional angiographic "improvement," many of these lesions appear no better or sometimes worse after stand-alone balloon therapy; a recent small study (90) suggested that perfusion balloons do not change the incidence of ultrasonically detected dissections after balloon angioplasty. These lesions may best be treated with stenting or IVUS-guided directional atherectomy.

D. Optimal Use of Serial Devices

A recently proposed strategy for the treatment of selected target coronary lesions is the use of sequential interventional devices. With this approach, preprocedural ultrasound imaging is used to select the initial transcatheter therapy and, in selected cases, a second (or third) device, again based on the ultrasound findings. In theory, the ultrasonic assessment of the effects of each sequential device would allow the operator to maximize lumen size at the end of the procedure, and, since percent cross-sectional narrowing is considered to be the most important predictor of outcome, would reduce the incidence of restenosis (91,92). For example, rotablation may be used to remove a heavy, superficial "cap" of calcium; if the target vessel is large, the decalcification could be followed by directional atherectomy to debulk most effectively the residual soft plaque.

Although many interventional operators often use the strategy of ultrasound guidance of serial devices to reduce restenosis, it is important to remember that an improvement in long-term clinical outcome as a result is as yet unproven and it undoubtedly results in a substantial increase in procedural costs. The single study that has tested this approach prospectively did not show a benefit for ultrasound guidance of serial devices (93), although it may have been underpowered to detect moderate differences due to its small enrollment (154 lesions).

VII. FUTURE DIRECTIONS

Although the clinical value of routine ultrasound imaging before and after mechanical revascularization is only now being tested in randomized trials, it seems likely that the morphology of the vessel wall following interventions will provide valuable insights into phenomena such as elastic recoil, pathologic dissection, abrupt occlusion, and restenosis. In certain patients, "restenosis" may represent a failure to adequately augment luminal area at the time of the initial procedure, rather than an overabundant proliferation of smooth muscle cells. If this is indeed the case, ultrasound assessment of the residual lumen may be able to predict which patients have a higher likelihood of poor long-term clinical results. Ultrasound may also be able to predict which patients have a higher probability of acute postinterventional complications. Preliminary studies demonstrate that ultrasound can supplement angiography in the triage of patients to the appropriate form of revascularization and can successfully identify subsets of patients likely to manifest suboptimal long-term results. Of course, interventional cardiologists will need large-scale, prospective trials with large numbers of patients to validate these observations from nonrandomized series.

Important technical advances in intravascular imaging technology will continue to emerge during the next few years. An imaging guidewire is currently in clinical testing; this device will allow simultaneous imaging during revascularization procedures. Combination devices with both ultrasound imaging and balloon or atherectomy capability will be refined, permitting on-line guidance during the procedure. For example, an angioplasty balloon with an ultrasound transducer (the Endosonics Oracle Focus) (35,94,95) is now commercially available and may be particularly valuable if the data from the CLOUT pilot are validated in a larger, randomized trial. A transducer within an atherectomy cutter has been developed by Guidant and Hewlett-Packard. Several investigators have demonstrated three-dimensional reconstruction of cross-sectional ultrasound images (96–101), but use of this technique for clinical decision making is limited to a few centers with the experience to overcome the technical difficulties of this procedure. Forward-looking ultrasound probes are also under development; these devices could have important potential applications for safely crossing difficult total occlusions with stiff guidewires, lasers (Laserwire, Spectranetics Corp.), or ultrasound catheters (Sonicross, Guidant Corp.).

VIII. SUMMARY

Our initial experience supports an important potential role for intravascular ultrasound in the evaluation of PTCA results in selected patients and as a research tool. The cross-sectional perspective of IVUS is ideally suited for precision measurements of coronary luminal diameter and cross-sectional area. Luminal size after transcatheter therapies is often smaller and stenosis severity worse by IVUS than by angiography. The augmentation of the "apparent" angiographic diameter by extraluminal contrast within cracks, fissures, or dissection planes is probably responsible for these differences. In the presence of complex alterations in the vessel wall, tomographic measurements by intravascular ultrasound are theoretically superior.

REFERENCES

1. Farb A, Virmani R, Atkinson JB, Kolodgie FD. Plaque morphology and pathologic changes in arteries from patients dying after coronary balloon angioplasty. J Am Coll Cardiol 1990: 16(6):1421–1429.

2. Block P, Myler R, Stertzer S, et al. Morphology after percutaneous transluminal coronary angioplasty. N Engl J Med 1981; 35:382–385.

3. Waller BF. Anatomy, histology, and pathology of the major epicardial coronary series relevant to echocardiographic imaging techniques. J Am Soc Echocardiogr 1989; 2(4):232–252.

4. Waller BF, Orr CM, Slack JD, Pinkerton CA, Van Tassal J, Peters T. Anatomy, histology, and pathology of coronary arteries: a review relevant to new interventional and imaging techniques. Part IV. Clin Cardiol 1992; 15(9):675–687.

5. Holmes D, Vliestra R, Mock M, et al. Angiographic changes produced by percutaneous transluminal coronary angioplasty. Am J Cardiol 1983; 51: 678–683.

6. Waller B. Morphologic correlates of coronary angiographic patterns at the site of percutaneous transluminal coronary angioplasty. Clin Cardiol 1988; 11: 817–822.

7. Tobis JM, Mahon DJ, Moriuchi M, Honye J, McRae M. Intravascular ultrasound imaging following balloon angioplasty. Int J Card Imaging 1991; 6(3–4): 191–205.

8. Honye J, Mahon DJ, Jain A, et al. Morphological effects of coronary balloon angioplasty in vivo assessed by intravascular ultrasound imaging. Circulation 1992; 85(3):1012–1025.

9. Losordo DW, Rosenfield K, Pieczek A, Baker K, Harding M, Isner JM, How does angioplasty work? Serial analysis of human iliac arteries using intravascular ultrasound. Circulation 1992; 86(6):1845–1858.

10. The SH, Gussenhoven EJ, Zhong Y, et al. Effect of balloon angioplasty on femoral artery evaluated with intravascular ultrasound imaging. Circulation 1992; 86(2):483–493.

11. Fitzgerald PJ, Ports TA,Yock PG. Contribution of localized calcium deposits to dissection after angioplasty. An observational study using intravascular ultrasound. Circulation 1992; 86(1):64–70.

12. Potkin BN, Keren G, Mintz GS, et al. Arterial responses to balloon coronary angioplasty: an intravascular ultrasound study. J Am Coll Cardiol 1992; 20(4): 942–951.

13. Lee RT, Richardson SG, Loree HM, et al. Prediction of mechanical properties of human atherosclerotic tissue by high-frequency intravascular ultrasound imaging. An in vitro study. Arteriosclerosis Thromb 1992; 12(1):1–5.

14. De Franco AC, Nissen S, Tuzcu E, et al. Ultrasound plaque morphology predicts major dissections following stand-alone and adjunctive balloon angioplasty. Circulation 1994; 90(4 Part 2):I-59. Abstract.

15. Mintz GS, Popma JJ, Pichard AD, et al. Limitations of angiography in the assessment of plaque distribution in coronary artery disease: a systematic study of target lesion eccentricity in 1446 lesions. Circulation 1995; 93(5):924–931.

16. Lee RT, Loree HM, Cheng GC, Lieberman EH, Jaramillo N, Schoen FJ. Computational structural analysis based on intravascular ultrasound imaging before in

vitro angioplasty: prediction of plaque fracture locations. J Am Coll Cardiol 1993; 21(3):777–782.

17. Leimgruber P, Roubin G, Anderson H, et al. Influence of intimal dissection on restenosis after successful coronary angioplasty. Circulation 1985; 72:530–535.

18. Matthews B, Ewels C, Kent K. Coronary dissection: a predictor of restenosis? Am Heart J 1988; 115:547–554.

19. Nishioka T, Luo H, Eigler N, Berglund H, Kim CJ, Siegel RJ. Contribution of inadequate compensatory enlargement to development of human coronary artery stenosis: an in vivo intravascular ultrasound study. J Am Coll Cardiol 1996; 27: 1571–1576.

20. Mintz G, Popma J, Pichard A, et al. The dimorphic pathology of vein graft lesions effects acute procedural and late angiographic outcomes. J Am Coll Cardiol 1995; 79A. Abstract.

21. Timmis S, Davidson C, Hermiller J, Parker M, McPherson D, Bonow R. Influence of coronary atherosclerotic remodeling on the mechanism of balloon PTCA. Circulation 1996; 94:I-92. Abstract.

22. Mintz GS, Pichard AD, Kent KM, Satler LF, Popma JJ, Leon MB. Axial plaque redistribution as a mechanism of percutaneous transluminal coronary angioplasty. Am J Cardiol 1996; 77:427–429.

23. Kearney P, Erbel R, Rupprecht H, et al. Differences in the morphology of unstable and stable coronary lesions and their impact on the mechanisms of angioplasty. An in vivo study with intravascular ultrasound. Eur Heart J 1995; 17:721–730.

24. Cao N, Werns S, Moscucci M, Bates E, Muller D. Relationship between quantitatively determined lesion density and mechanism of coronary balloon dilatation. Circulation 1995; 92:I-401. Abstract.

25. De Scheerder I, De Man F, Herregods MC, et al. Intravascular ultrasound versus angiography for measurement of luminal diameters in normal and diseased coronary arteries. Am Heart J 1994; 127(2):243–251.

26. Tobis JM, Mallery JA, Gessert J, et al. Intravascular ultrasound cross-sectional arterial imaging before and after balloon angioplasty in vitro. Circulation 1989; 80(4):873–882.

27. Nissen SE, Gurley JC, Grines CL, et al. Intravascular ultrasound assessment of lumen size and wall morphology in normal subjects and patients with coronary artery disease. Circulation 1991; 84(3):1087–1099.

28. Nissen SE, Grines CL, Gurley JC, et al. Application of a new phased-array ultrasound imaging catheter in the assessment of vascular dimensions. In vivo comparison to cineangiography. Circulation 1990; 81(2):660–666.

29. Siegel RJ, Chae JS, Forrester JS, Ruiz CE. Angiography, angioscopy, and ultrasound imaging before and after percutaneous balloon angioplasty. Am Heart J 1990; 120(5):1086–1090.

30. Werner GS, Sold G, Buchwald A, Kreuzer H, Wiegand V. Intravascular ultrasound imaging of human coronary arteries after percutaneous transluminal an-

gioplasty: morphologic and quantitative assessment. Am Heart J 1991; 122(1 Pt 1):212–220.

31. Tobis JM, Mallery J, Mahon D, et al. Intravascular ultrasound imaging of human coronary arteries in vivo. Analysis of tissue characterizations with comparison to in vitro histological specimens. Circulation 1991; 83(3):913–926.

32. Davidson CJ, Sheikh KH, Kisslo KB, et al. Intracoronary ultrasound evaluation of interventional technologies. Am J Cardiol 1991; 68(13):1305–1309.

33. De Franco AC, Tuczu EM, Abdelmeguid A, et al. Intravascular ultrasound assessment of PTCA results: insights into the mechanisms of balloon angioplasty. J Am Coll Cardiol 1993; 21(2):485. Abstract.

34. De Franco A, Tuzcu E, Moliterno D, et al. Overestimation of lumen size after coronary interventions: implications for randomized trials of new devices. Circulation 1994; 90(4 Part 2):I-550. Abstract.

35. Hodgson JM, Reddy KG, Suneja R, Nair RN, Lesnefsky EJ, Sheehan HM. Intracoronary ultrasound imaging: correlation of plaque morphology with angiography, clinical syndrome and procedural results in patients undergoing coronary angioplasty. J Am Coll Cardiol 1993; 21(1):35–44.

36. Nissen SE, Tuzcu EM, De Franco AC, et al. Intravascular ultrasound evidence of atherosclerosis at "normal" reference sites predicts adverse clinical outcomes following percutaneous coronary interventions. J Am Coll Cardiol 1994; 271A. Abstract.

37. Mintz GS, Painter JA, Pichard AD, et al. Atherosclerosis in angiographically "normal" coronary artery reference segments: an intravascular ultrasound study with clinical correlations. J Am Coll Cardiol 1995; 25(7):1479–1485.

38. Mintz GS, Painter JA, Pichard AD, et al. Atherosclerosis in angiographically "normal" coronary artery reference segments: an intravascular ultrasound study with clinical correlations. J Am Coll Cardiol 1995; 25(7):1479–1485.

39. Nissen SE, De Franco AC, Raymond R, Franco I, Eaton G, Tuzcu EM. Angiographically unrecognized disease at "normal" reference sites: a risk factor for sub-optimal results after coronary intervention. Circulation 1993; 88:I-412. Abstract.

40. Stone G, Linnemeier T, Frey A, et al. Incidence and implications of coronary dissection after PTCA using oversized balloons with intravascular ultrasound guidance. The CLOUT trial. Circulation 1996; 94:I-261. Abstract.

41. Kuntz R, Gibson C, Nobuyoshi M, Baim D. Generalized model of restenosis after conventional balloon angioplasty, stenting and directional atherectomy. J Am Coll Cardiol 1993; 21:15–25.

42. Kuntz R, Safian R, Carrozza J, Fishman R, Mansour M, Baim D. The importance of acute luminal diameter in determining restenosis after coronary atherectomy or stenting. Circulation 1992; 86:1827–1835.

43. Austin , Ratliff N, Hollman J, Tabei S, Phillips D. Intimal proliferation of smooth muscle cells as an explanation for recurrent coronary artery stenosis after percutaneous transluminal coronary angioplasty. J Am Coll Card 1985.

44. Nobuyoshi M, Kimura T, Ohishi H, et al. Restenosis after percutaneous transluminal coronary angioplasty: pathologic observations in 20 patients. J Am Coll Cardiol 1991; 17:433–439.

45. Forrester JS, Fishbein M, Helfant R, Fagin J. A paradigm for restenosis based on cell biology: clues for the development of new preventive therapies. J Am Coll Cardiol 1991; 17:758–769.

46. Schwartz RS, Holmes D Jr, Topol E. The restenosis paradigm revisited: an alternative proposal for cellular mechanisms. J Am Coll Cardiol 1992; 20:1284–1293.

47. Miller DD, Rivera FJ, Garcia OJ, Palmaz JC, Berger HJ, Weisman HF. Imaging of vascular injury with 99mTc-labeled monoclonal antiplatelet antibody S12. Preliminary experience in human percutaneous transluminal angioplasty. Circulation 1992; 85:1354–1363.

48. Miller DD, Boulet AJ, Tio FO, et al. In vivo technetium-99m S12 antibody imaging of platelet alpha-granules in rabbit endothelial neointimal proliferation after angioplasty. Circulation 1991; 83:224–236.

49. Ellis SG, Bates ER, Schaible T, Weisman HF, Pitt B, Topol EJ. Prospects for the use of antagonists to the platelet glycoprotein IIb/IIa receptor to prevent post-angioplasty restenosis and thrombosis. J Am Coll Cardiiol 1991; 17:89B–95B.

50. den Heijer P, van Dijk R, Hillege H, Pentinga M, Serruys P, Lie K. Serial angioscopic and angiographic observations during the first hour after successful coronary angioplasty: a preamble to a multicenter trial addressing angioscopic markers for restenosis. Am Heart J 1994; 128:656–663.

51. Rensing BJ, Hermans WRM, Beatt KJ, et al. Quantitative angiographic assessment of elastic recoil after percutaneous transluminal coronary angioplasty. Am J Cardiol 1990; 66:1039–1044.

52. Rensing B, Hermans W, Deckers J, de Feyter P, Tijssen J, Serruys P. Lumen narrowing after percutaneous transluminal coronary balloon angioplasty follows a near gaussian distribution: a quantitative angiographic study in 1,445 successfully dilated lesions. J Am Coll Cardiol 1992; 19:939–945.

53. Rensing BJ, Hermans WRM, Vos J, et al. Angiographic risk factors of luminal narrowing after coronary balloon angioplasty using balloon measurements to reflect stretch and elastic recoil at the dilatation site. Am J Cardiol 1992; 69:584–591.

54. Rensing BJ, Hermans WRM, Vos J, et al. Luminal narrowing after percutaneous transluminal coronary angioplasty. Circulation 1993; 88:975–985.

55. Koenig M, Gilmore P, Kelsey R, Jordan T, Bass T. Immediate vs delayed intravascular ultrasound (IVUS) assessment of PTCA: Is there further loss following coronary angioplasty as assessed by IVUS? Circulation 1995; 92:I-76. Abstract.

56. Jain R, Ramee SR, Mesa J, Collins TJ, White CJ. Intracoronary thrombus: chronic urokinase infusion and evaluation with intravascular ultrasound. Cathet Cardiovasc Diagn 1992; 26(3):212–214.

57. Comess K, Fitzgerald PJ, Yock PG. Intracoronary ultrasound imaging of graft thrombosis. N Engl J Med 1992; 327(23):1691–1692. Letter.

58. Mintz GS, Potkin BN, Cooke RH, et al. Intravascular ultrasound imaging in a patient with unstable angina. Am Heart J 1992; 123(6):1692–1694.

59. Chemarin-Alibellli MJ, Pieraggi MT, Elbaz M, et al. Identification of coronary thrombus after myocardial infarction by intracoronary ultrasound compared with histology of tissues sampled by atherectomy. Am J Cardiol 1996; 77(5):344–349.

60. Mintz GS, Popma JJ, Pichard AD, et al. Intravascular ultrasound predictors of restenosis after percutaneous transcatheter coronary revascularization. J Am Coll Cardiol 1996; 27(7):1678–1687.

61. Luo H, Nishioka T, Eigler N, et al. Coronary artery restenosis after balloon angioplasty in humans is associated with circumferential coronary constriction. Arterioscler Thromb Vasc Biol 1996; 16:1393–1398.

62. Mitsuo K, Degawa T, Nakamura S, et al. Serial intravascular ultrasound evaluation of the mechanism of restenosis after directional coronary atherectomy. Circulation 1995; 92(8):I-149. Abstract.

63. Manyari D, Knudtson M, Kloiber R, et al. Sequential thallium-201 myocardial perfusion studies after successful percutaneous transluminal coronary artery angioplasty: delayed resolution of exercise-induced scintigraphic abnormalities. Circulation 1988; 77(1):86–95.

64. Guide Trial Investigators. IVUS-determined predictors of restenosis in PTCA and DCA: an interim report from the GUIDE trial, Phase II. Circulation 1994; 90(suppl I):I-23. Abstract.

65. Wijns W, Serruys PW, Reiber JH, et al. Early detection of restenosis after successful percutaneous transluminal coronary angioplasty by exercise-redistribution thallium scintigraphy. Am J. Cardiol 1985; 55(4):357–361.

66. Stuckey T, Burwell L, Mygaard T, et al. Quantitative exercise thallium-201 scintigraphy for predicting angina recurrence after percutaneous transluminal coronary angioplasty. Am J Cardiol 1989; 63:517–521.

67. Vlay SC, Chernilas J, Lawson WE, Dervan JP. Restenosis after angioplasty: don't rely on the exercise test. Am Heart J 1989; 117(4):980–986.

68. Leimgruber PP, Roubin GS, Hollman J, et al. Restenosis after successful coronary angioplasty in patients with single-vessel disease. Circulation 1986; 73: 710–717.

69. Laarman G, Luijten HE, van Zeyl LG, et al. Assessment of "silent" restenosis and long-term follow-up after successful angioplasty in single vessel coronary artery disease: the value of quantitative exercise electrocardiography and quantitative coronary angiography. Am Coll Cardiol 1990; 16(3):578–585.

70. Breisblatt W, Weiland F, Spaccavento L. Stress thallium-201 imaging after coronary angioplasty predicts restenosis and recurrent symptoms. J Am Coll Cardiol 1988; 12:1199–1204.

71. Duerr RL, Topol EJ. Dissociation between minimal lumen diameter and clinical outcome at 6 month follow-up randomized trials of percutaneous revascularization. J Am Coll Cardiol 1995; 25:37A. Abstract.

72. Peters R, for the PICTURE Study Group. Prediction of the risk of angiographic restenosis by intracoronary ultrasound imaging after coronary balloon angioplasty. J Am Coll Cardiol 1995; 25:35A. Abstract.

73. Topol E, Nissen S. Our Preoccupation with coronary luminology: the dissociation between clinical and angiographic findings in ischemic heart disease. Circulation 1995; 92:2333–2342.

74. Hirzel H, Nuesch K, Gruentzig A, Luetolf UM. Short- and long-term changes in myocardial perfusion after PTCA assessed by thallium-201 exercise scintigraphy. Circulation 1981; 63:1001–1007.

75. Wijns W, Serruys PW, Simoons ML, et al. Predictive value of early maximal exercise test and thallium scintigraphy after successful percutaneous transluminal coronary angioplasty. Br Heart J 1985; 53(2):194–200.

76. Hardoff R, Shefer A, Gips S, et al. Predicting late restenosis after coronary angioplasty by very early (12 to 24 h) thallium-201 scintigraphy: implications with regard to mechanisms of late coronary restenosis. J Am Coll Cardiol 1990; 15:1486–1492.

77. Tenaglia AN, Buller CE, Kisslo KB, Phillips HR, Stack RS, Davison CJ. Intracoronary ultrasound predictors of adverse outcomes after coronary artery interventions. J Am Coll Cardiol 1992: 20(6):1385–1390.

78. Waller BF, Orr CM, Pinkerton CA, Van Tassel J, Peters T, Slack JD. Coronary balloon angioplasty dissections: "the good, the bad and the ugly." J Am Coll Cardiol 1992; 20(3):701–706. Editorial; comment.

79. Hausmann D, Sudhir K, Mullen W, et al. Contrast-enhanced intravascular ultrasound: validation of a new technique for delineation of the vessel wall boundary. J Am Coll Cardiol 1994; 23(4):981–987.

80. Isner J, Kishel J, Kent K. Accuracy of angiographic determination of left main coronary arterial narrowing. Circulation 1981; 63:1056–1061.

81. Hermiller JB, Buller CE, Tenaglia AN, et al. Unrecognized left main coronary artery disease in patients undergoing interventional procedures. Am J Cardiol 1993; 71(2):173–176.

82. De Franco AC, Tuzcu EM, Eaton G, et al. Detection of recognized LMCA disease by intravascular ultrasound in patients undergoing interventions: prevalence and severity. Circulation 1993; 88:I-411. Abstract.

83. Mintz GS, Pichard AD, Kovach JA, et al. Impact of preintervention intravascular ultrasound imaging on transcatheter treatment strategies in coronary artery disease. Am J Cardiol 1994; 73(7): 412–430.

84. Kearney P, Erbel R, Ge J et al. Assessment of spontaneous coronary artery dissection by intravascular ultrasound in a patient with unstable angina. Cathet Cardiovasc Diagn 1994; 32(1):58–61.

85. Wolff MR, Resar JR, Stuart RS, Brinker JA. Coronary artery rupture and pseudoaneurysm formation resulting from percutaneous coronary angioscopy. Cathet Cardiovasc Diagn 1993; 28(1):47–50.

86. Ritter M, Rickli H, Jakob M, Amann FW, Jenni R. Coronary pseudoaneurysm: diagnosis by intravascular ultrasonography. J Am Soc Echo 1995; 8(2):215–216.

87. Ennis BM, Zientek DM, Ruggie NT, Billhardt RA, Klein LW. Characterization of a saphenous vein graft aneurysm by intravascular ultrasound and computerized three-dimensional reconstruction. Cathet Cardiovasc Diagn 1993; 28(4): 328–331.
88. Garrand TJ, Mintz GS, Popma JJ, Lewis SA, Vaughn NA, Leon MB. Intravascular ultrasound diagnosis of a coronary artery pseudoaneurysm following percutaneous transluminal coronary angioplasty. Am Heart J 1993; 125(3):880–882.
89. Gorge G, Haude M, Ge J, Zamorano J, Erbel R. How does a continuous coronary perfusion catheter work in coronary artery dissection? Assessment by intravascular ultrasound. Eur Heart J 1996; 17(1):151–152. Letter.
90. Timmis S, Hermiller J, Burns W, et al. A randomized intracoronary ultrasound trial of perfusion balloon vs. conventional balloon PTCA. Circulation 1996; 92:I-317. Abstract.
91. Mintz GS, Pichard AD, Kent KM, et al. Transcatheter device synergy: preliminary experience with adjunct directional coronary atherectomy following high-speed rotational atherectomy or excimer laser angioplasty in the treatment of coronary artery disease. Cathet Cardiovasc Diagn 1993; 1:37–44.
92. Jackson JD Jr, Hermiller JB, Sketch MH Jr, et al. Combined rotational and directional atherectomy guided by intravascular ultrasound in an occluded vein graft. Am Heart J 1992; 124(1):214–216.
93. Tobis J, Colombo A, Almagor Y, et al. Intravascular ultrasound guidance of multiple interventions does not reduce restenosis. Circulation 1995; 92:I-148. Abstract.
94. Violaris AG, Linnemeier TJ, Campbell S, Rothbaum DA, Cumberland DC. Intravascular ultrasound imaging combined with coronary angioplasty. Lancet 1992; 339(8809):1571–1572.
95. Cacchione JG, Reddy K, Richards F, Sheehan H, Hodgson JM. Combined intravascular ultrasound/angioplasty balloon catheter: initial use during PTCA. Cathet Cardiovasc Diagn 1991; 24(2):99–101.
96. Cavaye DM, White RA, Kopchok GE, Mueller MP, Maselly MJ, Tabbara MR. Three-dimensional intravascular ultrasound imaging of normal and diseased canine and human arteries. J Vasc Surg 1992; 16(4):509–517.
97. Coy KM, Park JC, Fishbein MC, et al. In vitro validation of three-dimensional intravascular ultrasound for the evaluation of arterial injury after balloon angioplasty. J Am Coll Cardiol 1992; 20(3):692–670.
98. Evans JL, Ng KH, Wiet SG, et al. Accurate three-dimensional reconstruction of intravascular ultrasound data. Spatially correct three-dimensional reconstructions. Circulation 1996; 93(3):567–576.
99. Rosenfield K, Kaufman J, Pieczek A, Langevin R Jr, Razvi S, Isner JM. Real-time three-dimensional reconstruction of intravascular ultrasound images of iliac arteries. Am J Cardiol 1992; 70(3):412–415.
100. Rosenfield K, Kaufman J, Pieczek AM, et al. Human coronary and peripheral arteries: on-line three-dimensional reconstruction from two-dimensional intravascular US scans. Work in progress. Radiology 1992; 184(3):823–832.

101. Weissman NJ, Palacios IF, Nidorf SM, Dinsmore RE, Weyman AE. Three-dimensional intravascular ultrasound assessment of plaque volume after successful atherectomy. Am Heart J 1995; 130(3 Pt 1):413–419.

102. Gorge G, Liu F, Ge J, Haude M, Baumgart D, Caspary G. Intravascular ultrasound variables predict restenosis after PTCA. Circulation 1995; 92:I-148. Abstract.

103. Gussenhoven E, for the EPISODE study group (Evaluation Peripheral Intravascular Sonography on Dotter Effect). Prediction by intravascular ultrasound of failure after peripheral balloon angioplasty. Circulation 1995; 92:I-600. Abstract.

12

Use of Combined Intravascular Ultrasound and PTCA Catheter: Clinical Utility

Kathleen Quealy   *University Hospitals of Cleveland, Cleveland, Ohio*

Ravi Nair   *Case Western Reserve University and University Hospitals of Cleveland, Cleveland, Ohio*

I. INTRODUCTION

Intracoronary ultrasound has emerged as an extremely useful complement to both diagnostic coronary angiography as well as coronary angioplasty, by providing information not obtainable by any other means (1–6). Although coronary angiography has been the "gold standard" for evaluating the severity of coronary artery stenoses, it provides only a silhouette of the vessel lumen. Intravascular ultrasound, on the other hand, demonstrates the important "details" of these stenoses; including composition of plaque and vessel architecture. In addition, by virtue of its tomographic images, intravascular ultrasound has the ability to accurately quantitate *true* lumen size, to define lumen geometry (concentric vs. eccentric plaque), and to identify vessel wall dissections, and is a tool to quantify plaque volume. By identifying these vessel and lesion characteristics, the choice of an appropriate, correctly sized interventional device can be made, ensuring optimum results and ultimately improving patient outcome (7,8).

To effectively use intracoronary ultrasound as a means to guide angioplasty, evaluation of the angioplasty site both before and after therapy is necessary. With the available dedicated ultrasound catheter, this would involve at least three catheter exchanges after coronary angiography is performed. First, evaluation with a standard intravascular ultrasound catheter needs to be done. Second, the intravascular ultrasound catheter needs to be exchanged for a standard angioplasty balloon catheter/device. Finally, another catheter exchange needs to be performed to repeat the intravascular ultrasound evaluation postprocedure. In addition, any further interventions (e.g., repeat balloon inflations, stent, etc.) would require further catheter exchanges.

These multiple catheter exchanges can be cumbersome as well as time-consuming. It would be ideal, therefore, to have an ultrasound transducer present on the treatment catheter in order to avoid these exchanges. Whereas transducers on nonballoon interventional devices are being developed (9), they are not yet available for clinical use. A combination angioplasty and intravascular ultrasound catheter has undergone clinical evaluation and is currently commercially available (10,11). This catheter enables the operator to evaluate vessels and atherosclerotic lesions just prior to balloon inflation. Information obtained from this on-line evaluation can be used to guide further decisions about balloon inflations without the need for multiple catheter exchanges.

II. CATHETER DESIGN

The combination intravascular ultrasound and angioplasty balloon catheter presently available (Endosonics, Oracle MicroPLUS) incorporates a compliant (nominal pressure = 6 atm) angioplasty balloon (2.0, 2.5, 3.0, 3.5 mm diameter in 20-mm length) with a 20-MHz synthetic aperture array ultrasound transducer. The shaft is 3.5 F along its entire length and has radiopaque markers at the center of the balloon and at the transducer (Fig. 1).

The aperture array transducer system allows for maintenance of a flexible, steerable catheter (12) without mechanically driven parts. The transducer is placed on the shaft, proximal to the angioplasty balloon. The catheter allows for a guidewire (.014" or smaller) through its central lumen, has a monorail design, and behaves essentially like any other balloon dilatation catheter.

A. Catheter Use

After the lesion is crossed with a wire, the combination catheter is advanced over the wire with the balloon portion beyond the lesion and the transducer positioned across the lesion (Fig. 2). Measurement of the true luminal area/ diameter of the reference vessel segment and the segment containing the lesion, eccentricity definition, and identification of plaque characteristics (soft, fi-

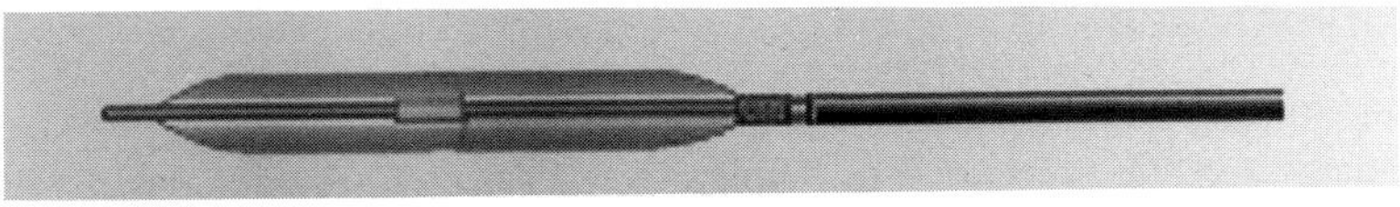

Figure 1   Oracle MicroPLUS catheter. The imaging transducer is located on the shaft of the catheter just proximal to the angioplasty balloon. (Courtesy Endosonics Corp., Pleasanton, CA.)

brous, hard) can be performed. The angioplasty balloon is then positioned over the identified lesion by partially withdrawing the catheter, and inflations are performed. The segment with the transducer is then advanced across the angioplasty site for a second time, and immediate intravascular ultrasound evaluation can be performed. If any further inflations become necessary, repeat inflations and evaluation of the results can be performed by advancing or withdrawing the catheter system.

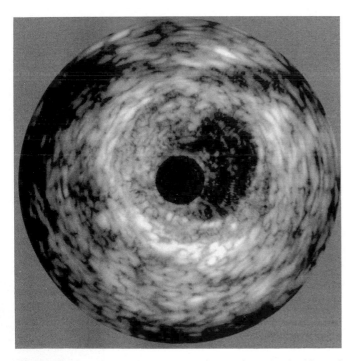

Figure 2   Image of an atherosclerotic lesion obtained with an Oracle MicroPLUS. (Courtesy Endosonics Corp., Pleasanton, CA.)

B. Advantages

The combination intravascular ultrasound/angioplasty balloon catheter allows for evaluation of the vessel wall integrity, residual plaque volume, and post-procedure luminal diameter immediately after balloon dilatation. In the presence of a large dissection, the decision to proceed to further balloon inflations and/or the deployment of an intravascular stent can be made without the delay inherent in using two separate catheters for angioplasty and intravascular ultrasound.

Intravascular ultrasound evaluation of postdilatation luminal diameter and residual plaque volume may reveal the need for a larger balloon to obtain optimal results. In this instance, the combination catheter must be exchanged for a larger-size angioplasty balloon and then reinserted to evaluate with ultrasound after dilatation with the larger balloon.

In elective stent procedures, the combination catheter can be used as the initial dilatation balloon, and, based on luminal diameter, stent and postdeployment balloon of the appropriate size can be chosen. This measurement is critical, since postdeployment inflations are done at high pressures, and larger balloon-to-lumen ratios could result in complications such as dissections or perforations. On the other hand, small balloon-to-lumen ratios may result in an underdeployed stent, increasing the incidence of stent thrombosis (13).

C. Limitations

Though visual estimates, caliper measurements, and quantitative angiography are traditional methods, it is clear that the more accurate method for choosing the appropriately sized angioplasty balloon is through the measurement of the true vessel luminal diameter via intravascular ultrasound. In using the combination catheter, the balloon size used for angioplasty must be chosen prior to ultrasound evaluation, using only the angiogram for sizing. This obviates one of the more beneficial components of intravascular ultrasound evaluation.

Intravascular ultrasound can "miss" dissections that are seen by angiogram, as a result of the catheter holding the vessel open, and/or the dissection being obscured by shadowing from heavily calcified vessels. In these instances, prior to demonstration by angiography or clinical symptoms, the operator may develop a false sense of security about the integrity of the vessel.

The combination intravascular ultrasound catheter currently available has its transducer proximal to the angioplasty balloon. In distal, narrow or tortuous vessels, advancement of the distal, balloon-containing segment of the catheter past the stenosis to perform ultrasound evaluation may be difficult, and transient occlusion of the vessel may occur.

III. GOALS FOR FUTURE DESIGNS

Intravascular ultrasound has had a major impact on the optimal deployment of intracoronary stents, reducing complications and reducing the need for aggressive poststent anticoagulation (14). Incorporating an ultrasound transducer either on a noncompliant balloon, on the balloon for high-pressure inflations poststent deployment, or, even better, on a noncompliant, high-pressure stent deployment balloon would make stent deployment faster and less cumbersome by avoiding multiple catheter exchanges. This would result in shorter procedure times, possibly improving patient outcomes and decreasing overall cost.

Placing the transducer in the center of the angioplasty balloon (15) would eliminate the need to cross the entire lesion before being able to image the segment of interest. This would be especially important in severe, tubular stenoses or lesions that are in tortuous segments, where the balloon cannot be passed beyond the lesion without compromising distal flow.

IV. SUMMARY

The combination ultrasound/angioplasty balloon catheter allows for immediate interchange between its diagnostic and therapeutic capability. Appropriate decisions on balloon sizing can be made, and, depending on postdilatation appearance, further strategy can be planned without multiple catheter exchanges. This makes the important information achieved from ultrasound evaluation of angioplasty results much more convenient to use. In the era of widespread stent use, this catheter can be used as an ideal predilatation catheter for elective stent cases. With further advancements in catheter technology/design, as proposed above, the use of such a device is likely to be vastly enhanced.

REFERENCES

1. Mallery JA, Tobis JM, Griffith J, et al. Assessment of normal and atherosclerotic arterial wall thickness with an intravascular ultrasound imaging catheter. Am Heart J 1990; 199:1392–1400.
2. Tobis JM, Mallery JA, Gessert, J, et al. Intravascular ultrasound cross-sectional arterial imaging before and after balloon angioplasty in vivo. Circulation 1989; 80:873–882.
3. Tobis JM, Mallery J, Mahon D, et al. Intravascular ultrasound imaging of human coronary arteries in vivo; analysis of tissue characterizations with comparison to in vitro histological specimens. Circulation 1991; 83:913–926.
4. Nissen SE, Gurley JC, Grines C, et al. Intravascular ultrasound assessment of

lumen size and wall morphology in normal subjects and patients with coronary artery disease. Circulation 1991; 84:1087–1099.

5. Yock PG, Fitzgerald PJ, Linker DT, Angelsen AJ. Intravascular ultrasound guidance for catheter-based coronary interventions. J Am Coll Cardiol 1991; 17: 39B–45B.

6. Wolfe CL, Klette MA, Trask RV, et al. Assessment of the results of percutaneous transluminal coronary angioplasty using an integrated ultrasound imaging-angioplasty catheter. Cathet Cardiovasc Diagn 1994; 32:108–112.

7. Lee DY, Eigler N, Luo H, et al. Effect of intracoronary ultrasound on clinical decision making. Am Heart J 1995; 129:1084–1093.

8. Honye J, Mahon DJ, Jain A, et al. Morphological effects of coronary balloon angioplasty in vivo assessed by intravascular ultrasound imaging. Circulation 1992; 85:1012–1025.

9. Fitzgerald PJ, Belef M, Connolly AJ, Sudhir K, Yock PG. Design and initial testing of an ultrasound-guided directional atherectomy device. Am Heart J 1995; 129:593–598.

10. Cacchione JG, Reddy K, Richards F, Sheehan H, Hodgson JMcB. Combined intravascular ultrasound/angioplasty balloon catheter: initial use during PTCA. Cathet Cardiovasc Diagn 1991; 24:99–101.

11. Hodgson JM, Nair R. Efficacy and usefulness of a combined intracoronary ultrasound-angioplasty balloon catheter: results of the Multicenter Oracle trial. (abstract) Circulation 1992; 84(suppl I):321.

12. Hodgson JM, Cacchione JG, Berry J, Savakus A, Eberle M. Combined intracoronary ultrasound imaging and angioplasty catheter: initial in vivo studies. Circulation 1990; 82(suppl III):2686.

13. Nakamura S, Colombo A, Gaglione MD, et al. Intracoronary ultrasound observations during stent implantation. Circulation 1994; 89:2026–2034.

14. Colombo A, Hall P, Nakamura S, et al. Intracoronary stenting without anticoagulation accomplished with intravascular ultrasound guidance. Circulation 1995; 91: 1676–1688.

15. Isner JM, Rosenfield K, Losordo DW, et al. Combination balloon-ultrasound imaging catheter for percutaneous transluminal angioplasty—validation of imaging, analysis of recoil and identification of plaque fracture. Circulation 1991; 84:739–754.

13

Use of Intravascular Ultrasound in Excimer Laser Angioplasty and Rotational Atherectomy

Rainer Hoffmann, Gary S. Mintz, Augusto D. Pichard, Kenneth M. Kent, and Lowell F. Satler *Washington Hospital Center, Washington, D.C.*

Jeffrey J. Popma and Martin B. Leon *Cardiology Research Foundation, Washington, D.C.*

I. INTRODUCTION

New devices, such as excimer laser angioplasty and rotational atherectomy, have been developed to overcome some of the limitations of conventional balloon angioplasty (1–8). Intravascular ultrasound (IVUS) allows transmural imaging of coronary arteries in humans in vivo, providing unique insights into the pathology of coronary artery disease by defining vessel wall geometry and the major components of the atherosclerotic plaque (9–11). IVUS has been used to study the mechanisms and the acute and chronic results of angioplasty devices. While IVUS is useful in selecting and monitoring the efficacy of new device angioplasty procedures, the operators cannot ignore the angiographic findings. For example, numerous studies have shown increased complications after both excimer laser angioplasty and rotational atherectomy in bendpoint lesions or tortuous vessels; current IVUS techniques are incapable of providing information about the spatial geometry of the coronary arteries.

II. EXCIMER LASER ANGIOPLASTY

The term LASER is an acronym for Light Amplification by the Stimulated Emission of Radiation, and EXCIMER is an acronym for EXCIted diMER. Specific properties characterize lasers. Laser light is monochromatic, which means that it is produced at a single, specific wavelength. Laser photons are characterized by spatial and temporal coherence due to collimation and synchronization of the photons. These properties result in constancy of energy density of the laser beam regardless of distance to the laser source.

Excimer is a pulsed laser, meaning that energy is emitted at brief bursts separated by relatively long periods of silence during which laser emission is switched off. Cardiovascular excimer lasers currently emit photons having a 308-nm wavelength. Two types of coronary laser catheters are available: concentric and eccentric, which vary in their distribution of laser fibers relative to the guidewire lumen. A total occlusion catheter is under investigation.

There are three types of laser tissue effects: thermal ablation, photoacoustic ablation, and photodecomposition. Photodecomposition results in direct molecular bond breaking. *In vitro* studies have suggested that lasers (such as the 308-nm excimer laser) that work via photodecomposition can achieve precise, scalpel-like excision and ablation of tissue. This is in sharp contradistinction to the first generation of vascular lasers (e.g., CO_2 or Nd-YAG lasers) which primarily caused thermal ablation and resulted in imprecise and disrupted lesion surfaces.

A. Mechanisms

However, serial IVUS studies in human coronary arteries *in vivo* have also been used to study the mechanism of lumen enlargement after excimer laser coronary angioplasty (12–14). Based on the in vitro validation of cross-sectional measurements by IVUS, measurement of the external elastic membrane cross-sectional area (representing the area within the border between the hypoechoic media and the echoreflective adventitia) is used as a reproducible measure of total arterial cross-sectional area; also, recognizing that IVUS cannot measure media thickness accurately, plaque+media cross-sectional area (calculated as external elastic membrane minus lumen cross-sectional area) is used as a measure of plaque mass. Mintz et al. (12) studied the effect of excimer laser coronary angioplasty in 49 lesions finding that lumen cross-sectional area increased (from preintervention to postexcimer laser angioplasty) by both atheroablation and vessel expansion. The main mechanism of lumen enlargement from 1.4 ± 0.5 mm^2 before intervention to 2.7 ± 0.8 mm^2 after excimer laser coronary angioplasty was tissue ablation, accounting for

76% of the increase of lumen area. This was indicated by a decrease of plaque+media area from 16.8 ± 7.1 to 15.9 ± 6.7 mm². The contribution of vessel expansion averaged 24% and was indicated by an increase of the vessel area from 18.2 ± 7.1 to 18.6 ± 6.8 mm² (Table 1). Possible mechanisms of excimer laser angioplasty induced vessel expansion are intraluminal laser-induced shock waves and forceful expansion of vapor bubbles into tissue.

It should be noted, though, that there was substantial varability from lesion to lesion; in some lesions lumen enlargement was almost entirely the result of tissue ablation while in other lesions lumen enlargement was almost entirely the result of vessel expansion (Fig. 1). Nevertheless, the overall increase of lumen area and reduction in plaque area after excimer laser angioplasty in all lesions was modest, and the residual plaque burden was substantial. This resulted in the need for adjunctive therapy in most cases.

Serial IVUS analysis failed to demonstrate evidence of calcium ablation by either quantitative (an absolute decrease in the measured arc of calcium) or qualitative (increased visualization of deep-vessel wall structures) criteria. Dissections were present in 39% of lesions after laser angioplasty. They almost always occurred within superficial fibrocalcific plaque. Superficial calcific deposits developed a "shattered" appearance that was not seen after other devices (Fig. 2). These findings would also be explained by intraluminal laser-induced shock waves and forceful expansion of vapor bubbles into tissue.

B. Indications and Results

The results of two multicenter studies (15,16) involving 764 and 3000 patients indicated favorable success rates in saphenous vein graft lesions, long lesions, ostial lesions, calcified stenoses, total occlusions, and after unsuccessful PTCA (15–17). Procedural success (defined as final stenosis ≤50% without in-hospital Q-wave myocardial infarction, coronary artery bypass surgery or death) was 90%. However, adjunctive balloon angioplasty was necessary in the

Table 1   Quantitative IVUS Analysis in 49 Lesions Before and After ELCA

	pre-ELCA	post-ELCA	P
External elastic membrane CSA (mm²)	18.2 ± 7.1	18.6 ± 6.8	<.05
Lumen CSA (mm²)	1.4 ± 0.5	2.7 ± 0.8	<.0001
Plaque+media CSA (mm²)	16.8 ± 7.1	15.9 ± 6.7	<.0001

Source: Mintz et al. (12).
Abbreviations: CSA, cross-sectional area; ELCA, excimer laser coronary angioplasty.

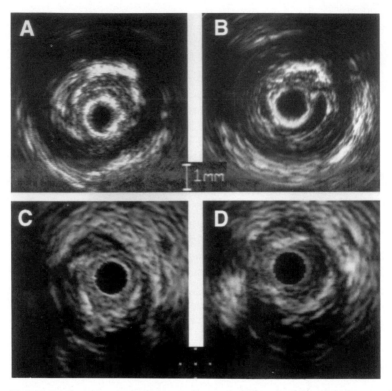

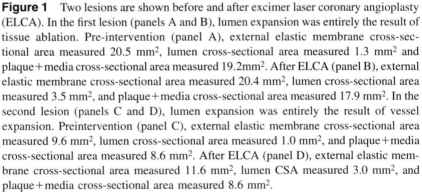

Figure 1 Two lesions are shown before and after excimer laser coronary angioplasty (ELCA). In the first lesion (panels A and B), lumen expansion was entirely the result of tissue ablation. Pre-intervention (panel A), external elastic membrane cross-sectional area measured 20.5 mm², lumen cross-sectional area measured 1.3 mm² and plaque+media cross-sectional area measured 19.2mm². After ELCA (panel B), external elastic membrane cross-sectional area measured 20.4 mm², lumen cross-sectional area measured 3.5 mm², and plaque+media cross-sectional area measured 17.9 mm². In the second lesion (panels C and D), lumen expansion was entirely the result of vessel expansion. Preintervention (panel C), external elastic membrane cross-sectional area measured 9.6 mm², lumen cross-sectional area measured 1.0 mm², and plaque+media cross-sectional area measured 8.6 mm². After ELCA (panel D), external elastic membrane cross-sectional area measured 11.6 mm², lumen CSA measured 3.0 mm², and plaque+media cross-sectional area measured 8.6 mm².

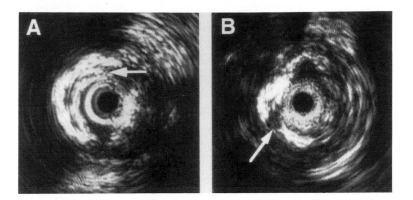

Figure 2 Postexcimer laser angioplasty IVUS images in these two lesions show dissection of superficial fibrocalcific plaque. Panel A shows fragmentation (arrow) of a large superficial calcific deposit with sharp edges demarcating the margins of the dissected calcium. Panel B shows an "onion skin" separation of the circumferential dissection planes (arrow).

majority of cases to achieve an optimal result. Conversely, major complications occurred in 6.4% to 7.6% (15,17).

C. IVUS Imaging Before Laser Angioplasty

In general, IVUS is useful preintervention for determining reference vessel size and reference disease segment measuring lumen dimensions and lesion length, assessing plaque composition (especially calcification) and plaque distribution (eccentricity), and evaluating unusual lesion morphology. In total occlusions or in many other lesions treated with excimer laser angioplasty (e.g., long diffuse disease in small vessels), preintervention intravascular ultrasound imaging may not be feasible.

Laser angioplasty has proven to be effective in soft, fibrous, and mildly calcific lesions; conversely, excimer laser angioplasty is limited in the presence of severe lesion calcium. Thus, if it can be performed, preinterventional intravascular ultrasound imaging should focus on 1. determining whether a guidewire which has crossed a total occlusion is intraplaque, intramural, or intraluminal 2. detecting severe superficial lesion calcification (in which the effectiveness of excimer laser angioplasty may be limited), and 3. detecting severe lesion eccentricity (in which case the eccentric laser catheter should be used preferentially, rather than the concentric laser catheter). On the other hand, while excimer laser angioplasty is useful in treating thrombus-containing lesions, IVUS has a limited ability to differentiate thrombus from nonthrombotic hypoechoic plaque elements.

Laser angioplasty techniques continue to evolve. Different strategies include single vs. multiple passes, slow pass vs. fast pass, and the use of saline flush. These have been based on reducing angiographic complications such as dissections. There is incomplete information on IVUS imaging in different laser angioplasty strategies.

The laser catheter size should be larger than the lumen dimensions preintervention. This is important for proper laser catheter size selection to maximize plaque ablation.

In treating in-stent restenosis, preintervention IVUS imaging is useful to confirm full stent expansion prior to laser ablation.

D. IVUS Imaging After Laser Angioplasty

Similarly, IVUS is useful postintervention for determining residual plaque burden (an important IVUS predictor of restenosis), final lumen dimensions, and resultant tissue disruption. Studies comparing IVUS and quantitative angiographic measurements of minimum lumen dimensions after excimer laser angioplasty in our laboratory have shown no significant correlation ($r = .190$, $P = .0971$), hence the value of relying on IVUS to determine procedural success.

Because of the only modest increase of lumen area after excimer laser therapy alone, adjunctive therapy is almost always necessary (12–14). The mechanism of adjunct PTCA is additional vessel expansion and dissection with no evidence of plaque compression. In large vessels the use of directional atherectomy has shown to result in a better lumen area than adjunctive PTCA. The mechanism of adjunctive directional atherectomy is a combination of vessel expansion and tissue removal. After adjunctive directional atherectomy or PTCA, the frequency of dissections increased to 73%; dissections occur at the junction of calcified and noncalcified plaque. Finally, adjunctive stenting results in a larger lumen area than either adjunctive PTCA or directional atherectomy. IVUS imaging is useful for determining reference vessel size for correctly sizing the adjunctive device.

III. ROTATIONAL ATHERECTOMY

Percutaneous rotational atherectomy uses a high-speed (160,000 to 190,000 rpm), diamond-coated metal burr to abrade and pulverize the atheromatous plaque into fine microparticles (5 to 10 μm in size). Unlike other devices, rotational atherectomy removes harder, calcific-fibrous atherosclerotic plaque while deflecting more elastic, normal tissue. In vitro studies (18,19) showed that the damage to normal arterial wall was largely confined to the intima without evidence of medial dissection, while noncompliant plaque material, especially calcium, is selectively removed. The resulting vessel surface after rotational atherectomy is smooth, shiny, and polished.

A. Mechanism of Rotational Atherectomy

Serial IVUS imaging has also been used to quantify the mechanism of lumen enlargement by rotational atherectomy. In a study on 48 lesions, the increase of lumen area from 1.8 $\pm$ 0.9 to 3.9 $\pm$ 1.1 mm^2 was the result of a decrease of plaque+media area from 15.7 $\pm$ 4.1 to 13.0 $\pm$ 4.7 mm^2, while the target lesion arterial area was unchanged (Table 2; 20). Serial IVUS imaging has also shown that rotational atherectomy ablates both calcified and noncalcified plaque. Although the plaque lumen surface is smooth, especially in calcified plaque (21), a significant plaque burden averaging 74% remains. The lumen after rotational atherectomy may be larger than the largest burr tip used. This finding has been explained by wire biasing or by spontaneous or nitroglycerin-induced postrotablator vasodilatation. However, postrotablator vasospasm (decrease in target lesion and reference segment arterial cross-sectional area) has also been noted, especially in noncalcified plaque. In our series, the arc of calcification decreased from 227 $\pm$ 107° to 209 $\pm$ 107° (P < .048; Fig. 3).

Dissections were reported to occur in only 26% to 32% of lesions after rotational atherectomy (20,21). This is in sharp contrast to the IVUS findings after PTCA of highly calcified lesions, which show dissections in up to 100% of lesions.

Table 2 Quantitative IVUS Analysis Before and After Rotational Atherectomy and After Adjunctive PTCA

	pre-RA	post-RA	post-PTCA	P ANOVA
External elastic membrane CSA (mm^2)	17.3 $\pm$ 5.9	16.7 $\pm$ 4.8	18.8 $\pm$ 5.6	<.0001
Lumen CSA (mm^2)	1.8 $\pm$ 0.9	3.9 $\pm$ 1.1	5.2 $\pm$ 1.2	<.0001
Plaque+media CSA (mm^2)	15.7 $\pm$ 4.1	13.0 $\pm$ 4.7	13.7 $\pm$ 5.0	<.0001

Source: Adapted from Kovach et al. (20).
Abbreviations: CSA, cross-sectional area; RA, rotational atherectomy.

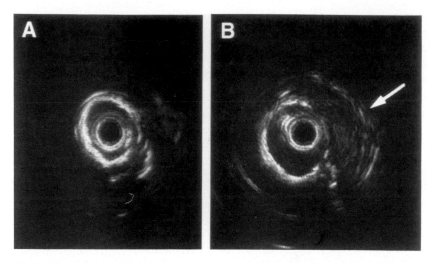

Figure 3   Before rotational atherectomy (panel A) there was circumferential superficial calcification of this circumflex lesion. After stand-alone rotational atherectomy with a 2.5 mm burr, there was lumen enlargement with full thickness calcium removal to reveal deeper adventitial structures (white arrow) with a significant reduction in the total arc of calcium.

B.   Indications and Results

Complex lesions such as calcified lesions, ostial lesions, and long lesions have been found to be successfully treated by rotational atherectomy. Success rates of 95% for type B lesions and 91% for type C lesions have been reported (22–28). Thrombotic lesions and saphenous vein grafts are thought to be inappropriate for rotational atherectomy. Evolving indications include in-stent restenosis.

Microembolization can result in severe wall motion abnormalities (26,27, 29). Further potential sequelae of distal embolization are the "slow" and "nonreflow" phenomena and microinfarction with resulting CPK elevation. In addition, rotational atherectomy applied to eccentric, tortuous, and calcified lesions is associated with an increased risk of dissection (22,30).

C.   IVUS Imaging Before Rotational Atherectomy

As with excimer laser angioplasty, IVUS is useful preintervention for determining reference vessel size and reference segment disease, measuring lumen dimensions and lesion length, assessing plaque composition (especially calcification) and plaque distribution (eccentricity), and evaluating unusual lesion morphology. With most conventional IVUS catheters preintervention imaging is feasible in over 90% of lesions regardless of severity. The two exceptions are vessel tortuosity just proximal to a stenosis (especially using short monorail catheters, which tend to prolapse) and lesions containing significant amounts of superficial calcium. The rotablator is the only device that removes calcium from lesions, and IVUS detects target lesion calcification approximately twice as often as does fluoroscopy. Conversely, while rotational atherectomy should be avoided in thrombus-containing lesions, not all angiographic filling defects are thrombi. Some are calcified "masses."

The initial burr selected should be larger than the minimum lumen diameter on preintervention imaging. The initial burr should be only *slightly* larger than the minimum lumen diameter *in long calcified lesions*; a more liberal choice of initial burr size is possible in shorter noncalcified lesions.

D. IVUS Imaging After Rotational Atherectomy

After passage of the rotational atherectomy burr, the lumen/plaque border will be more sharply defined. The lumen area should have increased. The resultant minimal lumen diameter may be useful in selecting the next burr size.

Pullback of the intravascular ultrasound catheter might show a step up in lumen diameter and abrupt decrease in plaque burden at the place where rotational atherectomy was stopped. This finding had been called a "stop lesion," and it suggests that the distal end of the lesion was not completely ablated. Complete calcium removal is rare if it occurs at all. To demonstrate a quantitative decrease in the IVUS arc of target lesion calcium, there must be full-thickness calcium removal. However, fissuring within the calcium may create a slitlike window for ultrasound penetration into the deeper arterial structures; this finding has been likened to a "headlight." IVUS imaging is also useful in excluding dissection, thrombus, deep wall hematoma, or vessel spasm as mechanisms of "no reflow." Lesion and reference segment media-to-media diameter should be similar to prerotational atherectomy. Smaller diameters indicate spasm of the artery; larger diameters indicate that stretching of the artery wall may have occurred.

Conventionally, the final burr is targeted to be 80% of the angiographic reference lumen dimension; however, the IVUS measurement of the reference lumen may be more reliable. Importantly, significant target lesion and reference segment plaque burden may suggest that an even larger final burr can be used safely.

After rotational atherectomy, the minimal lumen diameter should be close to the average of the reference segment minimum lumen diameters. If not, a decision must be made as to the use of a larger burr or an adjunctive device like PTCA, directional atherectomy, or stent placement.

For example, if IVUS shows significant residual calcification, more rotational atherectomy (with a larger burr) or adjunct PTCA at low pressures may be preferred. Kovach et al. (20) evaluated the mechanisms of adjunctive balloon angioplasty; additional increases in lumen areas were the result of a combination of plaque dissection and arterial expansion (Table 2). Alternatively, directional coronary atherectomy may be useful in the presence of a large residual plaque burden, especially if the plaque is eccentric without significant residual superficial calcium. It should be noted, however, that serial IVUS studies have shown that pretreatment of a lesion with rotational atherectomy will change its characteristics so that adjunctive directional atherectomy can remove superficial calcium (Fig. 4). Therefore, residual superficial target lesion calcium does not preclude the use of adjunctive directional atherectomy. After adjunct directional atherectomy, increases in lumen dimensions are the result of additional plaque removal as well as vessel expansion (31,32). Compared to adjunctive PTCA, directional atherectomy resulted in larger lumen dimensions, smaller residual plaque burden, and reduced target lesion revascularization. However, recent studies have shown that adjunctive stenting may result in a larger lumen than either adjunctive PTCA or directional atherectomy (33).

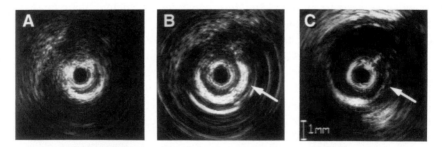

Figure 4 Sequential intravascular ultrasound images—preintervention (panel A), postrotational atherectomy (panel B), and postadjunct directional atherectomy (panel C)—of an ostial right coronary artery lesion are shown. After adjunct directional atherectomy there is almost complete removal of target lesion calcium (white arrow) with a marked increase in lumen cross-sectional area.

ACKNOWLEDGMENTS

This study was supported in part by the Cardiology Research Foundation, Washington, DC, and the Heinrich-Hertz Stiftung, Dusseldorf, Germany.

REFERENCES

1. Faxon DP, Kelsey SF, Ryan TJ, McCabe CH, Detre K. Determinants of successful percutaneous transluminal coronary angioplasty: report from the National Heart, Lung, and Blood Institute Registry. Am Heart J 1984; 108:1019–1023.
2. Tan K, Sulke N, Taub N, Sowton E. Clinical and lesion morphologic determinants of coronary angioplasty success and complications: current experience. J Am Coll Cardiol 1995; 25:855–865.
3. Detre K, Holubkov R, Kelsez S, et al. Percutaneous transluminal coronary angioplasty in 1985–86 and 1977–81 the National Heart, Lung, and Blood Institute Registry. N Engl J Med 1988; 318:265–270.
4. Gruentzig AR, King SB III, Schlumpf M, Siegenthaler W. Long-term follow-up after percutaneous transluminal coronary angioplasty: the early Zurich experience. N Engl J Med 1987; 316:1127–1132.
5. Leimgruber PP, Roubin GS, Hollman J, et al. Restenosis after successful coronary angioplasty in patients with single-vessel disease. Circulation 1986; 73:710–717.
6. Hirshfeld JW Jr, Schwartz JS, Jugo R, et al. Restenosis after coronary angioplasty: a multivariate statistical model to relate lesion and procedure variables to restenosis. J Am Coll Cardiol 1991; 18:647–656.
7. Ellis S, Roubin G, King S, et al. Angiographic and clinical predictors of acute closure after native vessel coronary angioplasty. Circulation 1988; 77:372–379.
8. Lincoff AM, Popma JJ, Ellis SG, Hacker JA, Topol EJ. Abrupt vessel closure complicating coronary angioplasty: clinical, angiographic and therapeutic profile. J Am Coll Cardiol 1992; 19:926–935.
9. Nissen SE, Gurley JC, Grines CL, et al. Intravascular ultrasound assessment of lumen size and wall morphology in normal subjects and patients with coronary artery disease. Circulation 1991; 84:1087–1099.
10. Nishimura RA, Edwards WD, Warner CA, et al. Intravascular ultrasound imaging: in vitro validation and pathologic correlation. J Am Coll Cardiol 1990; 16: 145–154.
11. Gussenhoven EJ, Essed CE, Lancee CT, et al. Arterial wall characteristics determined by intravascular ultrasound imaging: An in vitro study. J Am Coll Cardiol 1989; 14:942–952.
12. Mintz GS, Kovach JA, Javier SP, et al. Mechanism of lumen enlargement after excimer laser coronary angioplasty. An intravascular ultrasound study. Circulation 1995; 92:3408–3414.
13. Honye J, Mahon DJ, Nakamura S, et al. Intravascular ultrasound imaging after excimer laser angioplasty. Cathet Cardiovasc Diagn 1994; 32:213–222.

14. Schmid KM, Xie D, Voelker W, et al. Intracoronary ultrasound following excimer-laser angioplasty. An in-vitro study in human coronary arteries. Eur Heart J 1995; 16:188–193.

15. Bittl JA, Sanborn TA, Tcheng JE, Siegel RM, Ellis SG. Clinical success, complications and restenosis rates with excimer laser coronary angioplasty. Am J Cardiol 1992; 70:1533–1539.

16. Litvack F, Eigler N, Margolis J, et al. Percutaneous excimer laser coronary angioplasty: results in the first consecutive 3000 patients. J Am Coll Cardiol 1994; 23:323–329.

17. Cook SL, Eigler NL, Shefer A, Goldenberg T, Forrester JS, Litvack F. Percutaneous excimer laser coronary angioplasty of lesions not ideal for balloon angioplasty. Circulation 1991; 84:632–643.

18. Fourrier J, Stonkowiak C, Lablance J, Prat A, Brunetaund J, Bertrand M. Histopathology after rotational angioplasty of peripheral arteries in human beings. J Am Coll Cardiol 1988; 11:109.

19. Ahn S, Auth DC, Marcud D. Removal of focal atheromatous lesions by angiographically guided high-speed rotary atherectomy. J Vasc Surg 1988; 7:292.

20. Kovach JA, Mintz GS, Pichard AD, et al. Sequential intravascular ultrasound characterization of the mechanisms of rotational atherectomy and adjunct balloon angioplasty. J Am Coll Cardiol 1993; 22:1024–1032.

21. Mintz GS, Potkin BN, Keren G, et al. Intravascular ultrasound evaluation of the effect of rotational atherectomy in obstructive atherosclerotic coronary artery disease. Circulation 1992; 86:1383–1393.

22. Leon M, Kent K, Pichard A, et al. Percutaneous transluminal coronary rotational angioplasty of calcified lesions. Circulation 1991; 84:II-521.

23. Warth D, Bertrand M, Buchbinder M, et al. Percutaneous transluminal coronary rotational ablation: six-month restenosis rate. Circulation 1991; 84:II-82.

24. Koller P, Freed M, Niazi K, et al. Success, complications and restenosis following atherectomy of coronary ostial stenosis. J Am Coll Cardiol 1992; 19:333A.

25. Teirstein PS, Warth DC, Haq N, et al. High speed rotational coronary atherectomy for patients with diffuse coronary artery disease. J Am Coll Cardiol 1991; 18:1694–1701.

26. Bertrand ME, Lablanche JM, Leroy F, et al. Percutaneous transluminal coronary rotary ablation with rotablator (European experience). Am J Cardiol 1992; 69:470–474.

27. MacIssac AI, Bass TA, Buchbinder M, et al. High speed rotational atherectomy: outcome in calcified and noncalcified coronary artery lesions. J Am Coll Cardiol 1995; 26:731–736.

28. Stertzer S, Rosenblum J, Shaw R, et al. Coronary rotational ablation: initial experience in 302 procedures. J Am Coll Cardiol 1992; 21:287–295.

29. Fourrier JL, Bertrand ME, Auth DC, Lablanche JM, Gommeaux A, Brunetaud JM. Percutaneous coronary rotational angioplasty in humans: preliminary report. J Am Coll Cardiol 1989; 14:1278–1282.

30. Satler LF, Warth D. Dissections after high-speed rotational atherectomy: frequency, predictive factors and clinical consequences. Circulation 1992; 86:I-3124.
31. Dussaillant GR, Mintz GS, Pichard AD, et al. Mechanism and immediate and long-term results of adjunct directional coronary atherectomy after rotational atherectomy. J Am Coll Cardiol 1996; 27:1390–1397.
32. Mintz GS, Pichard AD, Popma JJ, Kent KM, Satler LF, Leon MB. Preliminary experience with adjunct directional coronary atherectomy after high-speed rotational atherectomy in the treatment of calcified coronary artery disease. Am J Cardiol 1993; 71:799–804.
33. Mintz GS, Dussaillant GR, Wong SC, et al. Rotational atherectomy followed by adjunctive stents: the preferred therapy for calcified lesions in large vessels? Circulation 1995; 92:I-329.

14

Role of Intravascular Ultrasound in Intracoronary Stent Deployment

Steven L. Goldberg   *Los Angeles County, Harbor–UCLA Medical Center, Torrance, and University of California, Los Angeles, School of Medicine, Los Angeles, California*

Antonio Colombo   *New York University Medical Center, New York, New York, and Columbus Hospital, Milan, Italy*

I. INTRODUCTION

An explosion in the use of intracoronary stents has revolutionized the transcatheter treatment of obstructive coronary artery disease. Stents were initially found to be useful in the treatment of acute or threatened closure complicating coronary angioplasty (1–3), resulting in fewer myocardial infarctions and less need for emergent coronary artery bypass surgery. With the completion of the STRESS and BENESTENT trials the stent has also been shown to be the first device to lower restenosis compared to standard balloon angioplasty in selected populations of patients (4,5). However, the strategies of stent deployment used in those studies were associated with important complications of stent thrombosis (occurring in around 3.5% of cases) and bleeding/vascular complications due to the aggressive anticoagulation regimens used to minimize the risk of stent thrombosis (which occurred in 7% to 13.5% of cases) (4,5). In addition, the problem of restenosis, although significantly lowered, was still present in 22% to 32% of patients receiving stents (4,5).

265

II. HISTORICAL SIGNIFICANCE

The introduction of intravascular ultrasound (IVUS) imaging into the stent deployment procedure has revealed the limitations of angiography in the identification of optimal stent expansion. It was common to achieve an angiographic result within a stented lesion which was quite acceptable by standards that had been applied to balloon angioplasty. When the result was evaluated by intravascular ultrasound the stent would appear poorly expanded, as identified by poor stent apposition to the arterial wall or stent compression by eccentric, resistant plaque, and a relative stenosis was frequently present compared to the distal lumen (Fig. 1). In our initial series of patients in whom intravascular ultrasound imaging was used inside intracoronary stents, suboptimal stent expansion was identified approximately 85% of the time, similar to the experience reported by others in native coronary arteries as well as saphenous vein grafts (6–10). This information became a key element in understanding possible mechanisms of stent thrombosis as well as providing a potential explanation for certain episodes of stent restenosis previously felt to be due to stent recoil.

A. Stent Thrombosis

A stent is a metal foreign body that has thrombogenic potential when inside a vascular system (11). When a stent is not well apposed to the arterial wall, more

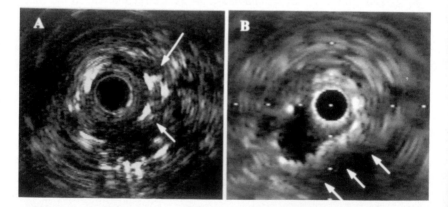

Figure 1 IVUS images of suboptimally expanded stents. (A) Asymmetric stent expansion with stent struts poorly apposed to the arterial wall. Arrows point to stent struts that are not apposed. (B) Asymmetric stent expansion due to calcific plaque compressing a section of stent. Distal shadowing is present characterizing calcified plaque (arrows).

thrombogenic surface area is exposed to the circulating blood. Furthermore, while laminar blood flow inhibits thrombus formation, the turbulence, which occurs from a foreign body within the bloodstream, allows for regions of slower flow and increased thrombus potential. Similarly, a partially compressed stent also will lead to turbulent blood flow with the potential for stagnant blood (11–13).

B. Stent Restenosis

Chronic stent recoil used to be considered a mechanism of in-stent restenosis. However, information from IVUS imaging suggests this probably does not occur with rigid stents, but reflects instead inadequate inital stent implantation (14). If a stent is not fully expanded during deployment, the lesion may recur as the arterial wall recoils back to the unexpanded stent. The initial angiogram may appear optimal, due to contrast present behind the stent struts (Fig. 2). If

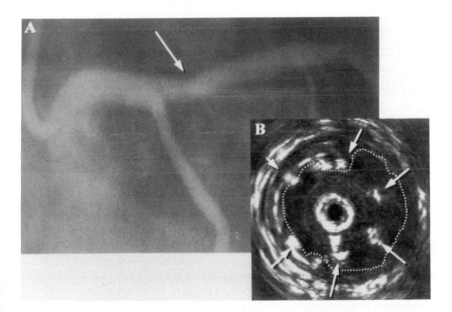

Figure 2 An adequate angiographic result poststenting with a segment of suboptimal stent expansion due to poor stent apposition. Contrast may pass on outside of stent and provide an angiographic illusion of adequate stent expansion. (A) Angiographic image after stenting of an ostial left anterior descending coronary artery lesion. Arrow points to the site of the intravascular ultrasound image. (B) Intravascular ultrasound image demonstrating suboptimal stent expansion with poor strut apposition. Arrows point to stent struts. Dotted line outlines the lumen border.

IVUS is performed only at the time of restenosis, this may give an impression of stent recoil, although the true mechanism is one of inadequate stent expansion. In a serial study of stented lesions with intravascular ultrasound, Painter et al. have demonstrated a lack of chronic recoil of Palmaz-Schatz stents (14). Whether other, less rigid stents, such as coil stents, manifest the same resistance to recoil has not been examined.

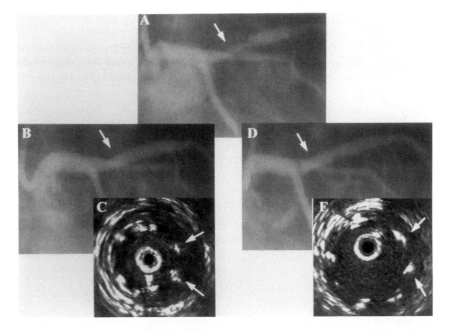

Figure 3   Same lesion seen in Figure 2. Using intravascular ultrasound guidance an improved stent expansion is achieved. (A) Preintervention angiogram. Arrow points to the lesion. (B) Poststenting a good angiographic result is obtained. Arrow points to the lesion and the site of the intravascular ultrasound imaging. (C) Intravascular ultrasound image of the site identified in B. Poor stent apposition to the arterial wall is seen. Arrows point to stent struts, which are poorly apposed. (D) Angiographic image after the area is treated with a larger balloon. Modest improvement in angiographic appearance may be appreciated. Arrow points to the site of the intravascular ultrasound imaging. (E) Intravascular ultrasound image of the site identified in D. Good strut apposition and full stent expansion are now seen. Arrows point to stent struts, which are now well apposed.

C. Anatomic Improvements in Stent Dimensions with IVUS Guidance

The achievement of the largest minimal lumen diameter possible during a coronary intervention has been proposed as important in minimizing the likelihood of restenosis (15). Intravascular ultrasound identifies those stents in which further expansion may safely achieve larger minimal lumen diameters; this additional information may lead to lower restenosis.

Not only is it important to identify suboptimal stent expansion, but it is also necessary to be able to act upon this information to achieve better anatomic results. To achieve anatomic improvements both larger balloons and higher-pressure inflations within the stented segments have been used. These strategies have been shown to improve intrastent area by an average of 34% compared to dimensions when angiographic guidance is used alone (Figs. 3, 4) (6,7,9). In part because of the lack of reliable high pressure balloons at that time, an early strategy was to use progressively larger balloons until the intravascular ultrasound images were considered to be acceptable. Because this strategy occasionally led to the devastating complication of vessel rupture (6), it was altered such that minimally oversized balloons were inflated to high pressures (>12 atm) until optimal stent expansion was achieved, or no improvements in stent expansion could be seen. This strategy was associated with a lower acute complication rate and higher clinical success rate compared with traditional stenting techniques and IVUS-guided stenting with oversized balloons, when a retrospective analysis was performed of 725 consecutive stenting procedures in Centro Cuore Columbus Hospital in Milan (Fig. 5; unpublished data).

III. CLINICAL OUTCOMES USING IVUS GUIDANCE OF STENT DEPLOYMENT

A. Stent Thrombosis

With the use of intravascular ultrasound imaging and techniques to maximize stent expansion, the incidence of stent thrombosis has diminished to less than 1% such that traditional anticoagulation regimens are no longer required (16). In a series of 28 patients undergoing IVUS imaging after stent implantation using standard techniques (non-oversized balloons inflated to 6 atm of pressure) Gorge et al. (8) described two patients with suboptimal stent expansion by IVUS imaging who developed subacute stent thrombosis. In the same study, using IVUS after high-pressure inflations inside stents, no cases of stent

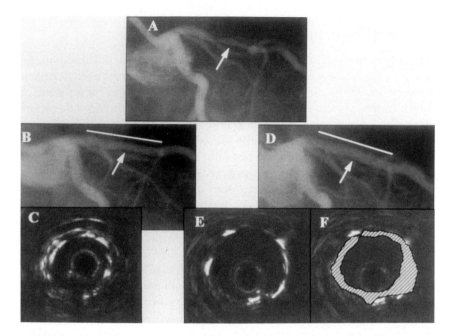

Figure 4 Angiographic and intravascular ultrasound images of a stented lesion in which ultrasound guidance led to improved anatomic benefit. (A) Angiogram preintervention. Arrow points to the lesion in the left anterior descending coronary artery. (B) Acceptable angiographic appearance after three Palmaz-Schatz stents are inserted and dilated with a 3.5-mm balloon to 12 atm. Line identifies the extent of the stented segment. Arrow points to the site of intravascular ultrasound image displayed in C. (C) IVUS image of the site identified in B. Good stent/arterial wall apposition is seen with a symmentrically expanded stent. However, the intrastent cross-sectional area was not as large as the distal reference lumen cross-sectional area, thus prompting further intervention. (D) Angiographic image after further inflations were performed with the same balloon at 16 atm. A modest angiographic improvement is seen. Line and arrow as in B. (E) Intravascular ultrasound image of the site identified in D. An improved intrastent cross-sectional area is seen. (F) A copy of E with the 33% increase in intrastent cross-sectional area identified by shaded area.

thrombosis were seen in 24 patients. Although this difference in stent thrombosis (7% vs. 0%) was not statistically significant, it is unlikely there will be future studies with intravascular ultrasound documentation of suboptimal stent expansion that is not acted upon.

Coincident to the recognition that stent thrombosis could be lessened by

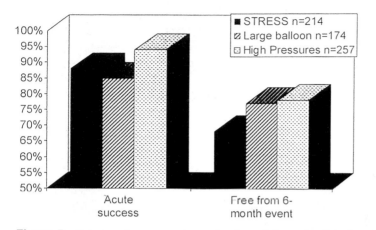

Figure 5 Retrospective comparison of early and 6-month clinical outcomes using three different strategies of stent deployment. The group on the left had "traditional" stent techniques, as used in STRESS: angiographic guidance without aggressive stent expansion and with postprocedure anticoagulation. The middle group had ultrasound guidance with predominantly oversized balloons used to optimize stent expansion. About half were treated with postprocedure anticoagulation and half with postprocedure antiplatelet therapy. The group on the right had ultrasound guidance with predominantly high-pressure inflations used to optimize stent expansion. The majority were treated without postprocedure anticoagulation therapy. Acute success (angiographic successfully deployed stents without the development of a clinical complication) was greater in the group receiving stents with ultrasound guidance, high-pressure inflations and no postprocedure anticoagulation. Freedom from 6-month clinical events was greater in the groups having IVUS-guided procedures than the group receiving stents using the strategy employed for the STRESS trial.

optimizing stent expansion was the burgeoning use of the antiplatelet agent ticlopidine. Preliminary reports with this agent have suggested low rates of stent thrombosis with and without intravascular ultrasound guidance (17–19). It has been proposed that intravascular ultrasound might help identify lesions with suboptimal stent results in which anticoagulant, as opposed to antiplatelet, therapy would be of specific benefit. However, in a study by Schomig et al. (19), patients undergoing Palmaz-Schatz stent deployment who were randomized to antiplatelet therapy with aspirin and ticlopidine had fewer clinical events, including a lower incidence of stent thrombosis, than patients randomized to aspirin and phenprocoumon. Based on this information there may not be any role for anticoagulation after stenting, regardless of the intravascular ultrasound findings. If routine high-pressure inflations are performed inside a stent (with meticulous attention paid to the angiographic appearance) and the patient is treated with aggressive antiplatelet therapy including aspirin and ticlopidine, it is possible that only in the rare case of stent underexpansion due to an unrecognized displacement of the stent on the delivery balloon, such as seen in Figure 6, would the use of IVUS achieve further benefits in lowering the risk of stent thrombosis.

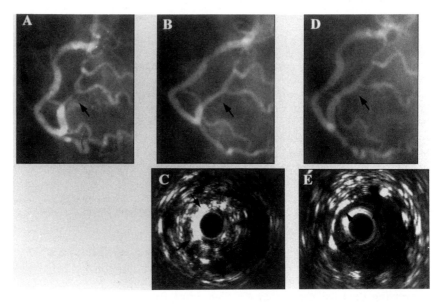

Figure 6   Angiographic and intravascular ultrasound images of a lesion in a postero-lateral branch of a right coronary. (A) Preintervention angiogram. Arrow points to the stenosis. (B) Angiographic appearance after a Palmaz-Schatz stent is inserted and dilated with a 3.0-mm balloon. Arrow points to the site of the IVUS imaging. (C) IVUS images of the stented lesion demonstrating a portion of unexpanded stent, not evident angiographically. Presumably the stent had slipped backward on the delivery balloon, leaving it partially unexpanded. Arrows point to the stent struts. (D) Angiogram after the stent was redilated with the same balloon to the same atmospheres. Arrow points to the site of the intravascular ultrasound image. (E) IVUS image of the site identified in D. Good stent-arterial wall apposition can now be appreciated. Arrows point to the stent struts.

B. In-Stent Restenosis

The risk of angiographic restenosis appears to be reduced by achieving the largest lumen possible in vessels undergoing balloon angioplasty, directional atherectomy, or intracoronary stent insertion (15). The use of IVUS guidance of stent deployment leads to greater acute gain than angiographic guidance (6,8,9), even when routine high-pressure balloon inflations are performed prior to IVUS imaging (20–22). It is not clear if this anatomic advantage ranslates into clinical reduction in restenosis.

The previous work of Kuntz et al. (15) suggests that "the bigger the better" concept applies in reducing restenosis, but there have been some concerns that the use of aggressive dilatation techniques may contribute to more intimal proliferation and an increase in late loss after stenting. This was examined in a retrospective analysis of 725 consecutive lesions receiving stents over a 2-year period in Centro Cuore Columbus Hospital (Fig. 5). The first 233 lesions (group A) had stents place without intravascular ultrasound guidance, using minimally oversized balloons and regular inflation pressures (approximately 6 to 8 atm)—i.e., the strategy used in the STRESS and BENESTENT trials. The second group, of 203 lesions (group B), had IVUS guidance with oversized balloons as the primary strategy in achieving optimal stent expansion (balloon/artery ratio of 1.25:1—c.g., a 3.75-mm balloon in a 3.0-mm lumen). The third group, of 289 lesions (group C), had intravascular ultrasound guidance with high-pressure inflations as the predominant means of achieving optimal stent expansion (balloon/artery ratio 1.1:1 and a mean 14.5 atm of inflation pressure).

The patients in group B had an important incidence of vessel rupture (3.4%) from the use of oversized balloons. Vessel rupture occurred with a mean balloon/artery ratio of 1.4:1—e.g. a 4.25-mm balloon in a 3.0-mm lumen. This occurrence was associated with a 43% (n = 3) need for emergent coronary artery bypass graft surgery and a 57% (n = 4) mortality rate, making this strategy unfavorable. However, the lesions in group B had the greatest increases in acute gain without significant increases in late loss, leading to the lowest rates of restenosis (Fig. 7). The group of lesions (group C) undergoing stent deployment with IVUS guidance but high-pressure inflations to optimize stent expansion (which had the less favorable baseline characteristic of longer mean lesion length) had intermediate increases in acute gain with intermediate rates of restenosis, supporting the theory that the greater the acute gain, the lower the restenosis—i.e., "the bigger the better." These data therefore support a role for IVUS guidance in lowering restenosis for stented lesions, although the relative benefit requires further analysis with prospective studies.

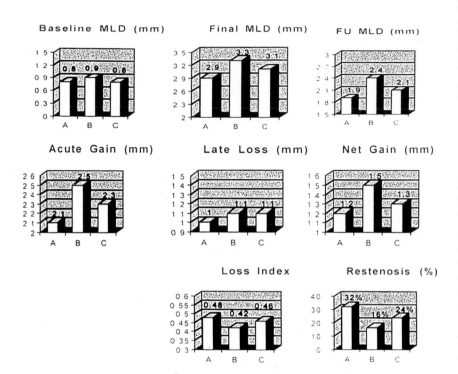

Figure 7 Angiographic dimensions of the three groups described in Figure 5. Group A represents the techniques used in the STRESS and BENESTENT trials. Group B represents the group undergoing ultrasound guided stenting with oversized balloons as the predominant means to optimize stent expansion. Group C represents the group undergoing ultrasound guided stenting with high-pressure inflations as the predominant means to optimize stent expansion. Baseline dimensions are identical across the three groups. Group B represents the most aggressive strategy of stent deployment and was associated with the greatest acute and net gain and the lowest rate of restenosis, with group C midway between the other groups. This suggests that aggressive stent expansion does not lead to more late loss but rather reduces restenosis.

This study suggests that the use of IVUS-guided stenting with high-pressure inflations is associated with the most favorable combination of early and long-term results. However, there appears to be the potential for further reduction in restenosis by using more aggressive stent expansion techniques, if markers for vessel rupture can be identified to avoid this complication. One such marker may be seen in Figure 8, where a weakening may be seen in a short normal

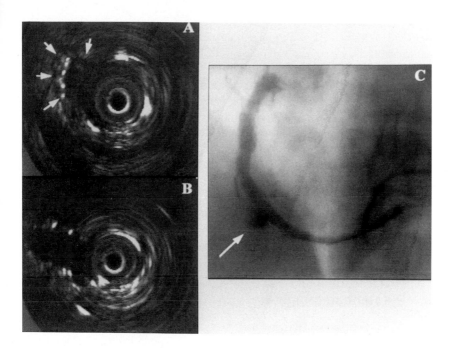

Figure 8 Vessel rupture predicted by intravascular ultrasound. (A) Intravascular ultrasound image after stent deployment. A short segment of thin, "normal" arterial wall is present with resistant plaque extending around the rest of the artery. The stent is expanding primarily in the thin segment (arrows) (B) After further inflations the stent can be seen prolapsing into a developing pseudoaneurysm. (C) Vessel rupture occurs (arrow).

segment of an arterial wall which is surrounded by resistant plaque. Frank pseudoaneurysm of the vessel and subsequent rupture occurred with further inflations.

IV. TECHNIQUES IN IVUS GUIDANCE OF STENT DEPLOYMENT

A. Techniques in Imaging

The IVUS catheter should be placed inside the artery, distal to the stented segment in order to image the entire segment including the distal bed. It is common to give intracoronary nitroglycerin prior to the insertion of the ultrasound catheter in the coronary artery to minimize catheter-induced spasm and to provide a framework for comparisons with subsequent studies. It is important to insert the ultrasound catheter carefully through the stent, particularly if there is a coil stent, without any force, which might deform it. A slow, continuous pullback should then be performed and recorded on videotape. If there is a specific region of interest to interrogate, the catheter may be reinserted to the area of interest and combined with angiography. This may be useful if questions arise, such as the angiographic location of an ultrasound-identified lesion or whether or not there is flow present in dissection plane. The ultrasound catheter should then be removed from the artery immediately and the videotape reviewed. It is useful to have present an assistant who can measure minimal intrastent dimensions as well as the proximal and distal reference segments, while the primary interventionalist is attending to the patient. Not uncommonly the decision to perform additional inflations depends on the careful performance of these measurements (Fig. 4), as opposed to reliance upon subjective impressions of stent expansion.

B. Prestenting Imaging

Intravascular ultrasound imaging may be used before as well as after a stent has been placed. Intravascular ultrasound may be of value prior to stenting to:

1. Evaluate the length of the lesion to select the appropriate length of stent and the true vessel size. This may also be important in deciding that the vessel is *not* suitable for stenting.

2. Evaluate the result following angioplasty to decide if a stent may be useful. Although restenosis is a vexing problem, less than half of patients undergoing balloon angioplasty are affected.

The identification of predictors of vessel renarrowing, either acutely or as restenosis, might allow for more selective use of stents and represent a potential cost saving. Currently there are no objective criteria to define which lesions are most likely to benefit from a stent. Lesions with excellent early anatomic results may not receive any additional benefit from the insertion of a stent (23). Rodriguez et al. have demonstrated that if there is acute recoil after balloon angioplasty, as assessed angiographically 24 hours after initial angioplasty, the insertion of a stent will reduce restenosis (24). This strategy is cumbersome, however, as it requires repeat angiography 24 hours after the initial procedure. The IVUS identification of dissection, or the absence of plaque fracture, has been related to a higher likelihood of restenosis or early event in some smaller trials, but not in others (25–30).

In the GUIDE trial, the only IVUS predictor of restenosis was related to the amount of residual plaque burden present after balloon angioplasty or directional atherectomy, with lesions that restenosed having a mean residual plaque burden of 69%, versus 60% in lesions that did not restenose. This is similar to data found by Mintz et al. (26,30). Other investigators have found a relationship between residual plaque burden and subacute recoil after balloon angioplasty (31). Therefore one potential strategy would be to place stents in those lesions with a suboptimal angiographic result, a residual plaque burden greater than 60% to 70%, or in the presence of an unfavorable dissection identified by IVUS (Fig. 9). This strategy has yet to be subjected to an appropriate randomized trial.

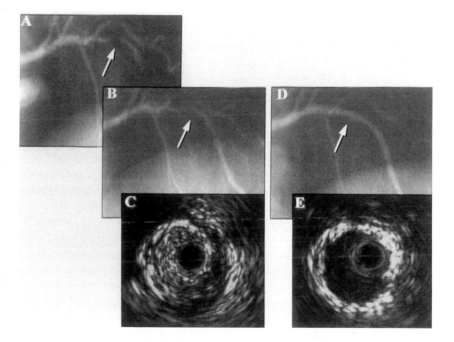

Figure 9 Angiographic and ultrasound images of a lesion that received a stent based partly on the intravascular ultrasound appearance after balloon angioplasty. (A) Preintervention angiogram. The lesion (arrow) is a functional total occlusion. (B) Acceptable angiogram after balloon angioplasty. Arrow points to the site of intravascular image seen in C. (C) IVUS image of the site identified in B. Plaque takes up nearly the entire lumen, surrounding the intravascular ultrasound catheter, representing a plaque burden > 85%. (D) Improved angiographic appearance after the insertion of a stent. Arrow points to the site of the intravascular image seen in E. (E) Intravascular image of the site identified in D. A much improved luminal cross-sectional area can be seen compared with C.

Preintervention intravascular ultrasound imaging may be useful in selecting an appropriate device prior to the insertion of a stent (32). Specifically, the identification of significant fibrocalcific plaque may be important because fibrocalcific plaque limits stent expansion even when identified only by intravascular ultrasound and not angiography (33,34). IVUS imaging is much more sensitive for the presence, location, and extent of vascular calcification than fluoroscopy (35). In order to achieve optimal lumen dimensions, there may be a role for rotational atherectomy to debulk the fibrocalcific lesion prior to stent insertion, particularly when the arc of calcium is extensive—e.g., greater than 180° (Fig. 10). Rotational atherectomy may in theory not only debulk the lesion but also modify the plaque to allow better balloon and stent expansion. This has yet to be validated with prospective trials, but the problem of fibrocalcific plaque limiting stent expansion is not uncommon and probably represents the most important element preventing the achievement of a maximal acute gain.

Preintervention IVUS imaging may also identify the presence of thrombus, although not as reliably as angioscopy (30,36–41). Thrombus may be treated with anticoagulants or antiplatelet therapy or with a device such as TEC atherectomy. This scenario, however, is much less common than fibrocalcific plaque.

Lesions that appear moderate angiographically frequently appear more significant by intravascular ultrasound imaging. In a study by Mintz et al. (32), 10% of lesions that appeared moderate by angiography appeared to be significant on IVUS imaging. Good flow going into and out of intracoronary stents is important to minimize the risk of a low-flow state in the thrombogenic milieu of the stent. The identification of unsuspected high-grade lesions in a vessel to be stented may assist in the planning of the stenting strategy by helping the interventionalist to decide how many stents to place and where they are needed. Because it is usually easier to stent distal segments first, and because it can be difficult to deliver a stent if there is a tight proximal lesion, the identification of significant lesions either proximal or distal to a segment of vessel in which stenting is planned can be valuable information.

C. Poststent IVUS Imaging

After a stent is implanted, intravascular ultrasound imaging can identify poor apposition of stent struts to the arterial wall, or a suboptimal intrastent lumen may be seen due to stent compression by fibrocalcific plaque (Fig. 1). In addition, the identification of significant stenoses at the boundaries of the stented segment which appear only moderate angiographically may be important. In a series of 288 lesions receiving stents and routine high-pressure balloon inflations poststent implantation (mean 14.8 atm) with good an-

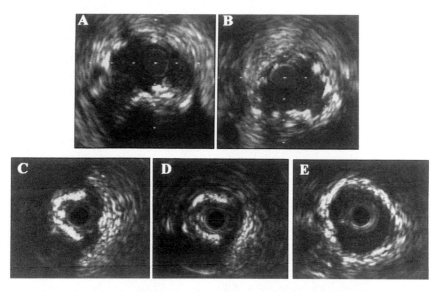

Figure 10   Intravascular ultrasound images of two lesions with calcification identified by intravascular ultrasound, not fluoroscopically. The lesion represented in A was not treated with prestenting rotational atherectomy, whereas the lesion in C was pretreated with rotational atherectomy. (A) Intravascular ultrasound image with a 100° arc of complex calcification. (B) After a stent is inserted, a persistent asymmetric, poorly expanded stent appearance is present despite the use of oversized balloons and high-pressure inflations. (C) Intravascular ultrasound image of a lesion in another patient with a 200° arc of calcium, identified by bright white echoes and distal shadowing. (D) After rotational atherectomy is performed, the calcified segment appears much less dense and more echoes may be seen distally, suggesting the plaque has been "modified." Only a modest improvement in luminal dimensions is seen. (E) After a stent is implanted, good stent expansion may be appreciated. In this case, the plaque was sufficiently "softened" by the rotational atherectomy to allow full stent expansion.

giographic results, we found only 45% of lesions to have an optimal appearance by IVUS imaging, which is similar to the results reported by others (42–48). Fifteen percent of vessels were considered to have significant lesions in the stent boundaries and received subsequent stents (see Fig. 11). This may be similar to the 10% of lesions found by Mintz et al. (32) on IVUS imaging which their group considered significant and led to subsequent intervention despite only moderate significance angiographically. Investigators at the Cleveland Clinic found that in nearly half of lesions with angiographic haziness in the

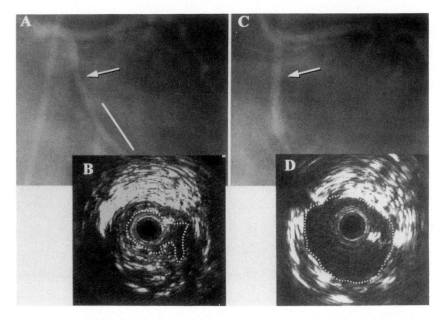

Figure 11 Angiographic and intravascular ultrasound images of a vessel receiving additional stents due to the intravascular ultrasound images. A stent was placed in the circumflex coronary artery electively for the treatment of a total occlusion. (A) Angiogram after the insertion of a Palmaz-Schatz stent (line demonstrates the extent of the stented segment). Arrow points to a 30% lesion proximal to the stented segment. (B) Intravascular ultrasound image of the site identified in A. Plaque surrounds the ultrasound catheter with an eccentric lumen present (dotted line), which provided an angiographic illusion of a large lumen and minimal disease. (C) Improved angiographic appearance after the insertion of an additional Palmaz-Schatz stent with high-pressure inflations throughout the entire stented segment. Arrow points to the site of the intravascular ultrasound image seen in D. (D) Improved luminal cross-sectional area after the insertion of a stent at the site seen in B. Dotted line identifies the lumen border.

persistent region (seen in 14% of cases), IVUS identified dissection and sonolucent plaque consistent with thrombus or lipid-laden atheroma, prompting the insertion of additional stents (49).

In our series described above, 55% of stented lesions were considered to have a suboptimal ultrasound appearance on the initial IVUS imaging despite the use of routine high-pressure balloon inflations and the attainment of an acceptable poststent angiographic appearance. However, with further inflations and the placement of additional stents, 91% of lesions achieved an optimal ultrasound appearance (22). Therefore, when suboptimal results were discovered by intravascular ultrasound, it was possible to act upon the information to achieve better results (22,46,50).

Different approaches to intravascular ultrasound guidance of stent deployment may be considered. The first strategy is to perform intravascular ultrasound imaging after routine high-pressure balloon inflations are employed with a minimally oversized balloon (balloon:artery ratio 1.1:1.2) and an acceptable angiographic appearance is obtained. An alternative approach is to dilate the stent with only moderate inflation pressures until an acceptable angiographic appearance is achieved and then perform intravascular ultrasound imaging— i.e., prior to high-pressure inflations. Selective high-pressure inflations can then be performed at sites of suboptimal stent expansion identified by the ultrasound images, with additional high-pressure inflations or the use of larger balloons used as necessary after sequential intravascular ultrasound imaging. The potential advantage of this approach is in avoiding unnecessary high-pressure inflations outside the stented segment and minimizing the risk of dissection at the stent border. This is most likely to be of benefit in tapering vessels, such as the left anterior descending coronary artery, in which the proximal stented segment may be 0.5 mm or more larger than the distal segment. If the stent were suboptimally deployed only in the proximal segment, a larger balloon could safely be inflated to high pressures in this area while further dilatations could be avoided in the smaller distal segment (see Fig. 12). It may be anticipated that in approximately 15% of cases, high pressure inflations may not be necessary (6).

Occasionally a fibrocalcific plaque may be particularly resistant to dilatation. Acute recoil may be present, as evidenced by full balloon expansion identified angiographically with suboptimal intrastent dimensions seen by IVUS (51). The insertion of a second stent inside the first one to provide additional radial support has been performed effectively when this occurs (51). When a short rim of normal vessel architecture is adjacent to nearly circumferential resistant fibrocalcific plaque, there is a risk of vessel rupture if very aggressive inflations are performed (Fig. 8). The recognition of this ultrasound pattern may be useful in limiting further, potentially dangerous inflations. In other instances full balloon expansion may not occur even if there is a lack of balloon indentation or waist visible fluoroscopically. We have observed this using an IVUS imaging wire during high-pressure balloon inflations (unpublished). Present rotational atherectomy should theoretically play a role in minimizing this situation.

There may be a role for IVUS in balloon sizing, although this remains an

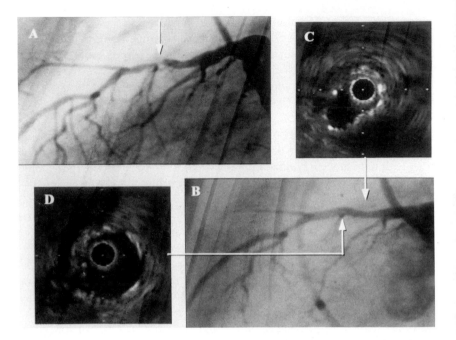

Figure 12   Angiographic and IVUS images of a lesion in which high-pressure inflations were used only selectively based on the IVUS information. (A) Preintervention
angiogram demonstrating a focal lesion in the left anterior descending coronary artery.
Distal to the lesion the artery measured only 2.0 mm. (B) A Palmaz-Schatz stent was
deployed with a 3.0-mm balloon to 8 atm with an acceptable angiographic appearance.
Two IVUS images are shown, identified by arrows. (C) IVUS image of the proximal part
of the stented segment, demonstrating a focal area of calcium compressing the stent.
(D) IVUS image of the distal part of the stented segment, demonstrating good stent
expansion. More aggressive dilatation could be limited to the proximal, suboptimally
expanded stented segment, thereby avoiding potential damage to the small-diameter
distal coronary bed.

area lacking sufficient data. The IVUS identification of *vessel* (as opposed to
lumen) dimensions has been proposed to be of value in selecting appropriate
balloon sizes (6,52). With this strategy, a balloon may be chosen with a
diameter that approaches, without exceeding, the vessel diameter (bounded by
the external elastic membrane) (Fig. 13). It is not clear how the amount or
quality of plaque burden should be factored in, as a balloon will push on the

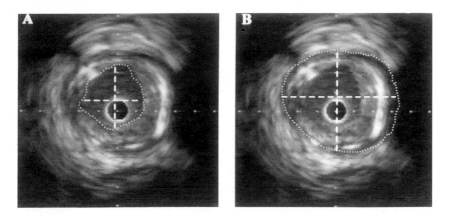

Figure 13 Vascular dimensions seen on intravascular ultrasound imaging. (A) Minimum and major *lumen* diameters and area. The lumen boundaries are defined by the lumen-intima interface. (B) Minimum and major *vessel* diameters and area. Vessel boundaries are defined by the external elastic membrane.

plaque and stretch the vessel even further, especially if a large amount of plaque is present. Using balloons larger than the measured vessel dimensions by IVUS is likely to increase the risk of vessel rupture and should be avoided. Studies are ongoing to address this issue (52).

D. Criteria for Optimal Stent Expansion

The criteria for optimal stent expansion are not well established or validated. All criteria to date have included the requirements that good stent strut vessel wall apposition be seen, and that the stent should have a round, symmetric appearance (ratio of minor axis diameter to major axis diameter >0.7) (6,7,10, 16,20,21,44–46,53). The desired lumen dimensions and the reference standards to be applied have varied among investigators and with time (6,7,16,20, 21,53). Our current strategy is to achieve an intrastent cross-sectional area that is at least as large as the closest normal proximal and distal reference lumen cross-sectional area. This strategy must be individualized for each lesion, because for tapering vessels the appropriate stent expansion will vary considerably from the proximal to the distal segment. The proximal segment should have an intrastent cross-sectional area that is similar to the proximal reference, whereas the distal stent should have lumen dimensions closer to the distal

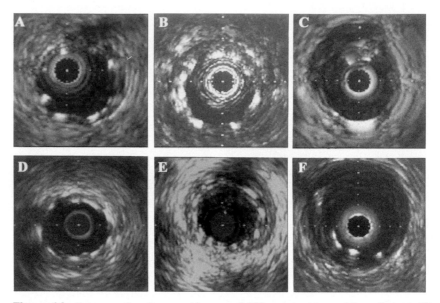

Figure 14   Intravascular ultrasound images of different stent types. The coil stents (C and F), especially the Gianturco-Roubin, are less visible by intravascular ultrasound owing to their smaller volume of metal. (A) Microstent by AVE. (B) Cordis stent. (C) Gianturco-Roubin stent. (D) NIR stent. (E) Wallstent. (F) Wiktor stent.

reference. An average of the proximal and distal reference lumen cross-sectional areas should be achieved in the midportion of the stented segment. This last criterion is often the most difficult to achieve because the midportion frequently corresponds to the center of the lesion, where the greatest plaque burden is present. Other strategies have proposed that optimal stent expansion is the achievement of a minimal intrastent cross-sectional area which is a percentage of the proximal and distal reference cross-sectional lumen or vessel area, or the achievement of a cross-sectional area which is 70% of the calculated balloon cross-sectional area at full inflation (6,7,20,44–46, 53). These criteria have the disadvantage of being cumbersome and difficult to achieve (54). A multicenter study, the MUSIC trial, is currently under way to evaluate the feasibility and value of achieving an intrastent cross-sectional area that is 90% of the average proximal and distal reference lumen area, with the allowance of 80% achievement provided the intrastent cross-sectional area is a minimum of 9.0 mm^2 (53).

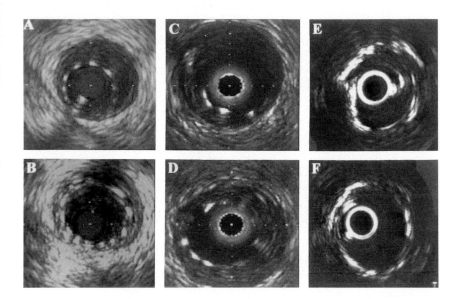

Figure 15 IVUS images demonstrating optimization of stent expansion with stent types other than Palmaz-Schatz stents. Acceptable angiographic images were seen prior to intravascular ultrasound imaging. (A) Wallstent at first intravascular ultrasound imaging. (B) Same Wallstent as in A after inflation with a larger balloon, demonstrating improvement in intra-stent cross-sectional area. (C) Wiktor stent demonstrating struts poorly apposed to the arterial wall. (D) Same Wiktor stent as in C after further inflation with the balloon to higher pressures, now demonstrating good strut-artery wall apposition. (E) Gianturco-Roubin stent partially compressed. (F) Same Gianturco-Roubin stent as in E after further inflation with the balloon to higher pressures, now demonstrating improved stent expansion.

E. Stent Types

Almost all of the work on intravascular ultrasound guidance of intracoronary stent deployment has focused on the Palmaz-Schatz stent. While it is likely that other rigid stents will be associated with similar benefits, it is much less clear how coil stents, such as Wiktor and Gianturco-Roubin stents, are impacted by intravascular ultrasound guidance (55). There is an increased risk in passing the ultrasound catheter through a coil stent as it can catch on part of the coil and deform the stent, adversely affecting the radial strength of the metal implant. The Gianturco-Roubin stent is more difficult to image, owing to the smaller relative volume of metal, and the tightest area within the stented segment often

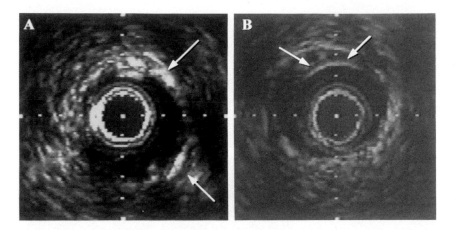

Figure 16 Intravascular ultrasound images of Gianturco-Roubin stents. (A) Cross section of metal gives the appearance of struts (arrows). (B) Tangential cut of metal gives appearance of a segment of ring (arrows).

does not demonstrate anything but plaque, without a stent clearly being present. However, this may reflect an important advantage of intravascular ultrasound imaging in a coil stent: the identification of plaque prolapsing through the stent, which may best be treated with the insertion of an additional stent.

V. CONCLUSION

Intravascular ultrasound has made important contributions to our understanding of proper stent deployment. Although excellent results with intracoronary stenting may be achieved without IVUS guidance, the use of this technology is still valuable in the stenting procedure. The ultimate contribution of intravascular ultrasound to stenting has yet to be determined. It is probably particularly valuable to the interventionalist with minimal experience at stent deployment as it is easier to identify inadequate stent expansion by intravascular ultrasound than by angiography. It is also valuable in identifying plaque morphology prior to stent deployment, which may be important in the choice of devices that may be used. Stenoses appearing moderate on angiography may be identified as more significant by IVUS and may be treated to ensure better inflow and outflow of the stented segment. Current retrospective data suggest restenosis may be lowered when IVUS is used to obtain greater improvements in acute gain. Finally, with intravascular ultrasound, the rare but important surprise, such as seen in Figure 6, may be identified.

The dramatic advances in interventional cardiology that have occurred in recent years have led to changes that often outpace our ability to provide definitive data from randomized trials. The use of intravascular ultrasound imaging as a guide to stent deployment has contributed to the rapid advances, and yet much of its potential value remains untested owing to the swift changes. Current and future trials will be important in defining the role of IVUS in achieving optimal stent deployment.

Despite the need for more definitive information we should never forget where we came from: small underdilated stents with prohibitive rates of stent thrombosis and mediocre incidences of stent restenosis. So far, IVUS-guided stent expansion has made a difference.

REFERENCES

1. Roubin GS, Cannon AD, Agrawal SK, et al. Intracoronary stenting for acute and threatened closure complicating percutaneous transluminal coronary angioplasty. Circulation 1992; 85:916–927.
2. Colombo A, Goldberg SL, Almagor Y, Maiello L, Finci L. A novel strategy for stent deployment in the treatment of acute or threatened closure complicating balloon coronary angioplasty. J Am Coll Cardiol 1993; 22:1887–1891.
3. George BS, Voorhess WD, Roubin GS, et al. Multicenter investigation of coronary stenting to treat acute or threatened closure after percutaneous transluminal coronary angioplasty: clinical and angiographic outcomes. J Am Coll Cardiol 1993; 22:135–143.
4. Serruys PW, de Jaegere P, Kiemeneij F, et al. A comparison of balloon expandable stent implantation with balloon angioplasty in patients with coronary artery disease. N Engl J Med 1994; 331:489–495.
5. Fischman DL, Leon MD, Baim DS, et al. A randomized comparison of coronary stent placement and balloon angioplasty in the treatment of coronary artery disease. N Engl J Med 1994; 331:496–501.
6. Goldberg SL, Colombo A, Nakamura S, Almagor Y, Maiello L, Tobis JM. Benefit of intracoronary ultrasound in the deployment of Palmaz-Schatz stents. J Am Coll Cardiol 1994; 24:996–1003.
7. Nakamura S, Colombo A, Gaglione A, et al. Intracoronary ultrasound observations during stent implantation. Circulation 1994; 89:2026–2034.
8. Gorge G, Haude M, Ge J, et al. Intravascular ultrasound after low and high inflation pressure coronary artery stent implantation. J Am Coll Cardiol 1995; 26:725–730.
9. Mudra H, Klauss V, Blasini R, et al. Ultrasound guidance of Palmaz-Schatz

intracoronary stenting with a combined intravascular ultrasound balloon catheter. Circulation 1994; 90:1252–1261.

10. Painter JA, Mintz GS, Wong SC, et al. Intravascular ultrasound assessment of biliary stent implantation in saphenous vein grafts. Am J Cardiol 1995; 75:731–734.

11. Palmaz JC. Intravascular stenting: from basic research to clinical application. Cardiovasc Intervent Radiol 1992; 15:279–284.

12. Mustard JF, Packham MA, Kinlough-Rathbone RL. Platelets, blood flow, and the vessel wall. Circulation 1990; 81(suppl I):I-24–I-27.

13. Falk E. Coronary thrombosis: pathogenesis and clinical manifestations. Am J Cardiol 1991; 68(suppl):28B–35B.

14. Painter JA, Mintz GS, Wong SC, et al. Serial intravascular ultrasound studies fail to show evidence of chronic Palmaz-Schatz stent recoil. Am J Cardiol 1995; 75: 398–400.

15. Kuntz RE, Safian RD, Carrozza JP, Fishman RF, Mansour M, Baim DS.The importance of acute luminal diameter in determining restenosis after coronary atherectomy or stenting. Circulation 1992; 86:1827–1835.

16. Colombo A, Hall P, Nakamura S, et al. Intracoronary stenting without anticoagulation accomplished with intravascular ultrasound guidance. Circulation 1995; 91: 1676–1688.

17. Morice MC, Breton C, Bunouf P, et al. Coronary stenting without anticoagulant, without intravascular ultrasound. Results of the French Registry. Circulation 1995; 92:796. Abstract.

18. Lablanche JM, Grollier G, Bonnet JL, et al. Ticlopidine aspirin stent evaluation (TASTE); a French multicenter study. Circulation 1995; 92:476. Abstract.

19. Schomig A, Schuhlen S, Blasini R, et al. Anticoagulation versus antiplatelet therapy after intracoronary Palmaz-Schatz stent placement—a prospective randomized trial. Circulation 1995; 92:280. Abstract.

20. Nunez BD, Foster-Smith K, Berger PB, et al. Benefit of intravascular ultrasound guided high pressure inflations in patients with a "perfect" angiographic result: the Mayo Clinic experience. Circulation 1995; 92:I-545–I-546. Abstract.

21. Caputo RP, Ho KKL, Lopez JJ, Stoler RC, Cohen DJ, Carroza JP. Quantitative angiographic comparison of Palmaz-Schatz stent implantation with and without intravascular ultrasound. Circulation 1995; 92:545. Abstract.

22. Goldberg SL, Hall P, Nakamura S, et al. Is there a benefit from intravascular ultrasound when high-pressure stent expansion is routinely performed prior to ultrasound imaging? J Am Coll Cardiol 1996; 27:306A. Abstract.

23. Serruys PW, Azar AJ, Sigwart U, et al. Long term follow-up of "stent-like" (≤30% diameter stenosis post) angioplasty: a case for provisional stenting. J Am Coll Cardiol 1996; 27:15A. Abstract.

24. Rodriguez AE, Sanaera O, Larribau M, et al. Coronary stenting decreases restenosis in lesions with early loss in luminal diameter 24 hours after successful PTCA. Circulation 1995; 91:1397–1402.

25. Honye J, Mahon DJ, Jain A, et al. Morphological effects of coronary balloon angioplasty in vivo assessed by intravascular ultrasound imaging. Circulation 1992; 85:1012–1025.

26. GUIDE Trial Investigators. IVUS-determined predictors of restenosis in PTCA and DCA: final report from the GUIDE trial, Phase II. J Am Coll Cardiol 1996; 27:156A. Abstract.

27. Jain SP, Jain A, Collins TJ, Ramee SR, White CJ. Predictors of restenosis: a morphometric and quantitative evaluation by intravascular ultrasound. Am Heart J 1994; 128:664–673.

28. Tenaglia AN, Buller CE, Kisslo K, Phillips HR, Stack RS, Davidson CJ. Intracoronary ultrasound predictors of adverse outcomes after coronary artery interventions. J Am Coll Cardiol 1992; 120:1385–1390.

29. Peters RJG, PICTURE Study Group. Predictions of angiographic restenosis by intracoronary ultrasound imaging after coronary balloon angioplasty. Eur Heart J 1995; 16:201. Abstract.

30. Mintz GS, Chuang YC, Popma JJ, et al. The final % cross-sectional narrowing (residual plaque burden) is the strongest intravascular ultrasound predictor of angiographic restenosis. J Am Coll Cardiol 1995; 35A. Abstract.

31. Kok WE, Peters RJG, Pasterkamp G, Liebergen RA, Kock KT, David GK. Subacute recoil in the first 60 minutes after balloon angioplasty: determinants found by intracoronary ultrasound imaging. Circulation 1995; 92:17. Abstract.

32. Mintz GS, Pichard AD, Kovach JA, et al. Impact of preintervention intravascular ultrasound imaging on transcatheter treatment strategies in coronary artery disease. Am J Cardiol 1994; 73:423–430.

33. Goldberg SL, Hall P, Almagor Y, et al. Intravascular ultrasound guided rotational atherectomy of fibro calcific plaque prior to intracoronary deployment of Palmaz-Schatz stents. J Am Coll Cardiol 1994; 23:290A. Abstract.

34. Fitzgerald PJ, STRUT Registry Investigators. Lesion composition impacts size and symmetry of stent expansion: initial report from the STRUT Registry. J Am Coll Cardiol 1995; 49A.

35. Mintz GS, Douek P, Pichard AD, et al. Target lesion calcification in coronary artery disease: an intravascular ultrasound study. J Am Coll Cardiol 1992; 20: 1149–1155.

36. Sherman CT, Litvack F, Grunfest WS, et al. Coronary angioscopy in patients with unstable angina pectoris. N Engl J Med 1986; 315:913–919.

37. Mizuno K, Satamura K, Miyamoto A, et al. Angioscopic evaluation of coronary artery thrombi in acute coronary syndromes. N Engl J Med 1992; 326:287–291.

38. Siegel RJ, Ariani M, Fishbein MC, et al. Histopathologic validation of angioscopy and intravascular ultrasound. Circulation 1991; 84:109–117.

39. Siegel RJ, Fishbein MC, Chae JS, Helfant RH, Hickey A, Forrester JS. Comparative studies of angioscopy and ultrasound for the evaluation of arterial disease. Echocardiography 1990; 7:495–502.

40. Pandian NG, Kreis A, Brockway B, Sacharoff A, Caro R. Intravascular high-frequency two-dimensional ultrasound detection of arterial dissection and intimal flap. Am J Cardiol 1990; 65:1278–1280.

41. Frimerman A, Miller HI, Hallman M, Laniado S, Keren G. Intravascular ultrasound characterization of thrombi of different composition. Am J Cardiol 1994; 73:1053–1057.

42. Goldberg SL, Almagor Y, Hall P, et al. Clinical and angiographic outcomes using different techniques in the deployment of Palmaz-Schatz stents. Submitted.

43. Prati F, di Mario C, Gil R, et al. Is quantitative angiography a surrogate of intravascular ultrasound for guidance of stent deployment? A comparison with 3-D quantitative reconstruction of intracoronary ultrasound. J Am Coll Cardiol 1996; 27:305A. Abstract.

44. Allen KM, Undemir C, Shaknovich A, Moses J, Strain J, Kreps E. Is there need for intravascular ultrasound after high-pressure dilatations of Palmaz-Schatz stents? J Am Coll Cardiol 1996; 27:138A. Abstract.

45. De Franco AC, Tuzcu EM, Ziada KM, et al. High-pressure inflations do not insure 'adequate' stent deployment: evidence from intravascular ultrasound. J Am Coll Cardiol 1996; 27:305A-3050. Abstract.

46. Werner GS, Diedrich J, Ferrari M, Buchwald A, Figulla HR. Can additional intravascular ultrasound improve the luminal area gain after high-pressure stent deployment? J Am Coll Cardiol 1996; 27:225A. Abstract.

47. Botas J, Elizaga J, Garcia E, et al. IVUS assessment of high pressure stent implantation. J Am Coll Cardiol 1996; 27:199A. Abstract.

48. Nunez BD, Holmes DR JR, Lerman A, Berger PB, Garratt KN, Higano ST. Detailed intravascular ultrasound analysis after routine high pressure assisted intracoronary stent implantation. J Am Coll Cardiol 1996; 27:199A. Abstract.

49. Ziada KM, Tuzcu EM, De Franco AC, et al. Angiographic 'haziness' following stent deployment: differential diagnosis using intravascular ultrasound. J Am Coll Cardiol 1996; 27:224A. Abstract.

50. Stone GW, Linnemeier T, St. Goar FG, et al. What is the optimal pressure for stent implantation (How high is high)? J Am Coll Cardiol 1996; 27:225A. Abstract.

51. Itoh A, Hall P, Maiello L, et al. Acute recoil of Palmaz-Schatz stent: a rare cause of suboptimal stent implantation—report of two cases with intravascular ultrasound findings. Cathet Cardiovasc Diagn 1996; 37:334–338.

52. Stone GW, Linnemeier T, St. Goar FG, Mudra H, Sheehan H, Hodgson JM. Improved outcome of balloon angioplasty with intracoronary ultrasound guidance—core lab angiographic and ultrasound results from the CLOUT study. J Am Coll Cardiol 1996; 27:155A. Abstract.

53. de Jaegere P, Mudra H, Almagor Y, et al. In-hospital and 1-month clinical results of an international study testing the concept of IVUS guided optimized stent expansion alleviating the need of systemic anticoagulation. J Am Coll Cardiol 1996; 27:137A. Abstract.

54. Hodgson JM, Mecca W, Nair R, Strony J, Comal D, Huck KB. Ultrasound-guided coronary stent implantation in routine practice: how realistic are the MUSIC and Milan criteria? Eur Heart J 1995; 16:290. Abstract.

55. Jain SP, Liu MW, Iyer SS, et al. Do high pressure balloon inflations improve acute gain within flexible metallic coil stents? An intravascular ultrasound assessment. J Am Coll Cardiol 1995; Feb:49A. Abstract.

15

Practical Use of Intravascular Ultrasound in the Cardiac Transplant Patient

Severin P. Schwarzacher   *Innsbruck University, Innsbruck, Austria*

Richard L. Popp and Alan C. Yeung   *Stanford University School of Medicine, Stanford, California*

I. INTRODUCTION

Short-term survival rates in cardiac transplantation have improved dramatically in the past decade, with a first year survival rate approaching 85% (1,2). Long-term survival remains limited primarily because of a unique form of coronary artery disease that develops early after transplantation (3–7). This entity, termed cardiac allograft vasculopathy (CAV), resembles the obliterative vascular diseases which are also seen in renal, lung, and liver transplantation. Early autopsy and experimental reports revealed a disease pattern of CAV distinctively different from common atherosclerotic coronary artery disease (8–10). Striking differences were found between CAV and native coronary disease, with CAV being more diffuse and involving smaller vessels in addition to the epicardial vessels. A higher percentage of CAV shows a concentric distribution and frequently encountered features of native atherosclerosis such as ulcerations, thrombosis, and calcifications are missing in CAV. The internal elastic lamina is often intact in CAV as well (11). In addition to the morphological changes of CAV, the clinical presentation of CAV has also been shown to be different compared to native coronary artery disease. Typical clinical signs of ischemia such as chest pain are frequently missing in transplant patients owing to partial or complete cardiac denervation (12–14).

Although a clear risk pattern for the development of CAV has not been established, several studies have shown that the presence of CAV correlates with poor graft outcome and impaired survival rates (15). It is therefore logical to seek diagnostic modalities with high sensitivity for the early detection of this detrimental disease process.

The following chapter describes several diagnostic tools for the detection of CAV emphasizing the practical utility of intravascular ultrasound.

II. CURRENT METHODS OF DETECTION

A. Conventional Stress Testing

The diffuse nature of CAV has resulted in limited specificity and sensitivity of traditional noninvasive diagnostic modalities for the detection of significant ischemic coronary artery disease. Conventional methods, such as ECG ST segment monitoring, echocardiographic wall motion, and nuclear medicine perfusion studies (16), have not shown reliability in the detection of CAV. Stress echocardiography has recently been performed to screen for the presence of CAV. The overall sensitivity was 25%, the specificity 86%, with a positive predictive value of 25% and a negative predictive value of 86%. The false-negative rate is especially high in patients with only moderate disease 16–19). These studies comprise only a limited number of patients and further studies need to be performed.

The unreliability of these methods in detecting CAV is in part due to the reliance of these tests on significant differences in regional blood supply of the myocardium and therefore they cannot assess a diffuse disease pattern, affecting the entire coronary tree.

B. Angiography

The inconsistent clinical signs and symptoms of CAV, the lack of reliable noninvasive testing, and the rapidity of CAV development have forced the adoption of annual coronary angiograms as the surveillance tool for CAV and as part of the standard of care.

Angiography demonstrated a very distinctive pattern of CAV in comparison to conventional coronary artery disease. In addition to the occurrence of proximal stenoses of the epicardial vessels, CAV commonly involves the primary, secondary, and tertiary branches, leading to angiographic "pruning" of the vasculature. This disease pattern, however, is often not appreciated until careful comparisons are performed among several studies. In cases of total occlusions, the lack of collateral development is commonly seen (20). The incidence of CAV ranges from 30% to ~50% at 5 years after transplantation (6).

The use of coronary angiography as the gold standard to detect CAV has several limitations. Angiography produces a luminal cast of the vessel, and the severity of stenoses is measured in relation to normal nondiseased adjacent vessel segments. This hampers the sensitivity of angiography in the detection of CAV, considering the diffuse character of the disease pattern. Year-to-year changes can be subtle and therefore could remain undiscovered. These limitations become clear in serial quantitative angiography (QCA) studies of transplant patients (21–23). In a series of 25 transplant recipients followed for 2 years, 515 coronary segments at year 1 and 353 segments at year 2 were studied by QCA. Only two transplant recipients developed a qualitative progression of disease at 1 year. However, by QCA lumen narrowing was seen in 21/25 patients (22). Histological studies have also revealed the presence of significant CAV despite normal angiograms (24,25). Almost every patient surviving 1 year after transplantation has CAV in varying degrees.

These studies clearly demonstrate the low sensitivity of conventional angiography in detecting CAV due to the diffuse pattern and rapid progression, especially within the first years after transplantation.

III. INTRAVASCULAR ULTRASOUND

Angiography has been used as the diagnostic study of choice for serial examinations in heart transplant recipients. Because of limitations mentioned above, new modalities such as intravascular ultrasound (IVUS) have been investigated for the detection of CAV. Two basic technical approaches are available (a mechanically rotating transducer and a phased array transducer) which show different capabilities of lateral resolution. Recent technical developments such as increased transducer frequency and miniaturization of the sheath-style catheters also allow inspection of small vessels and improved assessment of detailed structures.

In addition to standard lumen parameters such as diameter, IVUS provides on line information on plaque area, % area stenosis, and vessel wall characteristics, which are unattainable by conventional angiography. The sonographic information not only provides dimensional information but also elucidates plaque extent and composition in a cross-sectional format. Previous investigations have shown that the commonly employed 30-MHz probe can detect intimal thickening exceeding 150 to 180 μm in thickness (26).

IVUS studies in CAV elucidate why the angiographic disease pattern in these patients is different compared to native coronary artery disease. Sonographic imaging shows that the distribution of plaque stands in contrast to normal coronary artery disease. Typically, considerable concentric intimal thickening with a relatively homogeneous plaque type is seen in transplanted hearts, in contrast with a mixed plaque burden, which is eccentrically distributed in ~80% of hearts with atherosclerotic coronary artery disease (27).

Early work in using IVUS to study CAV has established the discrepancy between the angiographic and sonographic information regarding intimal thickening of coronary arteries in heart transplant patients (28,29) (Fig. 1). St. Goar and associates investigated patients 1 month and 1 year following transplantation with IVUS. The severity of CAV was graded regarding the thickness of intimal thickening (≤ 0.3 mm = minimal, to ≥ 0.5 mm = severe) and involvement of the vessel circumference ($\leq$ or $\geq$ than 180°). Only 7 of 20 patients studied 1 month after transplantation had no intimal thickening in their coronary segments by IVUS. In the other 13 patients with normal coronary angiograms, intimal thickening was clearly present by IVUS, and three patients had severe intimal thickening exceeding 0.5 mm in diameter. In a cohort of 60 patients 1 year posttransplantation, 42 patients had normal angiograms but intimal thickening was observed in every patient, 29 of whom had moderate to severe findings of CAV. In patients presenting with CAV by angiography, IVUS showed moderate or severe intimal thickening (28) (Fig. 2).

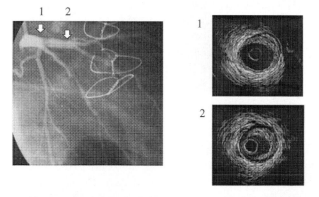

Figure 1 An angiogram of the left coronary descending artery is shown in the left panel. The white arrows indicate the image plane of IVUS cross sections, shown in the right panels. Intimal thickening as seen by ultrasound is not appreciated with angiography, which shows a smooth vessel contour.

Class (Severity)	Description
0 (none)	no visible intimal thickening (IT)
1 (minimal)	IT < 300 μm, < 180° vessel circumference
2 (mild)	IT < 300 μm , >180° vessel circumference
3 (moderate)	IT 300-500 μm , < 180° vessel circumference; or IT > 500 μm at any point
4 (severe)	IT 500-1000 μm, >180° vessel circumference; or IT > 1000 μm at any point

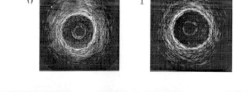

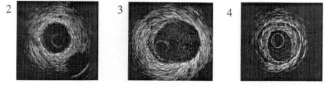

Figure 2 Examples of IVUS transplant images representing each class of the severity. The classification of intimal thickening in cardiac allograft vasculopathy, based on the experience of Stanford University, is shown.

The extensive experience with IVUS in heart transplantation in our center has led to the introduction of a grading system of intimal thickening, which is shown in Figure 3.

A. Incidence and Severity of CAV by IVUS

The incidence and severity of CAV as defined by IVUS has been clarified by several studies. Pinto and associates investigated 70 transplant patients with IVUS 1 year apart. The sites investigated annually were matched using anatomical landmarks such as branches. They found progression of intimal thickening in all patients, whether they had mild or severe CAV at the initial study (mild disease: progress 0.05 ± 0.13 mm; severe disease: progress 0.07 ± 0.15 mm increase in intimal thickening). Progression by ultrasound was identical in cases with and without angiographic evidence of disease (30). This study also demonstrated the feasibility to follow patients and respective coronary sites with disease over time with reliability. Another study investigated the incidence of CAV over time (up to 15 years) using ultrasound in 174 transplant recipients. The mean intimal thickening was significantly higher 1 year after transplantation with progression of disease within the first several years. Calcification in plaques of these patients, an entity rarely seen in the first years after transplantation, increased especially after the sixth year (31) (Fig. 4A,B). These observations have been confirmed by a recent multicenter study (32).

The advantage of IVUS over angiography in the diagnosis of CAV is also highlighted by Lowry et al. (33), who found good correlation of lumen area and diameter measurements between quantitative angiography and IVUS. How-

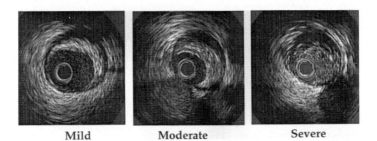

Mild   Moderate   Severe

Figure 3 Three IVUS cross sections within one coronary artery of a transplanted heart are shown representing severity classes of intimal thickening. While a reasonable lumen is still seen in the mild and moderate classes (left and middle), almost total occlusion by the plaque can be seen in the severe class of intimal thickening (right).

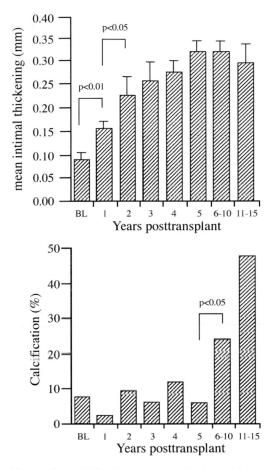

Figure 4 (A) The development of intimal thickening in transplant coronary arteries, as observed with IVUS, is shown in this graph. Within the first 2 years after transplantation, a significant increase in intimal thickening is observed reaching the maximum at ~10 years. (B) The incidence of calcification, as detected by IVUS, over time is shown. In the first years following transplantation, calcification is a rare entity to be seen. A significant increase in calcification of coronary intimal thickening can be seen late after transplantation.

ever, IVUS was able to provide information about the shape of the lumen and the intimal thickness. A recent study investigated the variability of CAV among the three coronary vessels in the same patients (34). They found significantly more CAV in the left anterior descending, followed by the circumflex and the right coronary artery. In 64% of the investigated patients the proximal segment showed a higher degree of CAV compared to the distal segment of the same artery.

B. Donor Disease Influencing CAV

Besides the individual development of CAV in transplant patients, recent investigations have tried to answer the question of whether preexisting coronary artery disease of the donor heart can influence the development of CAV in the transplant patient. In a serial IVUS study of our institution 30 patients had a baseline IVUS study (within 3 weeks following transplantation) and a follow-up exam 1 to 2 years later. At baseline, 9 of these 30 patients had preexisting donor disease (29%) by ultrasound. At the first annual follow-up examination, the patients with donor disease still had more intimal thickening than patients without donor disease. However, the progression of CAV in the group with preexisting disease was not significantly different from the group without donor disease. This was also true for patients receiving an additional IVUS exam later than 1 year following transplantation (35) (Fig. 5). These data suggest that preexisting donor disease does not accelerate CAV though sites that have donor disease will become angiographically apparent sooner owing to the larger burden of disease. Another study also found relevant intimal thickening in 56% of donor hearts immediately after transplantation by IVUS (36). The presence of donor disease correlated with donor age and male sex, and was predictive of the sonographic presence of CAV. The influence of this disease pattern on CAV was not studied in this patient cohort.

C. Remodeling

The phenomenon of compensatory vessel enlargement has been shown to occur in coronary artery disease. The increase in vessel size is directly related to the increase in plaque growth, delaying the loss in lumen area until the lesion area stenosis reaches approximately 30% to 40% (37). In general, this phenomenon is considered to be a compensatory mechanism, since the luminal encroachment is delayed and, occasionally, can be avoided. A lack of remodeling can increase the luminal narrowing, as has been shown by Pasterkamp et al., who found that in vessels with a lack of compensatory enlargement, area stenosis was higher than in vessels with compensatory enlargement (38).

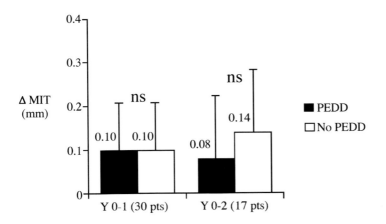

Figure 5 Bar graphs showing the change in intracoronary ultrasound parameters of mean intimal thickness (MIT), 1 year (Y 0–1) and 2 years (Y 0–2) after transplantation in the patients (pts) with (solid bars) and without (open bars) preexistent donor disease (PEDD). Patients transplanted with allografts having preexistent coronary artery lesions did not develop more, or accelerated, intimal vasculopathy compared with those patients without preexistent disease.

Whether this phenomenon is also a relevant factor in CAV is currently under investigation. A recent study in our institution investigated the effect of compensatory vessel dilatation in transplant coronary arteries using IVUS. One hundred fifty-one patients with progression of intimal area, matched by IVUS and angiography as previously described, were studied over 3 years. In 49% of segments, the relative increase in total vessel area was larger than the increase in intimal area. This occurred especially early after transplantation. In the remaining segments compensatory dilatation was absent or only partially present. In some segments actual decrease in vessel area was noted. This study reports that, as in ischemic heart disease, the development of CAV in transplant disease is obviously influenced by compensatory enlargement of the vessel. The clinical importance and whether compensatory enlargement affects prognosis in this patient group still needs to be shown.

D. Physiological Significance of Intimal Thickening

Although IVUS increases the insight into the morphology of CAV in epicardial vessels, it is not entirely clear how the resistance vessels and blood flow are affected by CAV. Additionally, the relationship between the morphology of

CAV and the function of the vascular endothelium is still under investigation. It has been assumed that the most important factor initiating the development of CAV is an immune-mediated damage to the vascular endothelium. This has been suggested in early studies, where endothelial dysfunction as tested by acetylcholine infusions was found to be impaired early after transplantation. When acetylcholine was injected into transplant coronary arteries showing a smooth, nondiseased contour on angiography there was almost no preservation of endothelium-dependent vasodilatation in these arteries. In arteries stenosed by angiography there was severe constriction following acetylcholine (40). Mugge and associates found a significant reduction of endothelium-dependent coronary blood flow increase in patients with sonographic evidence of CAV (41). In contrast, others have tried to establish a relation between the evidence of CAV and the presence of disturbed endothelium-dependent vasomotion (42). In these studies it was shown that intimal thickening by IVUS does not necessarily correlate with impaired vasodilatation, but this functional disturbance might precede the development of the intimal thickening process (43). Endothelium-independent vasodilatation, induced by nitroglycerin, was shown to be well preserved throughout a long period of time after transplantation, and intimal thickening as diagnosed by IVUS had no impact on this functional measure (41,44). A recent study also could not find a significant difference in maximal coronary flow response between transplant patients with and without sonographic evidence of CAV (45).

E. Risk Factors for CAV as Detected by IVUS

Several attempts to evaluate traditional risk factors of coronary artery disease and to characterize specific risk factors for the prediction of CAV have been difficult owing to controversial results gathered in a large number of studies. Hyperlipidemia, mainly induced by the immunosuppressive therapy, is present in almost every transplant patient and is clearly a risk factor for CAV, although studies showed controversial results (46–51). The increase of LDL in these patients shortly after transplantation has been shown to be specifically crucial, since treatment of transplant patients with pravastatin has been shown to result in the lowering of coronary plaque volume and improved outcome (52). Other possible nonimmune risk factors include diabetes mellitus (51,53) and also infections with cytomegalo- and herpesvirus (54,55).

Although immune-mediated mechanisms have been implicated for the development of CAV, improved immunosuppressive regimens have not decreased the occurrence of CAV. Therefore several investigators have tried to elucidate nonimmunological risk factors for CAV, using IVUS for the assessment of CAV over time. In a study of 101 patients, intravascular ultrasound studies were performed on an annual basis and patients were additionally investigated regarding nonimmunological risk factors for CAV. Separated into groups depending on the severity of CAV, independent risk factors or predictors for the occurrence and degree of CAV were found. Higher levels of total cholesterol and LDL cholesterol as well as elevated triglycerides, weight gain, and body mass index were predictors of severe intimal thickening. Additionally, the time after transplantation and the donor age also predicted the degree of intimal thickening in these patients (50).

Mehra et al. developed a computer model to assess both immunologic and non-immunologic risk factors for CAV. They also found the donor age > 35 and hypertriglyceridemia predictive for the development of CAV as assessed by IVUS (56). On the basis of IVUS findings, these studies for the first time were able to assess the development of CAV, depending on risk factors, which affect any transplant recipient due to the drug therapy regimen. A recent investigation highlighted the importance of hyperlipidemia in general and hypercholesterolemia especially as a risk factor for CAV (52). In transplant patients, a cholesterol lowering therapy with pravastatin (a blocker of the cholesterol-synthesizing enzyme HMG CoA reductase) was able to reduce plaque volume significantly as measured with IVUS.

In the above-mentioned studies, the age of the heart donor was predictive for CAV. This entity is totally unpredictable at the time of transplantation, as is the presence of coronary artery disease in the donor hearts. The influence of donor characteristics on the presence of CAV as detected by IVUS was presented by a recent investigation in our institution. One hundred sixteen heart transplant recipients were studied with quantitative coronary angiography and intravascular ultrasound for the presence of CAV and compared to demographic, clinical, and immunologic donor characteristics (57). Mainly nonimmunologic variables could be found to be predictive for CAV by angiography as well as by IVUS. Angiographic evidence of CAV was predicted by a higher donor age. In 39 of these patients, who were studied with IVUS exactly 1 year after transplantation, a history of donor smoking and the white race of donors predicted the development of CAV by IVUS. The fact that higher donor age predicted angiographic evidence of CAV supports earlier-mentioned data, that only CAV at a later stage can be picked up by angiography, indicating a higher burden of disease making an angiographic appearance earlier.

F. Safety

Annual investigations with intravascular ultrasound in patients prone to intimal thickening have raised concerns about the safety of this method. Two major studies (58,59) have addressed this issue in over 2000 patients showing an extremely low incidence of complications. The main complication is transient coronary spasm in ~3% of cases, which disappears immediately after intra-coronary nitroglycerin. Our institution has also shown that vessels repeatedly instrumented with IVUS catheters do not have greater progression of CAV than noninstrumented vessels over several years of follow-up (58).

IV. PROGNOSIS

It has been suggested earlier that any degree of angiographic CAV in transplant recipients implicates an increased risk for cardiac events and mortality in these patients (60). A recent study correlated the degree of CAV by angiography with the 2 year survival rate (61). When the angiographic luminal stenosis exceeded 40%, the survival rate at 2 years was only 50%. This relationship was even worsening when the percent stenosis grade was >70%.

Clearly, IVUS is more sensitive than angiography in detecting intimal thickening; however, whether the prognosis of heart transplantation is affected by the degree of CAV present as detected by IVUS is not entirely clear. A recent study from our institution established the importance of sonographically de-

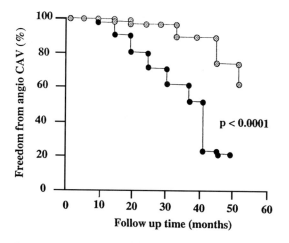

Figure 6 Predicted freedom of angiographic evidence of CAV according to the presence of intimal thickening by IVUS of <0.3 mm (striped symbols) and >0.3 mm (black symbols) is shown. When intimal thickening exceeds 0.3 mm in thickness soon after transplantation, the chance to have CAV by angiography at follow-up was signifi-cantly lower than in cases with evidence of intimal thickening of <0.3 mm in thickness.

tected intimal thickening for determining the long-term outcome of transplantation in 145 transplant recipients (62). In this study, intimal thickening was considered pathological when it exceeded 0.3 mm. This was based on pathological studies (15) and also on IVUS in vitro studies from our group (26). Intimal thickening of >0.3 mm correlated with decreased cardiac survival and also with reduced freedom from cardiac death and retransplantation (Fig. 6). Additionally, in cases in which IVUS could not detect any intimal thickening initially, this finding predicted freedom of CAV by angiography at follow up (63). The important message of this investigation is that intimal thickening of >0.3 mm by IVUS did predict worse outcome regardless of angiographic evidence of CAV. These results indicate the feasibility and importance of CAV detected by ultrasound and may suggest that this method be used for the annual investigation of transplant patients, since changes in therapeutic strategies could be drawn from ultrasound results.

V. PRACTICAL GUIDELINES

Intravascular ultrasound enables close and regular investigation of CAV in the transplant recipient. Numerous studies have revealed that this method is far more accurate than angiography and that follow-up investigations of transplant recipients with IVUS help to select patients with different degrees of CAV.

Two questions are raised by new insights into CAV using IVUS. Does every transplant recipient need IVUS investigations, and are annual IVUS follow-up investigations necessary?

These questions cannot be entirely answered from the literature available, and multicenter trials including a large number of patients are on-going. However, it can be suggested from the current literature that an IVUS investigation at baseline to document donor disease and at 1 year will have an impact on the treatment plan and eventually prognosis of the patient. If the initial and first-year IVUS exams show no significant intimal thickening, further IVUS exams in the next few years are probably not necessary, since most of the progression in this group is during the first year. If significant donor disease is present at the initial study, these patients should be treated aggressively with calcium channel blockers and lipid-lowering agents to retard further development of intimal thickening on top of these lesions. All patients should have IVUS examinations at year 5 since if the vessels are disease free, they are likely to have little progression over the next few years.

Despite the fact that the pathophysiology of CAV is not entirely understood, IVUS has improved our understanding of the disease process and serves as an ideal clinical tool for the follow-up investigation of heart transplant patients.

REFERENCES

1. Kriett JM, Kaye MP. The registry of the International Society for Heart Transplantation: seventh annual report—1990. J Heart Transplant 1990; 9:323–330.
2. Bourge RC, Naflel DC, Costanzo-Nordin M, et al. A multiinstitutional study: pretransplantation risk factors for death after cardiac transplantation. J Heart Lung Transplant 1993; 12:549–562.
3. Griepp RB, Stinson EB, Bieber CP, et al. Control of graft atherosclerosis in human heart transplant recipients. Surgery 1977; 81:262–269.
4. Bieber CP, Hunt SA, Schwinn DA, et al. Complications in long-term survivors of cardiac transplantation. Transplant Proc 1981; 8:207–211.
5. Hunt SA. Complications of heart transplantation. J Heart Transplant 1983; 3: 70–74.
6. Uretsky BF, Murali S, Reddy PS, et al. Development of coronary artery disease in cardiac transplant patients receiving immunosuppressive therapy with cyclosporine and prednisone. Circulation 1987; 76:827–834.
7. Barnhart GR, Pascoe EA, Mills S, et al. Accelerated arteriosclerosis in cardiac transplant recipients. Transplant Rev 1987; 1:31–46.
8. Kosek JC, Hurley EJ, Sewell DH, Lower RR. Histopathology of orthotopic canine cardiac allografts and its clinical correlation. Transplant Proc 1969; 1:311–315.
9. Thomson JG. Production of severe atheroma in a transplant human heart. Lancet 1969; 2:1088–1092.
10. Bieber CP, Stinson EB, Shumway NE, Payne R, Kosek J. Cardiac transplantation in man. VII. Cardiac allograft pathology. Circulation 1970; 41:753–772.
11. Billingham ME. Cardiac transplant atherosclerosis. Transplant Proc 1987; 19 (suppl 5):19–25.
12. Heroux AL, Silverman P, Costanzo MR, et al. Intracoronary ultrasound assessment of morphological and functional abnormalities associated with cardiac allograft vasculopathy. Circulation 1994; 89:272–277.
13. Rowe SK, Kleiman NS, Cocanougher B, et al. Effects of intracoronary acetylcholine infusion early versus late after heart transplant. Transplant Proc 1991; 23:1193–1197.
14. Theron HT, Mills RM, Hill JA, Lambert CR, Pepine CJ, Conti CR. Quantitative analysis of nitroglycerin-induced coronary artery vasodilation in transplanted hearts. J Heart Lung Transplant 1992; 11:886–891.
15. Velican D, Velican C. Comparative study on age-related changes and atherosclerotic involvement of the coronary arteries of male and female subjects up to 40 years of age. Atherosclerosis 1981; 38:39–50.
16. Smart FW, Ballantyne CM, Cocanougher B, et al. Insensitivity of noninvasive tests to detect coronary artery vasculopathy after heart transplant. Am J Cardiol 1991; 67:243–247.
17. Collings CA, Pinto FJ, Valantine HA, Popylisen S, Puryear JV, Schnittger I. Exercise echocardiography in heart transplant recipients: a comparison with an-

giography and intracoronary ultrasonography. J Heart Lung Transplant 1994; 13: 604–613.

18. Spes CH, Mudra H, Schnaack SD, et al. Dobutamine stress echocardiography for detection of transplant coronary vasculopathy; comparison with angiography and intracoronary ultrasound. Transplant Proc 1995; 27:1973–1974.

19. Ciliberto GR, Massa D, Mangiavacchi M, et al. High-dose dipyridamole echocardiography test in coronary artery disease after heart transplantation. Eur Heart J 1993; 14:48–52.

20. Gao SZ, Schroeder JS, Alderman EL, et al. Clinical and laboratory correlates of accelerated coronary artery disease in the cardiac transplant patient. Circulation 1987; 80(suppl V):V56–V61.

21. O'Neill BJ, Pfugfelder PW, Singh NR, Menkis AH, McKenzie FN, Kostuk WJ. Frequency of angiographic detection and quantitative assessment of coronary arterial disease one and three years after cardiac transplantation. Am J Cardiol 1989; 63:1221–1226.

22. Gao SZ, Alderman EL, Schroeder JS, Hunt SA, Wiederhold V, Stinson EB. Progressive coronary luminal narrowing after cardiac transplantation. Circulation 1990; 82(suppl IV):IV269–IV275.

23. Mills RM Jr., Hills JA, Theron HD, Gonzales JI, Pepine CJ, Conti CR. Serial quantitative coronary angiography in the assessment of coronary disease in the transplanted heart. J. Heart Lung Transplant 1992; 11:S52–S55.

24. Johnson DE, Alderman EL, Schroeder JS, et al. Transplant coronary artery disease: histopathologic correlations with angiographic morphology. J Am Coll Cardiol 1991; 17:449- 457.

25. Dressler FA, Miller LW. Necropsy versus angiography: how accurate is angiography? J Heart Lung Transplant 1992; 11:S56–S59.

26. Fitzgerald PJ, Goar FG, Connolly RJ, et al. Intravascular ultrasound imaging of coronary arteries. Is three-layer the norm? Circulation 1992; 86:154–158.

27. Waller BF. Anatomy, histology, pathology of the major coronary arteries relevant to echocardiographic imaging techniques. J Am So Echo 1989; 2:232–252.

28. St. Goar FG, Pinto FJ, Alderman EL, et al. Intracoronary ultrasound in cardiac transplant recipients: in vivo evidence of "angiographically silent" intimal thickening. Circulation 1992; 85:979–987.

29. Valantine H, Pinto FJ, Goar FG, Alderman EL, Popp RL. Intracoronary ultrasound imaging in heart transplant recipients: the Stanford experience. J Heart Lung Transplant 1992; 11(3):S60–S64.

30. Pinto FJ, Chenzbraun A, Botas J. et al. Feasibility of serial intracoronary ultrasound imaging for assessment of progression of intimal proliferation in cardiac transplant recipients. Circulation 1994; 90:2348–2355.

31. Rickenbacher PR, Pinto FJ, Chenzbraun A, et al. Incidence and severity of transplant coronary artery disease early and up to 15 years after transplantation as detected by intravascular ultrasound. J Am Coll Cardiol 1995; 25:171–177.

32. Yeung AC, Davis SF, Hauptman PJ, et al. Incidence and progression of transplant

coronary artery disease over 1 year: results of a multicenter trial with use of intravascular ultrasound. J Heart Lung Transplant 1995; 14:S215–S220.

33. Lowry RW, Kleiman NS, Raizner AE, Young JB. Is intravascular ultrasound better than quantitative coronary arteriography to assess cardiac allograft arteriopathy? Cathet Cardiovasc Diagn 1994; 31:110–115.

34. Klauss V, Mudra H, Ueberfuhr P, Theisen K. Intraindividual variability of cardiac allograft vasculopathy as assessed by intravascular ultrasound. Am J Cardiol 1995; 76:463–466.

35. Botas J, Pinto FJ, Chenzbraun A, et al. The influence of preexistent donor coronary artery disease on the progression of transplant vasculopathy: an intravascular ultrasound study. Circulation 1995; 92:1126–1132.

36. Tuzcu EM, Hobbs RE, Rincon G, et al. Occult and frequent transmission of atherosclerotic coronary disease with cardiac transplantation. Insights from intravascular ultrasound. Circulation 1995; 91:1706–1713.

37. Glagov S, Weisenberg E, Zarins CK, Stankunavicius R, Kolettis G. Compensatory enlargement of human atherosclerotic coronary arteries. N Engl J Med 1987; 316:1371–1375.

38. Pasterkamp G, Wensing PJ, Post MJ, Hillen B, Mali WP, Borst C. Paradoxical arterial wall shrinkage may contribute to luminal narrowing of human atherosclerotic femoral arteries. Circulation 1995; 91(5):1444–1449.

39. Lim TT, Liang DH, Botas J, et al. Role of compensatory enlargement and shrinkage in transplant coronary artery disease: serial IVUS study. Circulation 1997; 95:855–859.

40. Fish RD, Nabel EG, Selwyn AP, et al. Response of coronary arteries of cardiac transplant patients to acetylcholine. J Clin Invest 1988; 81:21–31.

41. Mugge A, Heublein B, Kuhn M, et al. Impaired coronary dilator responses to substance P and impaired flow-dependent dilator responses in heart transplant patients with graft vasculopathy. J Am Coll Cardiol 1993; 21:163–170.

42. Yeung AC, Anderson T, Meredith I, et al. Endothelial dysfunction in the development and detection of transplant coronary artery disease. J Heart Lung Transplant 1992; 11:S69–S73.

43. Anderson TJ, Meredith IT, Uehata A, et al. Functional significance of intimal thickening as detected by intravascular ultrasound early and late after cardiac transplantation. Circulation 1993; 88:1093–1100.

44. Pinto FJ, St. Goar FG, Fischell TA, et al. Nitroglycerin-induced coronary vasodilation in cardiac transplant recipients: evaluation with in vivo intracoronary ultrasound. Circulation 1992; 85:69–77.

45. Caracciolo EA, Wolford TL, Underwood RD, et al. Influence of intimal thickening on coronary blood flow responses in orthotopic heart transplant recipients. Circulation 1995; 92(suppl II):II-182–II-190.

46. Hess ML, Hastillo A, Mahanakumar T, et al. Accelerated atherosclerosis in cardiac transplantation: role of cytotoxic B-cell antibodies and hyperlipidemia. Circulation 1983; 68(suppl II):II94–II101.

47. Keogh A, Simons L, Spratt P, et al. Hyperlipidemia after heart transplantation. J Heart Lung Transplant 1988; 7:171–175.
48. Kemna MS, Valantine H, Hunt SA, Schroeder JS, Chen Y-D I, Reaven GM. Metabolic risk factors for atherosclerosis in heart transplant recipients. Am Heart J 1994; 128:68–72.
49. Bilodeau M, Fitchett DH, Guerraty A, Sniderman AD. Dyslipoproteinemias after heart and heart-lung transplantation: potential relation to accelerated graft arteriosclerosis. J Heart Transplant 1989; 8:454–459.
50. Escobar A, Ventura HO, Stapleton DD, et al. Cardiac allograft vasculopathy assessed by intravascular ultrasonography and nonimmunologic risk factors. Am J Cardiol 1994; 74:1042- 1046.
51. Eich D, Thompson JA, Ko DJ, et al. Hypercholesterolemia in long-term survivors of heart transplantation: an early marker of accelerated coronary artery disease. J Heart Lung Transplant 1991; 10:45–49.
52. Kobashigawa JA, Katznelson S, Laks H, et al. Effects of pravastatin on outcomes after cardiac transplantation. N Engl J Med 1995; 333:621–627.
53. Olivari MT, Homans DC, Wilson RF, Kubo SH, Ring WS. Coronary artery disease in cardiac transplant patients receiving triple-drug immunosuppressive therapy. Circulation 1989; 5(suppl III):III111–III115.
54. Min KW, Wickemeyer WJ, Chandran P, et al. Fatal cytomegalovirus infection and coronary arterial thromboses after heart transplantation: a case report. J Heart Lung Transplant 1987; 6:100–105.
55. Hajjar DP, Pomerantz KB, Flacone DJ, Weksler BB, Grant AJ. Herpes simplex virus infection in human arterial cells: implications in arteriosclerosis. J Clin Invest 1987; 80:1317–1321.
56. Mehra MR, Ventura HO, Chambers R, et al. Predictive model to assess risk for cardiac allograft vasculopathy: an intravascular ultrasound study. J Am Coll Cardiol 1995; 26:1537–1544.
57. Rickenbacher PR, Pinto FJ, Lewis NP, et al. Correlation of donor characteristics with transplant coronary artery disease as assessed by intracoronary ultrasound and coronary angiography. Am J Cardiol 1995; 76:340–345.
58. Pinto FJ, Chenzbraun A, Botas J, et al. Feasibility of serial intracoronary ultrasound imaging for assessment of progression of intimal proliferation in cardiac transplant recipients. Circulation 1994; 90:2348–2355.
59. Hausmann D, Erbel R, Alibelli-Chemarin M-J, et al. The safety of intracoronary ultrasound: a multicenter survey of 2207 examinations. Circulation 1995; 91:623–630.
60. Uretsky BF, Kormos RL, Zerbe TR, et al. Cardiac events of heart transplantation: incidence and predictive value of coronary arteriography. J Heart Lung Transplant 1992; 11:S45–S51.
61. Koegh AM, Valantine HA, Hunt SA, et al. Impact of proximal or midvessel discrete coronary artery stenoses on survival after heart transplantation. J Heart Lung Transplant 1992; 11:892–901.

62. Rickenbacher PR, Pinto FJ, Lewis NP, et al. Prognostic importance of intimal thickness as measured by intracoronary ultrasound after cardiac transplantation. Circulation 1995; 92:3445–3452.

63. Liang DN, Schwartzkopf A, Botas J, Alderman E, Yeung AC. Prediction of future angiographic disease by intravascular ultrasound findings in heart transplant recipients. J Heart Lung Transplant. In press.

16

Clinical Applications of Intravascular Ultrasound in Peripheral Vascular Disease

Donald B. Reid *Royal Infirmary, Glasgow, Scotland*

Edward B. Diethrich *Arizona Heart Institute, Phoenix, Arizona*

Peter Marx and Robert Wrasper *Columbia Medical Center Phoenix, Phoenix, Arizona*

I. INTRODUCTION

Ultrasound was introduced into clinical medicine over 40 years ago, and its initial use in gynecology and obstetrics was met by considerable skepticism (1,2). Over the years, however, ultrasound has proven itself and has gained credibility and acceptance in a variety of medical disciplines. Ultrasound now enjoys a reputation for being a safe, reliable, and inexpensive diagnostic method to assist in clinical decision making and alter patient management. At present, the use of intravascular ultrasound (IVUS) does not enjoy such acceptability and is regarded by many endovascular surgeons as a costly guidance system. However, the demonstrated benefit of IVUS in coronary angioplasty and stenting (3) has encouraged its use in peripheral vascular procedures where it is proving to have practical application and clinical value. In patients with peripheral vascular disease, IVUS is most frequently used following percutaneous transluminal angioplasty, intravascular stenting, atherectomy, and in the deployment of endoluminal grafts (ELGs) (4–7).

IVUS has two important clinical roles: first, in assessment following intervention, and second, in diagnostic evaluation of arterial disease. Its primary use is in the former, where it provides information about the success of intervention and the need for additional treatment. In the peripheral arteries, IVUS has a complementary role to angiography, which provides the endovascular surgeon with detail of collateral circulation, vessel contour, quality of flow, and inflow and outflow. IVUS allows appreciation of the vessel wall and lumen and can distinguish soft plaque and calcification (8). Intimal dissection flaps, thrombus formation, and ulceration are also visible with IVUS, and the luminal diameter and cross-sectional area can be measured (9). Occasionally, IVUS detects lesions missed on conventional arteriography (10). Hence, the ideal use of IVUS in peripheral interventions is in partnership with angiography.

This chapter outlines the clinical value of IVUS in the peripheral arteries and describes the technical aspects of its use in a variety of clinical situations. The results of a prospective study of the clinical utility of three-dimensional intravascular ultrasound (3D IVUS) in peripheral interventions are also presented.

II. TECHNICAL ASPECTS OF THREE-DIMENSIONAL IVUS IN PERIPHERAL INTERVENTIONS

A. Creating IVUS Images

In real-time imaging, conventional IVUS provides a two-dimensional (2D) image of the vessel similar to a CT scan cut (Fig. 1a). It is now possible, however, to reconstruct conventional 2D images into 3D images (11). Serial images are stacked by the computer during a single "pull-through" and reassembled into a 3D image. While 2D IVUS provides detail that is not possible with duplex, 3D IVUS allows imaging that is superior to 2D. Three-dimensional IVUS is a technological advance we have found particularly helpful in peripheral interventions (12).

Figure 1   (a) Axial 2D IVUS of an abdominal aortic aneurysm showing laminated mural clot. (b) "Longitudinal" 3D IVUS reconstruction of the aneurysm demonstrating a proximal neck, aneurysm with laminated thrombus and heavily calcified distal neck. (c) "Volume" 3D IVUS reconstruction showing the cylinder of the aorta with aneurysm and proximal and distal necks. (d) Aortogram of this patient's abdominal aortic aneurysm.

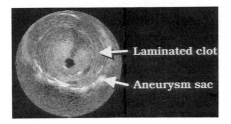

(a)

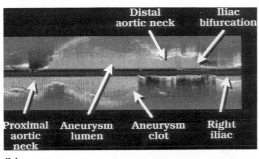

(b)

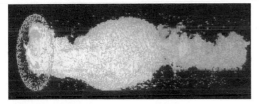

(c)

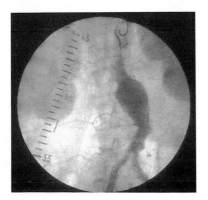

(d)

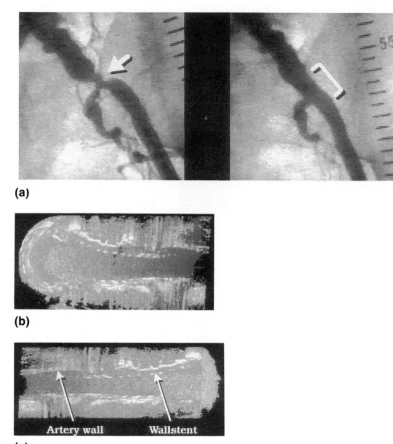

(a)

(b)

(c)

Figure 2   (a) Pre- and postprocedural angiograms of a stenosis at the common iliac artery bifurcation treated by angioplasty and stenting. (b,c) 3D IVUS "volume" image of the stented artery. The image has been hemisected along the longitudinal axis of the artery to demonstrate the luminal aspect with an incompletely deployed Wallstent.

Three-dimensional IVUS allows the whole length of the artery to be displayed at one time, and images may be examined from any angle, slice, or rotation. Three-dimensional IVUS images are presented either as "longitudinal" or "volume" views. The authors prefer the longitudinal images because they are immediately available in the operating room and enable the physician to make rapid clinical decisions following a pull-through (Fig. 1b). These views are similar in appearance to an angiogram but also define vessel wall morphology and may be rotated to provide a lateral perspective. Volume images take 2 to 3 min to create, but they provide a 3D cylindrical view of the vessel that can be turned over or revolved around (Fig. 1c,d). Computer software allows hemisection of the cylinder along its length for inspection of the luminal aspect of the artery (Fig. 2). Three-dimensional reconstruction provides the IVUS operator with a maximum of information in the operating room to assist him or her with clinical decisions and patient management.

B. Anatomic and Procedural Considerations

1. Carotid Artery

Carotid angioplasty and stenting are currently being evaluated as possible alternatives to carotid endarterectomy (13). IVUS has an important role in these procedures because it can detect inadequate stent deployment that may not be visible on the completion angiogram. It can also be used before angioplasty and stenting to help achieve accurate placement (14).

Following stent placement, a 3.5 F, 30-MHz IVUS catheter is advanced into the cephalic internal carotid artery on a 0.018-inch guidewire. The artery is usually free of disease at this level, and luminal diameters are measured (Fig. 3). The catheter is pulled through the stent so that deployment can be assessed and the minimum stent diameter measured. The deployed stent should be uniformly expanded along its length, and there should be no space between the stent and artery wall (Fig. 4). The IVUS operator should confirm that the stent covers the lesion and no proximal or distal disease is left untreated. A careful examination for any intimal dissection should also be made. In general, a

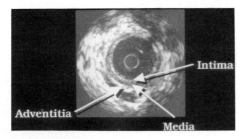

Figure 3 2D IVUS of a normal peripheral artery: the internal carotid, demonstrating the layers of the artery wall.

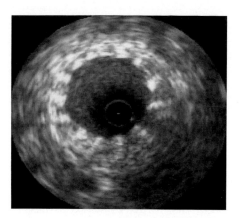

Figure 4 2D IVUS of a well-deployed carotid stent, fully expanded against the vessel wall.

minimum stent diameter of greater than 4 mm is recommended in the internal carotid artery.

Accurate stent deployment in the diseased carotid may be difficult to achieve because stenotic plaque is often heavily calcified (14). Calcifications and fibrotic tissue resist complete stent expansion, and this is often seen on IVUS as midstent "waisting" that usually responds to redilation with a larger balloon (Fig. 5). IVUS may also visualize incomplete apposition of the stent to the artery wall. The internal carotid artery is often wider at its origin than it is distally, and even a stent that is uniformly expanded in the majority of the carotid may not appose to the wider origin (Fig. 6a). This portion of the stent may be "trumpeted" with a larger balloon to expand the incompletely apposed section (Fig. 6b) (15).

IVUS can also be used for primary deployment of carotid stents, a procedure that eliminates preliminary angioplasty (Fig. 7). The IVUS catheter is carefully negotiated through the diseased artery to allow measurement of the minimum lumen diameter and an evaluation of the plaque morphology. This technique determines whether it is safe to deploy a stent primarily, but it is still experimental because the attachment of the guidewire to the IVUS catheter in a

---

Figure 5 (a) Angiogram of an internal carotid artery stenosis. (b) Satisfactory post-stent angiogram. (c) 2D and 3D IVUS demonstrate unsuspected incomplete deployment with midstent "waisting." (d) 3D IVUS showing improvement following reballooning. (Used with permission from the Journal of Endovascular Surgery.)

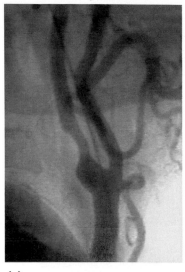

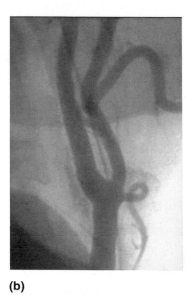

(a) **(b)**

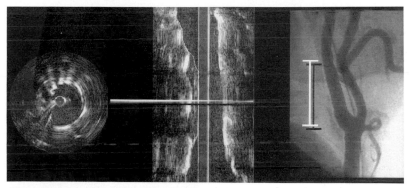

(c)

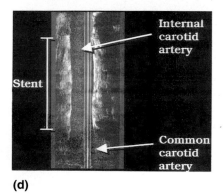

(d)

315

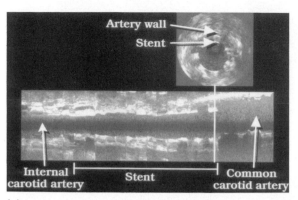

(a)

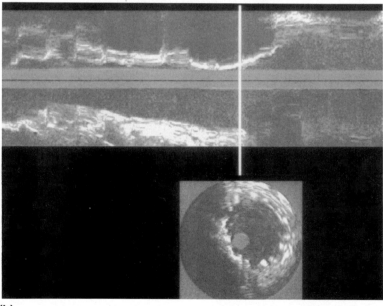

(b)

Figure 6   (a) 2D and 3D IVUS of a stent in the internal carotid artery which does not appose to the wider origin. (b) Caudal portion of the stent has been reballooned to a larger diameter, apposing it to the artery wall.

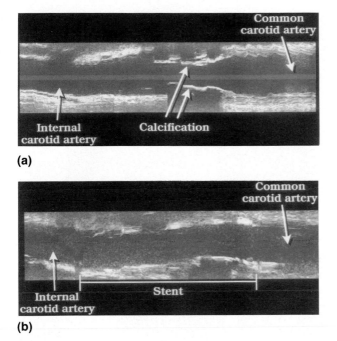

Figure 7 (a) "Longitudinal" image of an internal carotid artery stenosis assesses the plaque morphology and the minimum diameter before primarily deploying a stent. (b) Poststent 3D IVUS.

"side-saddle" configuration may increase the potential for dislodging emboli. Recently, we have preferred to use color flow Doppler ultrasound to provide a similar but safer assessment (16).

In the common carotid artery, disease is frequently present at the origin (Fig. 8). Accurate location of the origin is difficult with angiography alone because the aortic arch often covers and masks it. The IVUS catheter demonstrates the origin precisely, and its site may then be noted on fluoroscopy. IVUS examination of the distal common carotid artery may be achieved by placing the guidewire and IVUS catheter in the external carotid, avoiding instrumentation of the internal carotid (Fig. 9).

2. Subclavian and Innominate Arteries

IVUS allows a similar preliminary assessment of the subclavian and innominate arteries prior to stenting. Disease is most commonly found at the origins and is well suited to treatment with angioplasty and stenting. In this setting, a

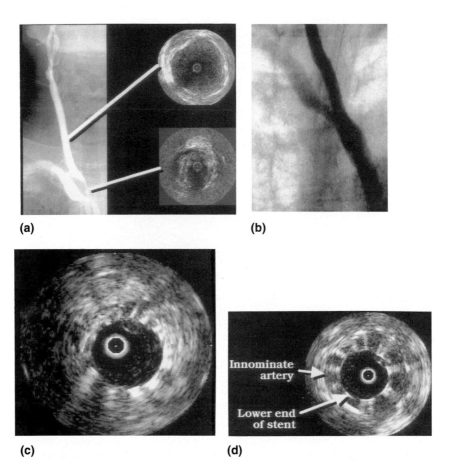

(a)   (b)

(c)   (d)

Figure 8 (a) Angiogram with IVUS images of a stenosis at the origin of the right common carotid artery. (b) Poststent angiogram. (c) 2D IVUS shows a well expanded stent against the artery wall. (d) 2D IVUS demonstrates that the lower end of the stent protrudes for 1 mm into the innominate artery. (Used with permission from the Journal of Endovascular Surgery.)

3.5 F, 30-MHz IVUS catheter is guided from a brachial artery approach. The pull-through is used to measure the artery diameter and the length of disease as well as to locate the vessel's origin (Fig. 10). The morphology of these lesions is usually soft, and stent expansion is generally satisfactory after the initial deployment (Fig. 11). When disease is present in the second part of the

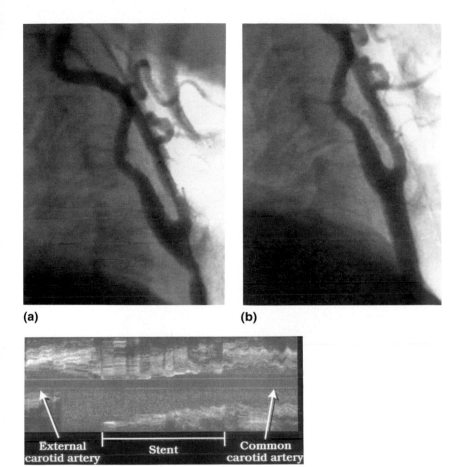

(a)   (b)

(c)

Figure 9   (a) Angiogram of a common carotid artery stenosis just proximal to the bifurcation. (b) Poststent angiogram. (c) 3D IVUS of common carotid artery stent demonstrating the bifurcation with the guidewire in the external carotid artery. (d) 2D IVUS of external carotid artery, which has a thicker media than the internal carotid. (e) 2D IVUS of the wider and more muscular common carotid artery.

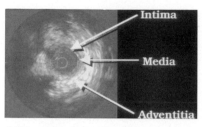

(d)

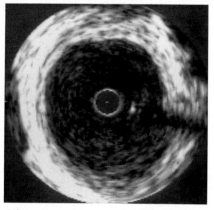

(e)

Figure 9   Continued

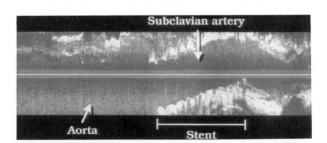

Figure 10   "Longitudinal" view of a stent at the origin of the left subclavian artery.

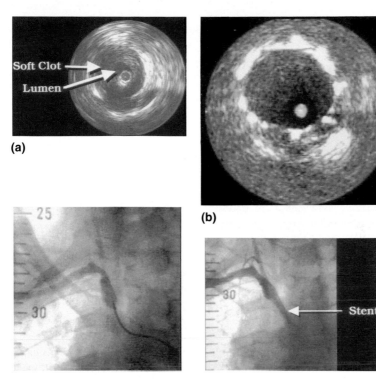

Figure 11 (a) 2D IVUS of a narrow proximal subclavian stenosis which is morphologically soft. (b) Poststenting IVUS shows satisfactory deployment. (c) Prestent angiogram. (d) Poststent angiogram.

subclavian artery, angioplasty and stenting may compromise a patent vertebral artery. The use of IVUS here can define the proximity of disease to the vertebral artery origin.

3. Aorta

In the aorta, a 6 F, 12.5-MHz catheter is most suitable for the large-vessel diameter. Accurate placement of stents or endoluminal grafts must avoid encroachment of the subclavian, celiac, renal, or iliac arteries (Fig. 12). In occlusive disease, IVUS demonstrates incomplete stent deployment and the need for additional ballooning (Fig. 13) or insertion of another stent (Fig. 14).

In abdominal aortic aneurysms, we have found IVUS particularly helpful in

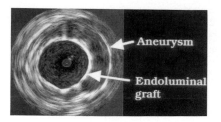

Figure 12   2D IVUS demonstrates a thoracic aneurysm excluded by an ELG. The aneurysm is highly calcified and is visible to IVUS through the ELG.

the preoperative assessment for endoluminal grafting (Figs. 15, 16). Under local anesthesia and fluoroscopic control, the IVUS catheter is advanced from the groin to a level just above the renal arteries. A steady and continuous pull-through allows 3D IVUS reconstruction. The proximal and distal necks of the aneurysm are measured together with the endoluminal length requiring grafting. The amount of calcification and mural clot are noted. An assessment of the shape of the proximal and distal necks often gives an indication of how well an ELG will exclude the aneurysm. The proximal neck is usually circular, and the distal neck is often oval and calcified. The volume 3D reconstruction indicates the shape and can assist in the decision to use a straight tube graft or bifurcated graft.

It is important that the pull-through be continued into the iliac artery on the side chosen to deliver the ELG (Fig. 17). Diameters are measured at the narrowest point to ensure the delivery system can advance safely through the iliac artery. We have, on more than one occasion, elected not to proceed to endoluminal grafting because of iliac disease found on IVUS.

4. Renal Artery

The value of IVUS in procedural decision-making was clearly demonstrated to us in the following situation. We treated a patient with severe renal failure in whom no x-ray contrast dye could be used. We successfully gained access to the stenosed renal artery and deployed a Palmaz stent using IVUS (Fig. 18) and fluoroscopy. The decision about where to place the stent, the choice of balloon and stent size, and the confirmation of accurate placement in the renal artery were all made using information obtained with IVUS.

5. Iliac Artery

In the iliac arteries, IVUS is useful in determining the success of balloon angioplasty and may indicate the need for stenting if intimal flap dissection or

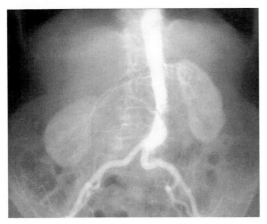

(a)

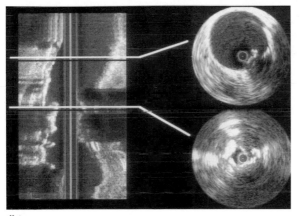

(b)

Figure 13 (a) Angiogram of aortic stenosis. (b) 2D and 3D IVUS demonstrating the highly calcified and tight stenosis. (c) 3D IVUS shows incomplete stent deployment. (d) Improved stent deployment following reballooning with larger balloon. (e) Completion angiogram.

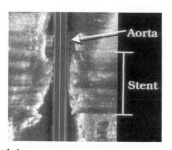

(c)

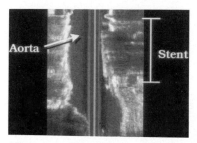

(d)

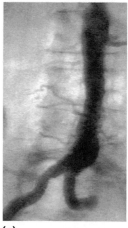

(e)

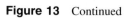

Figure 13 Continued

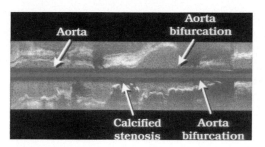

(a)

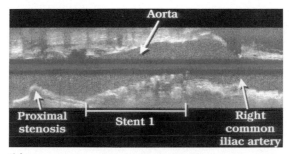

(b)

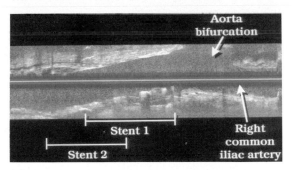

(c)

Figure 14 (a) 3D IVUS of aortic stenosis. (b) A residual proximal stenosis is demonstrated by 3D IVUS following stent placement. (c) A second stent treats the residual stenosis.

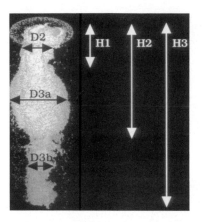

Figure 15 3D IVUS provides luminal measurements before endoluminal grafting of abdominal aortic aneurysm.

plaque recoil occurs. IVUS also indicates any inaccurate stent deployment requiring additional ballooning or placement of another stent (Figs. 2, 19). Occasionally, IVUS demonstrates a clinically suspected lesion that is not demonstrable with angiography.

6. Superficial Femoral, Popliteal, and Distal Arteries

In peripheral endoluminal grafting, IVUS provides preoperative assessment of the artery and allows determination of the balloon size required to expand the ELG. A long pull-through is usually necessary, and the IVUS operator must set the acquisition frame rate for 3D reconstruction accordingly. Following ELG deployment, IVUS detects any minor abnormalities in the graft's expansion; however, it is rarely necessary to treat these (Figs. 20, 21).

IVUS is also useful in peripheral atherectomy because it allows measurement of the luminal diameter and demonstrates residual plaque more accurately than angiography. It detects intimal flap dissection and also indicates the need for a larger burr (10).

III. CLINICAL VALUE OF THREE-DIMENSIONAL IVUS, A PROSPECTIVE STUDY

IVUS allows the clinician to confirm whether an intravascular stent has been placed correctly and, in some cases, detects incomplete stent deployment not apparent on a "satisfactory" completion angiogram. It can also confirm accu-

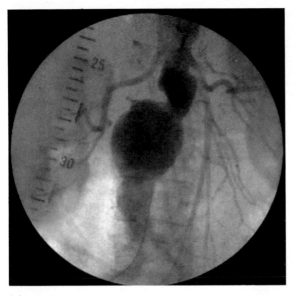

(a)

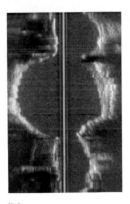

(b)

Figure 16 (a) Abdominal aortic aneurysm. (b) "Longitudinal" view of aneurysm—anteroposterior. (c) "Longitudinal" view—lateral: demonstrates a calcified stenosis at the proximal neck. (d) 3D IVUS "volume" view. (e) Angiogram following ELG deployment. (f) 2D IVUS following ELG deployment. (g) 3D IVUS following lELG deployment.

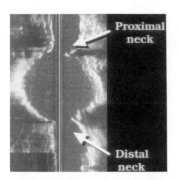

(c)

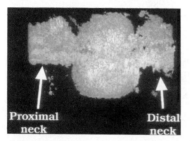

(d)

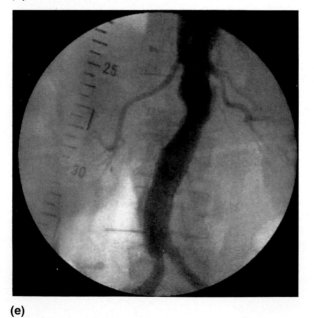

(e)

Figure 16 Continued

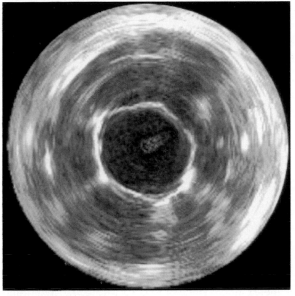

(f)

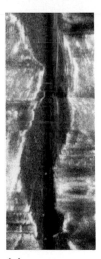

(g)

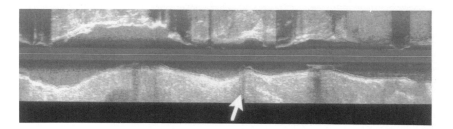

Figure 17 3D IVUS of a tortuous iliac artery demonstrated calcification with shadowIng of the ultrasound signal. Measurements provided a safe delivery of an aortic ELG.

rate placement of endoluminal grafts. The majority of endovascular surgeons, however, are not currently using intravascular ultrasound. Most perform pre- and postoperative angiography and measure arterial pressure gradients across the lesions before and after a procedure to determine the success of each intervention (17). Studies of the clinical value of IVUS are needed to determine whether it provides information that alters patient management and clinical

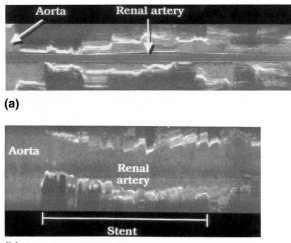

(a)

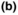

(b)

Figure 18 (a) 3D IVUS of a renal artery stenosis. IVUS was used with fluoroscopy to deploy a stent in a patient unable to tolerate x-ray contrast. (b) Poststent 3D IVUS confirmed satisfactory deployment.

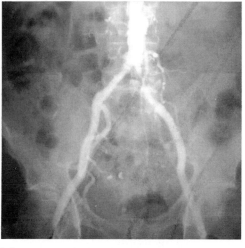

(a)

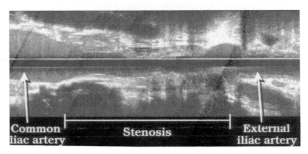

(b)

Figure 19 (a) Angiogram demonstrates left common iliac artery stenosis. (b) 3D IVUS of long stenosis. (c) Satisfactory poststent angiogram. (d) 3D IVUS demonstrates unsuspected residual stenosis following deployment of stent. (e) 3D IVUS following deployment of second stent demonstrates correction of stenosis.

outcome. With this in mind, we conducted a prospective study to evaluate the clinical value of 3D IVUS in peripheral vascular procedures.

A. Purpose

The purpose of this study was to determine the ability of 3D IVUS to detect inaccurate deployment of stents and endoluminal grafts following a satisfactory completion angiogram.

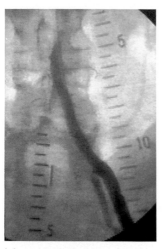

(c)

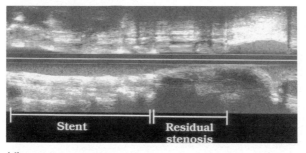

(d)

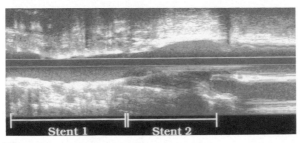

(e)

Figure 19 Continued

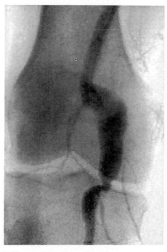

(a)

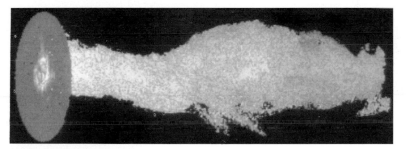

(b)

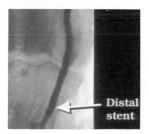

(c)

Figure 20 (a) Angiogram of tortuous popliteal aneurysm. (b) 3D IVUS "volume" view before endoluminal grafting. (c) Angiogram showing exclusion of popliteal aneurysm following ELG deployment. (d) 2D IVUS demonstrates uniform expansion of the ELG. (e) 3D IVUS demonstrates entire length of well-deployed ELG.

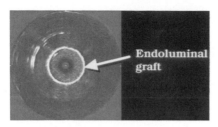

(d)

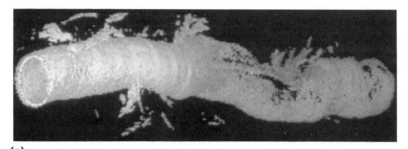

(e)

Figure 20   Continued

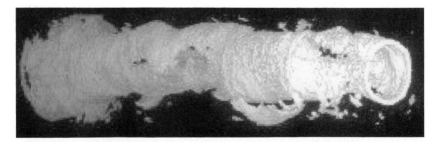

Figure 21   3D IVUS of ELG deployed for occlusive disease in the superficial femoral artery.

B. Materials and Methods

Between August 1995 and February 1996, 90 patients (54 male; mean age 70 years, range 42 to 83) underwent 103 separate endovascular procedures deploying intravascular stents and ELGs for treatment of occlusive or aneurysmal lesions (Table 1). Symptoms and indications for treatment are summarized in Table 2. A total of 100 stents were placed; 93 were Palmaz stents (Cordis, a Johnson & Johnson Company, Warren, NJ) [models P104 (n = 1), P154 (n = 13), P204 (n = 49), P294 (n = 14), P394 (n = 13), P308 (n = 3)] and 7 were Wallstents (Schneider USA Inc., Minneapolis, MN) [models 16×40 (n = 5), 16×60 (n = 1), 10×60 (n = 1)]. Fifteen endoluminal grafts were placed; each graft was custom-made for the individual patient. Eleven aortic endoluminal grafts were constructed using a self-expanding "Z" stent (Cook Inc., Bloomington, IN) covered with preexpanded polytetrafluoroethylene (PTFE), and four peripheral ELGs were made from an ultrathin PTFE tube graft 2 mm in diameter (18). The peripheral ELGs were balloon-expanded in the infrainguinal arteries, and Palmaz stents were used for their proximal and distal fixation. A preliminary balloon angioplasty prepared the artery for the deployment of three peripheral ELGs.

C. IVUS Assessment of Device Deployment

Following placement of the stents and endoluminal grafts, a completion angiogram was performed to assess deployment and patency of the artery. If the arteriogram indicated incomplete deployment, the stent was ballooned again until a satisfactory angiogram was obtained. IVUS examination of the stent followed.

A range of Sonicath ultrasound catheter sizes (Boston Scientific, Watertown, MA) was used; the size was chosen according to the caliber of the artery. A 3.5 F, 30-MHz catheter was most suitable for the narrow caliber vessels, while a 6 F, 12.5-MHz catheter was used in larger arteries. These IVUS catheters were guided over a 0.018-inch or 0.025-inch nitinol guidewire (Microvena, Whitebear Lake, MN) beyond the deployed device and then pulled back through the vessel across the area of investigation.

All images were processed by a 3D IVUS machine (Quinton Imaging, Sunnyvale, CA) connected to a Hewlett Packard IVUS machine (Hewlett Packard, Andover, MA). This provided longitudinal 3D gray-scale images that were immediately available in the operating room and allowed detection of any inaccurate device placement.

When IVUS showed satisfactory placement, the procedure was ended. In cases in which inaccurate stent deployment was detected, the stent was bal-

Table 1 Details of Endovascular Procedures

Artery	No. patients	No. procedures	No. stents	No. endoluminal grafts
Carotid artery	50	52	58	
Iliac artery	13	15	19	
Subclavian/innominate	9	10	10	
Aorta—occlusive	5	5	7	
Aorta—aneurysm	11	11	—	11
SFA	3	3	—	3
Renal	2	2	2	
Aortic graft	1	2	2	
Femoral vein	1	1	1	
Popliteal aneurysm	2	2	1	1

Table 2 Symptoms and Indications for Treatment

	No. patients	Symptoms/indications
Stents (lesions)		
Carotid artery stenosis	50	TIA, stroke, dizziness; stenosis >70%
Subclavian/innominate artery stenosis	9	Arm exercise pain, dizziness, subclavian steal
Iliac artery stenosis/ occlusion	13	Intermittent claudication, critical ischemia
Aortic stenosis	5	Intermittent claudication
Renal artery stenosis/ occlusion	2	Hypertension, deteriorating renal function
Vascular graft stenosis	1	Intermittent claudication
Femoral vein stenosis	1	Leg swelling
Endoluminal grafts (artery)		
Thoracic aorta	3	Aneurysm
Abdominal aorta	8	Aneurysm
Superficial femoral artery	3	Claudication
Popliteal artery	1	Aneurysm

looned again or another stent was placed as needed. Another completion angiogram and IVUS examination checked deployment. The minimum stent diameter was measured before and after any redeployment, and the percentage increase in the minimum stent diameter was calculated to assess any quantitative improvement.

D. Results

Three-dimensional IVUS detected unsuspected inaccurate deployment in 33 (34%) of 98 procedures with a satisfactory completion angiogram. In five cases, the completion angiogram indicated incomplete deployment that was confirmed by IVUS (Table 3). The inclusion of these five cases yielded a total IVUS detection rate of 37%.

In the procedures in which the completion angiogram was satisfactory, IVUS revealed incomplete expansion and stents not fully apposed to the vessel wall in 28 cases. In five patients, IVUS detected a ⩾ 50% stenosis proximal or distal to the stent, resulting from the device's failure to cover a long lesion. These five cases were treated by deploying a second stent. A total of 27 stents were successfully redilated, and the mean increase in the minimum stent diameter was 19%. In one patient, the guidewire position was lost from the internal carotid artery and additional ballooning was not possible.

E. Discussion

Three-dimensional IVUS revealed that approximately one-third of patients with apparently satisfactory stent deployment on angiography had inaccurate

Table 3 Details of Outcome in Patients Undergoing Endovascular Procedures

	Carotid	Iliacs	Subclavian innominate	Aorta	Others	ELG
Patients	50	13	9	5	5	15
Procedures	52	15	10	5	6	15
Satisfactory angiograms	50	14	9	5	6	14
Suboptimal on 3D IVUS	20	9	1	3	0	0
	(40%)	(64%)	(11%)	(60%)	(0%)	(0%)
Mean % increase in minimum stent diameter	19%	17%	10%	48%	—	—

stent deployment and required additional treatment. This altered the management of 32 patients in the operating room at the time of the procedure, and all had an improvement in their stent deployment following either additional ballooning or placement of another stent. Additional ballooning resulted in an increase in the minimum stent diameter of 19%. Such an increase is likely to be advantageous in reducing the risk of acute arterial occlusion and long-term restenosis.

Fifty-two patients undergoing carotid stenting in this study had routine duplex examination on their return to ICU. As anticipated, a highly significant association was found between the minimum stent diameter and the peak systolic velocity ratio across the stent ($r = -.5$, $P < .01$: Pearson's product moment correlation coefficient).

A recent multicenter study comparing the incidence of restenosis after balloon angioplasty and stenting in the coronary arteries found that the most accurate predictor of restenosis was the minimum lumen diameter immediately after the procedure, regardless of the intervention used (19). Hence, additional ballooning following 3D IVUS that allows an improvement in the minimum stent diameter is likely to be beneficial to the patient's clinical outcome.

When IVUS detects incomplete deployment, the decision to balloon again or place another stent needs to be undertaken with caution. This is particularly the case with carotid stenting, but it applies in other arteries as well. The advantages and possible complications must be weighed with an overall knowledge of the patient. Overinstrumentation may result in intimal dissection, spasm, thrombosis, or embolism. Clinical judgment is required.

The detection rate of incomplete stent deployment varied in different anatomic locations (Table 3). Three-dimensional IVUS had a high detection rate in carotid artery stenting with a subsequent improvement in stent diameter; however, the number of cases in this study is not large enough to allow us to draw any firm conclusions about its value in iliac, aortic, and arch vessels.

In this study, the use of 3D IVUS might initially appear inconsequential in the accurate placement of ELGs. It did not detect any inaccurate deployment in which the completion angiogram was satisfactory and, therefore, did not alter patient management in this setting. However, most of the ELGs were placed in the aorta, where the lumen and stent sizes were large. Minor abnormalities in the deployment of the self-expanding stents in the wide-bore artery appeared on IVUS to be clinically insignificant. The purpose of using an ELG in an aneurysm is to exclude it, and angiography demonstrates this result better than IVUS. Ultrasound signals penetrate PTFE poorly, often making the artery wall outside the ELG invisible and inaccurate deployment harder to diagnose.

Despite these problems, IVUS is of substantial help in the accurate placement of ELGs. Its role, however, is in the preoperative assessment and measurement of the artery. Additional information from 3D reconstruction also gives the IVUS operator maximum information to detect any inaccurate deployment. While we did not compare 2D and 3D IVUS, there were several instances in which the 2D pull-through missed an abnormality imaged with clarity by 3D IVUS.

IV. FUTURE OF IVUS

Improvements in the design of IVUS catheters may allow development of a catheter that is easier to maneuver and less likely to disturb plaque in the arterial wall. Currently, IVUS catheters are attached to the guidewire in a sidesaddle fashion that reduces "steerability" and may risk embolization or intimal dissection. A new catheter design (Spy catheter, Boston Scientific) incorporates a coaxial configuration that should be easier to maneuver safely through diseased or tortuous vessels.

Another advance is the Wise Wire (Boston Scientific). This device contains an IVUS transducer that is introduced through the central channel of an angioplasty balloon catheter. It allows accurate placement and real-time IVUS imaging during the intervention (Fig. 22). At present, however, the ultrasound signal does not pass completely through most balloon catheters. Enhancement of the ultrasound signal may be possible with technological improvement. Development of a "forward-looking" IVUS catheter is another innovation that

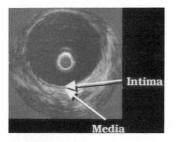

Figure 22 2D IVUS of a renal artery stenosis balloon angioplasty using a Wise Wire (Boston Scientific, Watertown, MA) which is placed inside the balloon catheter and allows real-time imaging during the procedure.

will allow accurate cannulation through total arterial occlusions and negotiation of tight stenoses (20). This technology is still experimental.

V. CONCLUSIONS

IVUS has clinical value in a wide variety of peripheral interventions. It is able to detect incomplete stent deployment in which the completion angiogram appears satisfactory. This alters the management of the patient with benefit because the deployment and stent diameter can be improved. IVUS also provides important information in the preoperative assessment of patients undergoing endoluminal grafting for aneurysmal or occlusive disease. Its use will increase among endovascular surgeons if the limiting factor of cost can be reduced. It then may become as common in endovascular procedures as conventional ultrasound has become in medical practice.

REFERENCES

1. Donald I. How and why medical sonar developed. Ann R Coll Surg Engl 1974; 54: 132–140.
2. Willocks J. Ian Donald and the birth of obstetric ultrasound. In: Neilson JB, Chambers SE, eds. Obstetric Ultrasound 1. Oxford: Oxford University Press, 1993:1–18.
3. Laskey WK, Brady ST, Kussmaul WG, et al. Intravascular ultrasonographic assessment of the results of coronary artery stenting. Am Heart J 1993; 125:1576–1583.
4. Gussenhoven EJ, van der Lugt A, Pasterkamp G, et al. Intravascular ultrasound predictors of outcome after peripheral balloon angioplasty. Eur J Vasc Endovasc Surg 1995; 10:279–288.
5. Cavaye DM, Diethrich EB, Santiago OJ, et al. Intravascular ultrasound imaging: an essential component of angioplasty assessment and vascular stent deployment. Int Angiol 1993; 12:212–220.
6. Katzen BT, Benenati JF, Becker GJ, et al. Role of intravascular ultrasound in peripheral atherectomy and stent deployment. Circulation 1991; 84:2152. Abstract.
7. White RA, Scoccianti M, Back M, et al. Innovations in vascular imaging; arteriography, three-dimensional CT scans, and two- and three-dimensional intravascular ultrasound evaluation of an abdominal aortic aneurysm. Ann Vasc Surg 1994; 8:285–289.
8. The SHK, Gussenhoven EJ, Zhong Y, et al. Effect of balloon angioplasty on femoral artery evaluated with intravascular ultrasound imaging. Circulation 1992; 86:483–493.
9. Kopchock GE, White RA, Guthrie C, et al. Intraluminal vascular ultrasound:

preliminary report of dimensional and morphological accuracy. Ann Vasc Surg 1990; 4:291–296.

10. Scoccianti M, Verbin CS, Kopchock GE, et al. Intravascular ultrasound guidance for peripheral vascular interventions. J Endovasc Surg 1994; 1:71–80.

11. Rosenfield K, Losordo DW, Ramaswamy K, et al. Three-dimensional reconstruction of human coronary and peripheral arteries from images recorded during two-dimensional intravascular ultrasound examination. Circulation 1991; 84:1938–1956.

12. Reid DB, Douglas M, Diethrich EB. The clinical value of three-dimensional intravascular ultrasound imaging. J Endovasc Surg 1995; 2:356–364.

13. Diethrich EB, Ndiaye M, Reid CB. Stenting in the carotid artery: initial experience in 110 patients. J Endovasc Surg 1996; 3:42–62.

14. Reid DB, Diethrich EB, Marx P, et al. Intravascular ultrasound assessment in carotid interventions. J Endovasc Surg 1996; 3:203–210.

15. Diethrich EB, Marx P, Wrasper P. Percutaneous techniques for endoluminal carotid interventions. J Endovasc Surg 1996; 3:182–202.

16. Reid DB, Diethrich EB, Chittick A, et al. Carotid morphological selection for endoluminal repair. J Endovasc Surg 1996; 3:332. Abstract.

17. Diethrich EB. Endovascular surgery: state of the art. In: Castellani LD, ed. Progress in Angiology and Vascular Surgery. Torino: Edizioni Minerva, 1995: 1–18.

18. Diethrich EB, Papazoglou K. Endoluminal grafting for aneurysmal and occlusive disease in the superficial femoral artery; early experience. J Endovasc Surg 1995; 2:225–239.

19. Fischman DL, Leon MB, Bain DS, et al. A randomized comparison of coronary-stent placement and balloon angioplasty in the treatment of coronary artery disease. N Engl J Med 1994, 331:496–501.

20. Back MR, Kopchock GE, White RA, et al. Forward looking intravascular ultrasonography: in-vitro imaging of normal and atherosclerotic human arteries. Am Surg 1994; 60:738–743.

17

Intravascular Ultrasound: Current Technological Limitations and Future Developments

John E. Abele, Yue-Teh Jang, and Robert J. Crowley
Boston Scientific Corporation, Natick, Massachusetts

I. INTRODUCTION

Although the concept of small-vessel intraluminal ultrasound imaging was anticipated in papers, patents, and prototypes in the 1960s and 1970s, intravascular ultrasound (IVUS) development did not begin in earnest until the mid-1980s (1,2). This was stimulated largely by the perceived need for better guidance for new interventional coronary techniques that were under development such as laser angioplasty and atherectomy. Because these new devices tended to rely on aggressive application of powerful tools, it was apparent that some type of improved imaging control would be needed that x-ray did not provide. At that time angiography led some physicians to believe that atherosclerosis was mainly a localized problem that would benefit from direct intervention at the site of severest stenosis. IVUS has since shown that atherosclerosis is significantly underestimated and that the interventional device approach generally treats only a late stage of its progression.

Bom et al. have described the early evolution of intraluminal measuring and imaging probes and catheters (2). These efforts were conducted long before the necessary imaging electronics and catheter technology were established, and when miniature transducers were virtually unknown. As digital signal processing and basic catheter technology did become available, researchers were better able to build IVUS systems with very costly, hand-built miniature transducers. At the same time, nonmechanical, synthetic aperture systems were also under serious development. By 1989 several competing mechanically scanned and all-electronic systems had been commercialized (3).

II. BASIC REQUIREMENTS FOR INTRAVASCULAR ULTRASOUND

To be clinically successful, catheter-based imaging must provide useful diagnostic and/or therapy guidance information that is not otherwise available to the practicing interventional cardiologist, and it must do so in a manner that minimizes patient risk and trauma as well as procedural time and cost. IVUS provided hope that the shadowgram view of x-ray or cine could be augmented by a more highly detailed image that would answer important clinical questions about choice of intervention and its follow-up. Other "intraluminal" ultrasound examples offered sources of encouragement; exquisite cross-sectional views of the heart, for example, could already be obtained with transesophageal ultrasound. It seemed reasonable that downsized ultrasound technology, if properly executed, would produce a similar view of a target blood vessel and the surrounding tissue. Designers of IVUS catheters and systems were challenged to provide detailed, reliable, high-quality images with these concerns in mind.

A good understanding of the key attributes of an IVUS system is essential to appreciate the evolution, limitations, and future potential for this modality.

III. IMAGE QUALITY

Image quality is difficult to quantify. Image characteristics must often be classified in "good, better, or best" terms which, over time, are certain to vary as improvements are made and users become more sophisticated and demanding with respect to the technical characteristics of the resulting image. Ultrasonographers frequently disagree about image quality as well as interpretation of images. The elements that make up the "quality" of an intravascular ultrasound image are similar to those for an optical image. They can be described in the following terms:

1. Spatial resolution
This refers to the smallest level of detail that can be resolved. It is influenced by the wavelength of the emitted energy (higher frequency means shorter wavelength). In the case of 30 MHz ultrasound, it is about 0.1 to 0.2 mm.

2. Contrast resolution
Also known as gray scale, this attribute refers to the intensity of the reflected

sound wave. It enables the user to differentiate between different types of tissue, clot, plaque, etc., by virtue of the differing densities of these materials.

3. Focus

Refers to the sharpness of the image and its level of definition. Small transducers tend to have a short range of focus. Spatial resolution may vary within a given image because focus is lost as the distance from the transducer increases.

4. Lack of distortion

Refers to the "spatial order" within the image or uniform sizing and perspective of the image compared to the object being imaged. Distortion can be measured by imaging a grid of uniform squares and looking for differences in the patterns between the image and the object.

5. Noise

Small, high-frequency transducers can be subject to interference from other electrical signals, resulting in "snow" or lines in the image. Noise can obscure details and reduce contrast resolution.

6. Artifacts

Other image distortions can be produced by friction on the rotating shaft of a mechanical transducer, "ring-down" signals close to the transducer, and other abnormalities (4).

All of these factors combine to determine image quality. Overall, good image quality could be defined as the successful display of all major features within the region of interest, without excessive noise, distortions, or artifacts. This "quality" can be measured by imaging phantoms which are constructed to simulate the shape and echo characteristics of the organ—in this case, a diseased coronary artery.

Each stage of the signal generation and display process is critical and must be designed carefully to produce an optimal image. One of the most important stages is the initial ultrasound signal acquisition "front end," consisting of the transducer, its cabling, and the ultrasound receiver, which contribute all of the information on which the subsequent image processing and display depend. It is nearly axiomatic for effective, high-quality imaging that as strong and pure a signal as possible be obtained by the imaging device. Accomplishing this provides an opportunity to further process and filter the signal, which can lead to additional image quality improvements.

IV. CATHETER CHARACTERISTICS

The handling characteristics of an IVUS catheter should be similar to a PTCA catheter. It must have pushability, trackability, and crossability, and its "feel" must be familiar to users. The subtleties of catheter manipulation can best be understood by looking more closely at the following critical parameters.

1. Trackability

Trackability refers to the characteristics of a catheter that allow it to flow over a guidewire through tortuous paths to its ultimate destination. It is a collection of "subcharacteristics" that include lateral flexibility of the shaft, lumen friction with the guidewire, and column strength (the ability to withstand axial force without compression or stretch). Catheters with varying degrees of stiffness must have very smooth and gradual transitions from one segment to another. Although smaller catheters tend to have greater flexibility, they tend to have lower column strength. Trackability is optimized when the guidewire and catheter are matched as a system for attributes such as axial and rotational friction, relative stiffness, and location and length of stiffness transition zones.

2. Crossability

The key subcharacteristics of crossability are the profile of the tip and the frictional properties of the surfaces. Tapered, smooth distal ends are usually best for crossing stenoses easily. Slippery materials can also be used to aid crossing.

3. Pushability

This refers to the ability to transfer axial force applied at the proximal end of the catheter to the tip. When there is tortuosity involved, as in distal coronary vessels with multiple "S" curves in three planes, the pushability characteristics is tested to its utmost. Catheters with good flexibility are more prone to be compressed when pushed, or to kink. Therefore, the most important subcharacteristic of pushability is column strength. Different materials, reinforced materials, laminated materials, lumen geometry, and gradually increased flexibility toward the tip tend to enhance this characteristic.

Early versions of IVUS catheters were too large and too stiff, and generally did not track very well. The key limitation in reducing the size of the catheter was the transducer. As catheters have become smaller, the challenge has been to maintain a strong, clean image signal in a structure that handles like an ideal PTCA catheter with high reliability, a safe failure mode, and reasonable cost.

Catheter connections to the imaging console and the inherently fragile nature of an assembly with a transducer and wires can add to the complexity of use. Mechanical systems require the user to fill the catheter tip with fluid for acoustic contact, or to flush the catheter prior to use. Array transducers require careful handling to avoid damage to the exposed elements.

Some of the earliest mechanical designs employed a reusable transducer and shaft and a disposable sheath. Early transducers were hand-built and too expensive to discard after a single use. This method was later abandoned as transducer costs moderated and because it was a time-consuming procedure that required assembly in the lab. Although modular systems tend to be more complicated with smaller sizes, the benefit of cost savings may warrant a reexamination of that approach (5).

V. RELIABILITY OF PERFORMANCE

Cardiovascular catheters are generally designed with a wide inherent tolerance for various use conditions and failure modes. Sterilization and shelf life of any components that might degrade over time or be changed by aggressive chemical sterilizing agents or radiation sterilization must be taken into account. High reliability can be achieved by design reliability analysis and the application of manufacturing processes that have been repeated many times and assigned probabilistic values that predict the likelihood and severity of failure of every part and assembly. The technology of designing and manufacturing for reliability is surprisingly new to medical devices but has recently been codified in a group of International Standards known as the ISO 9000 series.

Transducers in particular are prone to variations, and this tendency has contributed to their historically high cost. Small changes in dimensions, materials, and other factors can lead to drastic reductions in transducer efficiency. Imaging systems can also drift over time. Catheter and system must be designed together so that there is maximum latitude allowed to take into consideration the inherent variability. The U.S. Food and Drug Administration has mandated acoustic output power limits which must not be exceeded owing to drift or any other factor that might create a variation in output power (6). The need to make large numbers of transducers at a reasonable cost has stimulated the development of new manufacturing methods which, along with tight electrical and mechanical specifications and the application of statistical process control techniques, has resulted in the production of transducers that have virtually identical characteristics from unit to unit.

A. IVUS Economics

Ultrasound imaging probes used for external applications, including transesophageal cardiac evaluation, have traditionally been hand-built, individually tested, complex, and therefore very expensive. This is acceptable where reuse of the probe poses no additional performance or safety penalty, and cleaning can be effective. IVUS catheters, however, for both safety and performance reasons, are designed for single-use applications. This placed a burden on the designers to control the more costly components of IVUS catheters which tend to have many critical components. The cost impact of IVUS use can also be influenced by optimizing use protocols that reduce handling and procedure time. In addition, it is important to employ appropriateness-of-use criteria that ensure that the clinical and economic benefits of the additional information justify the cost. A number of studies have been conducted or are underway to obtain this information (7,8).

B. Limitations

With IVUS, as with the evolution of any new technology, there has been a great deal of interaction between the development of the technologies, understanding of the applications, and education of the users. All of these factors are strongly influenced by advancements in other fields that have nothing to do with ultrasound or even medicine. The tools for developing small transducers, for example, include nanotechnology (microasssembly techniques), rapid proto-typing, computer modeling and analysis (finite element analysis), and elec-tronic signal processing. All of these capabilities stem from other fields and in the last several years have enabled developers and manufacturers to reduce size and improve quality and reliability.

Most of the limitations of IVUS today relate to improving the performance attributes that have already been discussed. It is possible today to visualize vessel wall dimensions, monitor stent deployment, see most flaps and tears, and identify calcific deposits by size and location. It is generally possible to discriminate plaque deposits from healthy tissue. It is not yet possible to discriminate easily and precisely between thrombus and plaque or to identify and characterize ulcerative plaques and analyze their mechanical properties.

VI. IMPROVED IMAGE QUALITY: REQUIREMENTS AND DESIGN CONSIDERATIONS

Acquiring the scanned image is the first crucial step in the process of successful IVUS imaging, and it continues to be the most difficult stage in the develop-ment of both catheters and the imaging electronics. Understanding the basic limits and potential of single-element mechanical imaging has been essen-tial (8).

The acoustic appearance of a lumen under IVUS interrogation is somewhat similar to that of a histology specimen. The spatial relationships of all ele-ments, barring distortions, dropouts, or other artifacts, remain essentially the same for both. It must be remembered, however, that IVUS images are actually a sound map of reflections that occur with changes in mechanical properties of the coronary artery. Hardness, elasticity, water content, and other gross qualities of arterial tissue are primarily responsible for the brightness information that is displayed on the monitor.

The physical, acoustic, and electrical characteristics of the imaging transducer are most important for obtaining the information needed to create the sound map. Despite their complexity, nearly all of the critical dimensions that determine image performance can be described by the diagram shown in Figure 1. The physical thickness of the piezoelectric material has greatest effect on operating center frequency. Careful control of the material and thickness of the other layers is needed to avoid ring artifacts and for efficient power output and beam shape.

Figure 2 is an early IVUS image with a "ring-down" artifact in the near field. Better backing materials and other small improvements have cumulatively beaten down the ring artifact to the point where it is invisible in a typical mechanical IVUS image. Faster imaging electronics have also been essential to controlling the ring artifact to the point where it is rarely a problem in mechanical IVUS imaging.

As catheters have become smaller, so have the transducers. Figure 3a and b shows how resolution changes when the diameter of the transducer is varied. Typical IVUS images are characteristically sharp in the near zone and blurred in the far field. Sharper images are actually obtained by smaller transducers since most of the area of interest is within the near zone. The penalty for smaller size, however, is the loss of that sharp image as the distance from the transducer increases (Fig. 3a). Figure 3b shows how changing the frequency of operation can make up for this loss in sharpness at a greater distance. Focusing (Fig. 3c) can further sharpen the near field but has relatively little effect on the far field. Transducer designers have learned how to manipulate these variables for different catheter sizes, applications, and systems. However, there are practical limits today that may be improved tomorrow; frequencies of 50 MHz and higher may be used, for instance, to preserve sharpness in applications where very small transducers must be used or for better image clarity in present catheters (Fig. 4).

VII. TISSUE CHARACTERIZATION POSSIBILITIES

A. Requirements for Practical Acoustic Tissue Characterization

Quantitative spectral analysis of ultrasound images has been a dream for many years. The theory behind ultrasonic tissue characterization lies in the observation that various types of tissue reflect and attenuate ultrasonic energy differ-

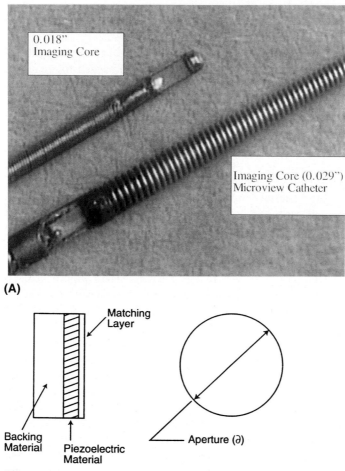

Figure 1   (A) Typical transducers used in catheter-based imaging: small rectangular or round elements are embedded in the ends of guidewire-like shafts. (B) The size of the transducer aperture affects the shape of the acoustic beam sent from the catheter, and contributes to the sharpness of the image. The thicknesses of the piezoelectric layer and the matching layer determine the frequency of operation.

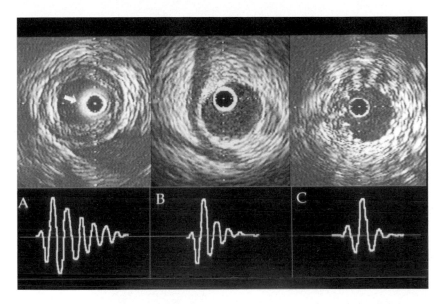

Figure 2 Ring artifact round the catheter: (A) The bright halo that surrounds the center of the image (arrow) is caused by prolonged "ringing" of the transducer. Ringing waveforms are shown below corresponding image. (B, and C) Successive shortening of the ringing duration results in a marked reduction of the artifact.

ently at different frequencies. Identifying tissue depends on recognizing signals that correspond to known tissue types (10).

There is hope that, given the limited number of tissue types expected and the nearness of the imaging transducer to the tissue, tissue characterization with IVUS will eventually become practical to perform. A convenient way to do this would be to superimpose a low-resolution, color-coded "spectral map" over the normal monochrome IVUS image, in the way color flow Doppler images are displayed today. There are, however, other potentially promising nonultrasound methods that discriminate tissue types. New, optically based instruments are being developed that use lightwave energy to interrogate and type tissue. Some of these instruments are being developed for cancer detection, but intravascular applications should be possible as well (11,12).

B. Use of Contrast Agents

In the normal, disease-free lumen of a coronary artery the luminal-intimal boundary can be seen quite easily with virtually all current IVUS systems. The

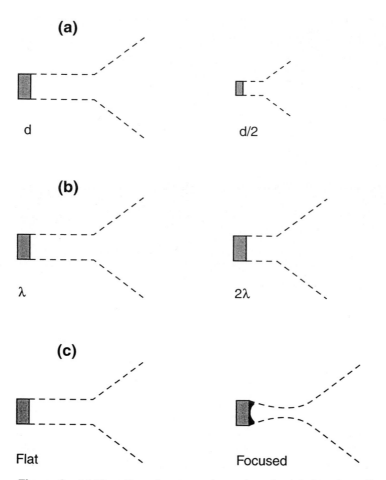

Figure 3 (a) The effect of aperture size on lateral resolution. A smaller transducer produces a narrower beam that corresponds roughly to the diameter of the transducer, however, the length of focus is much shorter. (b) The effect of frequency. The area of focus decreases by a factor of two when the wavelength is doubled and the frequency halved. Lower frequencies decrease the length of focus greatly. (c) A curved lens can sharpen the image close to the transducer but has little effect outside the length of focus.

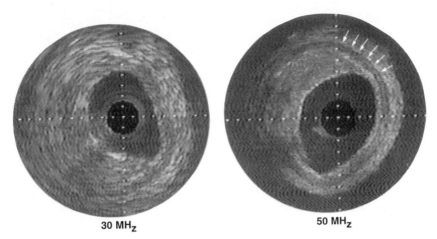

30 MH$_z$ 50 MH$_z$

Figure 4 Increasing the frequency of operation can improve sharpness. 30 MHz image (left) is compared with 50 MHz image (right). The 50 MHz image produces better detail, particularly at some distance from the catheter (arrows).

task becomes more difficult in diseased and disrupted vessels, since dissections, hard plaque, and hazy thrombus can obscure the image to the extent that it is difficult to ascertain the luminal boundary location. At higher frequencies blood scattering can usually be observed in motion, which provides a temporal contrast improvement. This strategy only works when the blood is flowing and when the system gain is high enough to detect the usually weak echoes from blood. The use of infused contrast agents to aid in delineating boundaries is being used clinically today. A first-generation agent is available and a number of second-generation materials are under investigation. These agents allow observation of cardiac perfusion abnormalities with transesophageal ultrasound or transthoracic ultrasound imaging (13). Its use with IVUS remains uncertain, but extending this use to IVUS might provide a better way to observe pre- and post-intervention flow.

C. Combined Imaging and Therapeutic Devices

It is ironic that the single most important reason for the numerous efforts in IVUS development in the mid-1980s was to guide laser angioplasty (14). IVUS has evolved and grown while laser angioplasty has all but disappeared.

Subsequently, there were and are efforts to combine imaging with other therapeutic devices. Directional atherectomy devices have been constructed with imaging capabilities (15), and a dilatation balloon with an integral transducer proximal to the balloon is available commercially (16).

In the vascular single-use world, however, the increased cost, fragility, and difference in handling that an integrated sensor entails make the development of a clinically useful device difficult.

D.   Ultrasound Imaging Guidewires

A potential solution to the cost and fragility problems of integrated imaging and therapy systems is the use of modular imaging components that are designed to work cooperatively. In this case, the modular imaging component is an ultrasound imaging guidewire (UIG). Even if the wire could not function as well as a state-of-the-art guidewire, being able to image a lesion through the balloon or distal to the catheter tip without having to exchange the catheter would provide several benefits compared to an integrated system:

1.   The handling would be familiar. The only change over normal practice would be a wire exchange.
2.   The cost would be less. The wire would be used only in cases where additional information was desired, not every one.
3.   The ability to handle a wide variety of different lesions would not be limited by a small selection of inherently more expensive balloon designs.

The UIG concept itself is not new; Omoto used an imaging wire to interrogate the heart and the aortic arch in the 1960s (16). An ideal UIG would look and perform like a primary coronary guidewire and provide the imaging function as well as the best IVUS catheters of today. Obviously, extreme miniaturization of the imaging components is required, and in the end the guidewire must still have good handling characteristics and be safe to use. Additionally, it would be complicated and expensive to try to duplicate all the varieties of present coronary guidewires and equip them with on-board imaging.

A possible alternative to the UIG that would be more realistic in the near future would be a rotating imaging core that is used in place of the primary wire during part of the interventional procedure. For this device to be used, guidewire swapping is required. The advantage is in being able to avoid a catheter exchange and monitor, in real time, procedures such as stent placement by imaging directly through sonolucent balloon material.

VIII. FUTURE

Continuing developments in computer power, imaging displays, materials, nanotechnology, and other technologies will increase the potential capabilities of IVUS. These developments will improve the ability to discriminate between the various arterial elements and ultimately, in conjunction with additional modalities and adjunctive techniques, to perform metabolic imaging to observe the biological response to various therapeutic strategies. Examples of some of these future possibilities include the following.

A. Real-Time 3D

At the present time, three-dimensional reconstructions are accomplished through a pullback technique which saves a series of 2D slices and compiles them into a 3D structure. The resulting cube of picture elements can be cut in any plane to show a section of the 3D object.

By employing a number of transducers displaced axially along the shaft— 10, for example—and feeding those data into high-speed processors, it should be possible to acquire and display a real-time, three-dimensional image. By employing "ghosting" software similar to what is used in the movies to create translucent objects (like ghosts), all parts of 3D real-time image can be seen in relationship to one another. Motion in a 2D-image improves the ability to discriminate between objects of varying elasticity or compliance (like plaque vs. tissue). Motion in three dimensions adds to that ability and allows one to see the connection between the subject and the structures surrounding it. This method of 3D imaging should also reduce the "stairstep" artifact of present reconstruction techniques and, in addition, show the correct spatial orientation of the artery over its length. Current techniques show a curved vessel as if it were straight because the display has no way of telling which direction the transducer is moved.

B. Elastic Imaging

Ultrasonographers frequently employ external compression as a technique to enhance visibility of a tumor or mass. Elastic imaging is a technique that uses software to aid in analyzing an image that is being perturbed in a controlled way. In an artery, for example, by applying controlled pressure pulses, one can quantify, in a relative sense, the varying shear moduli. Instead of an image that displays echogenic density, this technique produces a "compliance image" that can significantly enhance the ability to differentiate tissue types (13).

Compliance rather than density imaging can help in the discrimination of disease stages and should improve the ability to monitor the results of interventions that affect the mechanical properties of the tissue.

C. Flow

Color flow Doppler is well understood and widely used. The radial slice of the mechanical IVUS image is actually aimed slightly forward (about 10° off perpendicular), which allows the user to see blood flow with the gray-scale image (non-Doppler) in some instances. The addition of color flow Doppler to the high-frequency IVUS image should allow the user to see flow patterns or distribution in the vessel rather than the low-resolution information available from low-frequency transesophageal ultrasound or external ultrasound today. Whether this information has clinical utility is unknown, but it would be helpful for identifying jets, turbulence, and branch arteries, and useful in research—for example, into the origins and evolution of spiral dissections.

D.   Forward Viewing

A variety of forward viewing probes have been built over the years, but at this point the images are of much lower quality than radial ones, and, with extremely small probes, it is a much more difficult design challenge.

E.   Metabolic Imaging

It would obviously be desirable to be able to tag metabolites or chemicals the way one does in nuclear imaging. Ultrasound does not require nuclear licenses, and it is less expensive and less complicated to use. A number of companies make echogenic contrast agents, and some researchers have described versions that are taggable. Thrombus, for example, can be labeled and made to light up on an ultrasound image (18). One problem is that the contrast particles must be relatively large compared to target molecules. If there is adequate concentration, however, they become visible. And for those purposes it may be desirable to have very high ultrasound frequencies (100 to 200 MHz) to increase the resolution. If one could look at the real-time biological response to mechanical or chemical therapy, it might be possible to titrate that therapy to avoid restenosis.

F.   Multimodal Imaging/Image Fusion

Anybody who has a television with "picture-in-picture" capabilities knows that having multiple moving images simultaneously on a screen is technically easy to do. And anyone who has attended a live demonstration course knows the benefit of simultaneous images to improving the understanding of a case. Gastroenterologists performing ultrasound endoscopy sometimes employ multimodality screens with ultrasound, endoscopy, and fluoroscopy. These capabilities can and will be added to IVUS consoles. As 3D capabilities of other modalities such as fast CT and MRI increase, and as position sensors become more available (19), it will be possible to show the IVUS image in the proper perspective within the 3D image of another modality.

IX. CONCLUSION

Despite the skeptical predictions of many experts in the 1980s and before, small-diameter IVUS catheters with good-quality images are a reality today. Image quality will continue to improve as the technology advances, users become more familiar with the technique and its limitations, and procedures that include IVUS-guided interventions continue to evolve. With future enhancements such as those described here and others not anticipated, the application of intracoronary ultrasound imaging to improved lesion analysis and guidance of appropriate therapy should grow as an important tool in the interventional cardiologist's armamentarium.

REFERENCES

1. Gamble WJ, Innis RE. Experimental intracardiac visualization. N Engl J Med 1967; 276:1397–1403.
2. Born N, ten Hoff H, Lancee CT, Gussenhoven WJ, Bosch JG. Early and recent intraluminal ultrasound devices. Int J Card Imaging 1989; 4:79–88.
3. Intraluminal Ultrasound: A Physician's Guide. Kauai, Hawaii: Strategic Business Development, 1990.
4. Finet G, Maurincomme E, Tabib A, et al. Artifacts in intravascular ultrasound imaging: analyses and implications. Ultrasound Med Biol 1993; 19(7):533–547.
5. Crowley RJ. Ultrasound catheter imaging: a functional overview. SPIE Proc 1989; 1068:160.
6. Revised 510(k) Diagnostic Ultrasound Guidance for 1993. Washington: Food and Drug Administration, Center for Devices and Radiological Health, Feb. 1993.
7. Stone GW, Linnemeier T, St. Goar FG, Mudra H, Sheehan H, Hodgson JM. Improved outcome of balloon angioplasty with intracoronary ultrasound guidance: core lab angiographic and ultrasound results from the CLOUT study. JACC 1996; 27(2 suppl A).
8. Higano ST, Berger PB, Garratt KN, Reeder GS, Lerman A. Intravascular ultrasound and restenosis: a cost analysis. Circulation 1994; 90(1491):1–227.

9. Crowley RJ, von Behren PL, Couvillon LA, Mai DE, Abele JE. Optimized ultrasound imaging catheters for use in the vascular system. Int J Card Imaging 1989; 4:145–151.

10. Linker DT, Kleven A, Gronningsaether A, Yock PG, Angelsen BJ. Tissue characterization with intra-arterial ultrasound: special promise and problems. Int J Card Imaging 1989; 4:255–263.

11. Baraga R, Rava R, Fitzmaurice M, et al. Characterization of the fluorescent morphological structures in human arterial wall using ultraviolet-excited microspectrofluorimetry. Atherosclerosis 1991; 8:1–14.

12. Brezinski M. Tearney G, Bouma B, et al. Optical coherence tomography for optical biopsy: properties and demonstration of vascular pathology. Circulation 1996; 93:1206–1213.

13. Winkelmann JW, Kenner MD, Dave R, Chandwaney RH, Feinstein SB. Contrast echocardiography. Ultrasound Med Biol 1994; 20(6):507–515.

14. Webster WW. Catheter for removing arteriosclerotic plaque. U.S. Patent 4,576,177 (issued March 18, 1986).

15. Yock PG. Catheter apparatus, system and method for intravascular two-dimensional ultrasonography. U.S. Patent 4,794,931 (issued Jan. 3, 1989).

16. Omoto R. Intracardiac scanning of the heart with the aid of ultrasonic intravenous probe. Jpn Heart J 1962; 8:569–581.

17. Shapo BM, Crowe JR, Skovoroda AR, Eberle MJ, Cohn NA, O'Donnel M. Displacement and strain imaging of coronary arteries with intraluminal ultrasound. IEEE Trans Ultrasonics 1996; 43(2):234–246.

18. Wallace KD, Lanza GM, Scott MJ, et al. Intravascular ultrasound detection of thrombi after enhancement with novel site targeted acoustic contrast agent. Circulation 1995; 92(2800):1–585.

19. Aretz HT, Martinelli MA, LeDet EG. Intraluminal ultrasound guidance of transverse laser coronary atherectomy. Int J Card Imaging 1989; 4:153–157.

Index

About the Editor

ROBERT J. SIEGEL is the Director of the Cardiac Noninvasive Laboratory and a Staff Cardiologist at Cedars-Sinai Medical Center, Los Angeles, California, as well as a Professor of Medicine in Residence at the University of California, Los Angeles, School of Medicine. The editor of one book and the coauthor of more than 145 scientific publications and book chapters, he is a member of the American Heart Association, the Society for Cardiovascular Pathology, the American College of Cardiology, the American Society of Echocardiography, and the American College of Physicians, among others. Dr. Siegel received his B.A. degree (1971) from the University of California, Berkeley, and his M.D. degree (1974) from Baylor College of Medicine, Houston, Texas.